D0966218

Kidney for Sale by Owner

Human Organs, Transplantation, and the Market

MARK J. CHERRY

Georgetown University Press
Washington, D.C.

Georgetown University Press, Washington, D.C.
© 2005 by Georgetown University Press. All rights reserved.
Printed in the United States of America

10 9 8 7 6 5 4 3 2 1   2005

This book is printed on acid-free, recycled paper meeting
the requirements of the American National Standard
for Permanence in Paper for Printed Library Materials and those of the
Green Press Initiative.

. Library of Congress Cataloging-in-Publication Data

Cherry, Mark J.
    Kidney for sale by owner : human organs, transplantation, and the market /
Mark J. Cherry.
        p. cm.
    Includes bibliographical references and index.
    ISBN 1-58901-040-X (cloth : alk. paper)
    1. Procurement of organs, tissues, etc.—Economic aspects—United States. 2.
Procurement of organs, tissues, etc.—Moral and ethical aspects—United
States. 3. Transplantation of organs, tissues, etc.—Economic aspects—United
States. 4. Transplantation of organs, tissues, etc.—Moral and ethical aspects—
United States. I. Title.
    RD129.5.C448 2005
    617.9′54—dc22

                                                        2004022932

Contents

v

Acknowledgments

Throughout the writing of this manuscript, I benefited from numerous discussions and commentaries concerning various ancestral versions. I am in the debt of many for their critical comments and useful suggestions. In particular, this volume profited from my conversations with H. Tristram Engelhardt Jr., Baruch A. Brody, George Sher, and Gerald McKenny. Members of the Rice University Philosophy Department, especially Mark Kulstad, Richard Grandy, Donald Morrison, and Steven Crowell, as well as the Center for Medical Ethics and Health Policy at Baylor College of Medicine, especially Laurence McCullough, helped me to see many important issues in a new light. In addition, I wish to recognize the ongoing support and kindness of Saint Edward's University, the School of Humanities, the Departments of Philosophy and Religious Studies, and the Center for Ethics and Leadership, especially Donna M. Jurick, SND, Louis T. Brusatti, William J. Zanardi, Kelley Coblentz-Bautch, Richard Bautch, Edward Shirley, Peter Wake, and Phillip M. Thompson.

Many have read the manuscript in various stages or commented on its central arguments. Through the multitude of names, I will surely fail to remember them all. Here I can only mention a few among the many who have been so generous: B. Andrew Lustig, Joseph Boyle, Kevin Wm. Wildes, S.J., Nicholas Capaldi, Ana Iltis, Fabrice Jotterand, Lisa Rasmussen, Ruiping Fan, George Khushf, Christopher Tollesfsen, David Solomon, Griffin Trotter, Larry Temkin, Douglas den Uyl, Frederic J. Fransen, and Emilio Pacheco. The detailed comments of Richard Brown were integral to shaping the character of the final manuscript. I am deeply indebted to my friend H. Tristram Engelhardt Jr., whose encouragement was essential to the completion of this manuscript. Having acknowledged much excellent guidance, I must admit that I have not always followed it. Any mistakes and missteps are, of course, my own.

My deepest gratitude goes to Frank and Charlotte Cherry for their nurturing of intellectual skills as well as for unfailing encouragement, love, and support; to Carl and Lois Dorman for kindnesses too numerous to mention; to Jacob, Thaddeus, and Matthias for wonderful, exuberant, and never-ending distractions; and to Mollie, who besides possessing the virtues of faith, hope, joy, and love in great abundance has a wonderfully keen sense of humor. It is Mollie to whom this book is dedicated.

Introduction

To dismiss the idea of paid donors as the ethics of expediency is to deny these patients the right to live. We serve only the corrupt and the unscrupulous if we deny the patient benefit of a transplant that is medically indicated because of our fear that the paid donation process is too complex to be regulated.

—Dr. K. C. Reddy,
"Unconventional Renal
Transplantation in India"

In the United States, more than 44,308 patients died while waiting for organ transplants from 1992 through 2001.[1] An additional 6,385 patients died in 2002, and 6,509 in 2003.[2] Many others endured painful, life-sustaining measures, while queuing for available organs. Despite the significant potential of commercialization to increase the efficiency and effectiveness of organ procurement and distribution, to shorten waiting time, and thereby to reduce human suffering—while expanding the number of available organs—the possibility of creating a market in human organs for transplantation provokes in many feelings of deep moral repugnance, conjuring up nightmarish images of spare parts medicine. Others simply pronounce offense, anathema, and fear at the very possibility.[3] Indeed, an apparent global "consensus" holds such a market to be morally impermissible, if not fully indefensible, and actively promotes worldwide prohibition. In *Kidney for Sale by Owner: Human Organs, Transplantation, and the Market,* I critically reassess the arguments and assumptions that purportedly ground this alleged consensus.

Various policy statements have been broadly influential in shaping the global "consensus" against such a market. The Transplantation Society,[4] the World Health Organization,[5] the Nuffield Council on Bioethics[6] and the U.S. Task Force on Organ Transplantation[7] each has issued pronouncements condemning the creation of a for-profit market in human organs. The U.S. Congress, the National Kidney Foundation, the United Network for Organ Sharing (UNOS), the American Medical Association, the American Society of Transplant Surgeons, and the World Medical Association have similarly denounced proposals to broker human organs for transplantation. Professional organizations have, at times, resolved to expel members who were involved in such dealings.[8]

Condemnation of commercial organ markets is perceived as grounded in basic moral principles, such as "human dignity,"[9] "respect for persons," and the "sacredness of human life."[10] Such possible moral costs are believed to belie any potential the market may possess for increasing access to life-sustaining transplants and the concomitant reduction in human suffering. The underlying, taken-for-granted, but usually unexamined, assumption is that certain uses of human tissue are morally impermissible because they injure human beings, treating persons and their bodies as mere things, as less than fully human. A central and apparently forceful line of reasoning is that the unscrupulous would exploit the fact of poverty to compel or intimidate the poor into selling their redundant internal organs, which, given better circumstances, the poor would not have done. Whereas such conclusions purportedly evaluate the moral, social, and political theoretical parameters, as well as the medical costs and benefits of a market, human organ selling is often simply viewed with horror as gruesome.

Critically assessing such commonplace conclusions against commercialization, this study explores the underlying moral arguments and philosophical assumptions, as well as political and moral rhetoric that purportedly support this global consensus. Is such a global consensus and its promotion of worldwide legal prohibition morally justified?

Sympathetic articles and editorials exploring the various types of incentives (often even including financial remuneration) that might significantly alleviate the current organ shortage, while not necessarily leading to the purported laundry list of potential horrors, have begun appearing in many of the foremost medical journals—including the *Annals of Internal Medicine*, the *New England Journal of Medicine*, *Transplantation*, the *British Medical Journal*, and *The Lancet*.[11] Some commentators have begun suggesting that incentives to provide organs for transplantation need not lead to inappropriate treatment of body parts or to exploitation of the poor. Others have urged that insofar as one sets aside emotional reactions, most of the arguments put forward against even financial incentives do not stand up to careful scrutiny.[12]

Consider, for example, that the American Medical Association's Council on Ethical and Judicial Affairs adjusted its policy against all financial incentives, arguing that it is permissible for competent adults to enter into a futures contract, in which one agrees to the harvesting of organs after death, with one's family or estate receiving financial remuneration only once the organs are retrieved and judged medically suitable for transplant.[13] In 2002, the American Medical Association voted to promote studies to assess whether financial incentives would likely increase the pool of cadaver organ donors.[14] Insofar as a market system demonstrates significant potential to alleviate organ shortages and to decrease the time patients spend on waiting lists, thereby significantly reducing human suffering, prima facie more attention should be paid to its promise.

Despite such potential, the commercial market is denounced as inappropriately commodifying the human body. Selling human organs for profit is held to be necessarily degrading, as well as incompatible with basic human values, such as social justice and individual liberty, and important social goals, including equality and a spirit of altruism. The human body, it is urged, ought not be treated as mere property.[15] The market is viewed as corrosive of the "gift-of-life" sentiments, social beneficence, and community solidarity, which, it is claimed, ought to characterize organ procurement. On the one hand, altruistic donation is perceived as a free expression of important human values and community commitments. On the other hand, a market, it is claimed, would commodify human organs as a product for sale and trade, thereby ignoring and undermining the essential gift exchange dimensions of organ donation that purportedly bind a community together. The global "consensus" is thus marked by a view that organs should not be treated as commodities, but rather understood as a social resource to be distributed according to medical necessity. Organs are characterized as medical assets to be used to support public interests and social goods.

To emphasize, it is not just that organs are to be gifts, donated in the spirit of altruism and social solidarity; they are to be *nationalized* as a public resource. Human organs are to be understood as a *scarce public resource* and allocated on the basis of acceptable medical criteria and appropriate social goals, rather than private gain. A market for procurement and distribution of transplantable organs, it is believed, would lead to significant medical, social, and moral costs. The direct and indirect implications of the market, opponents conclude, create more harm than benefit.

In the following chapters, I assess the moral, ontological, and political theoretical concerns at issue in an organ market. The advantages and disadvantages of such markets are explored. In each chapter, I mark out the grounds for holding that the global consensus to proscribe organ sales does not have the force usually assumed.

Chapter 1 situates the moral debate within the medical practice of organ transplantation and the urgent public health care crisis. I consider the nature and scope of the global consensus against a for-profit market in human organs, together with the moral assumptions and arguments usually mustered in its support. I also critically assess claims that offering financial incentives to donate organs would undermine free and informed consent, as well as coerce the poor into offering their organs for sale; that such a market would exploit the poor, corrode important "gift of life" sentiments, and be morally repugnant. Moreover, I consider whether such a market would lead to increased inequality between the rich and the poor as well as worse medical outcomes than the current scheme of altruistic donation.

In chapter 2, I assess the conditions necessary and sufficient for a market in human organs to be morally licit. This analysis involves exploring basic foundational issues regarding the relationship between persons and their bodies, the senses in which organs can be property, the distinction between justified and unjustified moral repugnance, and the limits of society or governmental moral authority to interfere in consensual exchange of body parts. I consider, in addition, the standard of proof that must be met either to prohibit or to permit an organ market, as well as who should bear that burden of proof. Given the salience of particular constellations of factors, the moral licitness of an organ market will range from being rightfully forbidden, to prima facie permissibility, to the position that it clearly ought not be forbidden. The result of this analysis is a geography of considerations, which in different constellations will be sufficient to demonstrate that a market in human organs is morally permissible.

Chapter 3 turns to a more detailed evaluation of an organ market's costs and benefits, which tend to tip the balance in terms of one or another conclusion. I evaluate the advantages and disadvantages in terms of the market's impact on health care, the efficient and effective use of scarce resources, and whether such a market would lead to greater liberty, equality, and altruism. In addition, I gauge the impact of such a market on respect for sanctity of life, the exploitation of persons, social solidarity, and the pursuit of scientific excellence. The task of this chapter is to deepen the conceptual geographies of chapters 1 and 2, to consider particular instances of the foundational issues, and to determine under which circumstances a market in human organs advances health outcomes, as well as other special values and goals, more successfully then alternate organ procurement and allocation strategies. For example, I consider the ways in which an organ market would likely enhance a sense of community and raise scientific standards, as well as increase individual freedom and expressions of altruism. Given certain constellations of factors, the analysis will show that such values and goals are more successfully supported through an organ market.

Chapter 4 considers the historical and philosophical roots of the crucial moral intuitions, ontological considerations, and political theoretical premises, as well as understandings of special moral concerns, such as permissible uses of the body and its parts, which frame the purported "global consensus." I address the influential positions of Thomas Aquinas, John Locke, and Immanuel Kant, which would usually be interpreted as foreclosing a market in human organs. I consider, as well, the arguments of Robert Nozick's *Anarchy, State, and Utopia*, which would likely support such a market. Aquinas's principle of totality is the *locus classicus* of the view that preserving the body as a whole is a natural good, which may prohibit transplantation from living donors. The principle of totality has been widely influential in the West as forbidding the removal of healthy organs from living vendors. Locke's account of natural duties to oneself and others places constraints on the freedom one has to use one's body. Kant's arguments that selling one's body parts uses oneself as a means merely, rather than protecting oneself as an end, underlie many of the rationalizations that organ selling violates human dignity.

The concluding chapter brings these diverse sets of analyses together to show why the apparently strong consensus against the selling of human organs is misguided. It fails adequately to appreciate the phenomenological, physiological, and psychological distinctions among different body parts, the relative strength of ownership rights, and the significance in general secular society of forbearance and privacy rights. The purported "consensus" fails as well to take adequate account of the closeness of the analogy between dominion/possession/ownership of one's body and dominion/possession/ownership of other types of things, or the ground and extent of moral political authority. Moreover, I argue, maximizing health care benefits, promoting equality, liberty, altruism, and social solidarity, protecting persons from exploitation, and preserving regard for human dignity are more successfully supported through permitting a market rather than through its prohibition. The profit motive offers motivations to maintain both scientific excellence and moral virtue, which do not exist under other procurement and allocation schemes. Finally, with regard to Aquinas, Locke, and Kant, in each case the arguments on closer examination do not unequivocally preclude the selling of human organs, including redundant internal organs or those procured from cadaver sources. If certain critical premises are reexamined and recast in plausible ways, then their general positions support the permissibility of organ sales.

The arguments and assumptions rallied against the creation of a market for procurement and distribution of human organs are often rhetorically powerful, yet as this study concludes, they oversimplify the issues at stake. Throughout this book I respond to the central and forceful objections that are usually held to be decisive against such a market. At each step, my analysis considers whether and how commercialization may exploit persons in greatest need, violate human dignity, or otherwise harm other special moral goods, such as liberty, equality, and justice, or whether forbidding the sale of organs for transplantation itself exploits some to benefit others, violates basic dignity, and leads to significant moral harms. Perhaps some might find the sale of a redundant internal organ to be an acceptable, indeed valuable, means of improving their life circumstances and opportunities. In such cases, laws forbidding the sale of organs exploit those who would wish to sell an organ, or perhaps to enter into a futures contract, to support a very particular view of moral propriety, thereby denying those who wish to sell or those in need of a transplant this opportunity to choose freely on the basis of their own judgments regarding how best to advantage themselves. The outcome is not merely moral considerations against commercialization, or even reasons encouraging the poor and sick to forgo such opportunities, but robustly paternalistic legislation.

Whereas one might hope that legal and moral prohibition of commercialization is the result of sound rational moral argument, adequate scientific and medical data, and careful consideration of the likely costs and benefits, this study provides significant grounds for concluding that the global "consensus" proscribing organ sales fails to take adequate account of many of the issues central to the debate. Closer examination reveals significant grounds for concluding that a market would likely be more successful in preventing exploitation, preserving human dignity, and reducing needless human suffering than current governmental bureaucratic procedures for procuring and allocating organs for transplantation.

Moral reflections and public policies that regard human organs as a "public resource" and governmental legislation that nationalizes body parts coercively to support particular accounts of the "social good" themselves significantly contribute to the commodification of body parts, poor medical outcomes, and the dehumanization of persons. In this book I offer significant medical, moral, and social policy reasons for holding that legal prohibition of organ sales very likely causes more harm than benefit. Together, such considerations provide a well-founded basis critically to approach current national and international proscription of payments for human organs for transplantation. In short, the ubiquitous contemporary bioethical rhetoric of moral repugnancy, exploitation, coercion, sanctity of life, social justice, and human dignity, though prima facie appealing and politically fashionable, fails adequately to address or to resolve this urgent public health challenge. On balance the analysis supports a market in human organs, rather than its prohibition. Indeed, I argue, the market will prove to be the most efficient and effective, as well as morally justified, means of procuring and distributing organs for transplantation.

CHAPTER ONE

Human Organ Sales and Moral Arguments

The Body for Beneficence and Profit

INTRODUCTION

This study addresses a cluster of conceptually independent philosophical concerns. They are related by an urgent public health challenge: the considerable
disparity between the number of patients who could significantly benefit from
organ transplantation and the number of human organs available for transplant.
In August 2004, more than 86,000 patients in the United States waited on the
United Network for Organ Sharing lists for transplants. Yet, in all of 2003 fewer
than 26,000 organ transplants of all types were performed.[1] Organ availability is
not expected to increase significantly in the near future. Proposals to address this
crisis include national educational programs on the benefits of transplantation
and the pressing need to donate organs, as well as laws that range from requiring
physicians to ask families to donate organs from recently deceased relatives, to
those that make organ retrieval upon death mandatory or that reward those who
do donate, to the creation of a for-profit commercial market[2] in human organs.[3]

Such proposals elicit a number of questions: (1) What does it mean to own an
organ? (2) Under what circumstances do governments have moral authority to
regulate how persons utilize their own body parts? (3) What are the costs and benefits of a market in human organs, measured in terms of medical efficiency and
effectiveness, moral virtues and vices, as well as scientific integrity and community-directed altruism? Despite the apparent potential of a market in human
organs to increase the efficiency and effectiveness of organ procurement, as well as
the number of organs available for transplantation, an apparent global consensus
holds such a market to be morally impermissible and actively promotes worldwide
legal prohibition.

1

CHALLENGES FOR PUBLIC HEALTH CARE POLICY

Consider the extent of the medical challenges facing the transplantation field. In 1996, in the United States, 4,022 patients died while waiting for suitable organs; as noted, in 2002 this incidence had increased to 6,385. While there were 61,766 registrants for kidney transplants in August of 2004, only 15,123 renal transplants were performed in 2003. Similarly, there were 17,857 registrants for a liver transplant, but only 5,671 were performed during 2003. The data regarding pancreas and heart transplants are similar: there were 1,636 patients registered for a pancreas and 3,523 for a heart, with 502 pancreas transplants and 2,057 heart transplants performed in 2003. Table 1.1 summarizes this comparison with regard to various organs.[4]

Circumstances appear even more critical in other countries. For example, in Hong Kong, the rate of organ donation ranges from three to five per million. Throughout 2000, only 5.5 percent of the patients on the kidney transplant waiting list were transplanted, with an average waiting time for cadaver renal allografts exceeding seven years.[5] In India, reportedly more than 80,000 persons a year are diagnosed with end-stage renal failure. There are relatively few resources for kidney dialysis. Without organs, many such patients will die.[6]

The growing pool of potential transplant candidates is exacerbating waiting times. The median waiting time for a kidney transplant was 400 days for patients registered in 1988 compared to 1,121 days for patients registered in 1999, with

Table 1.1
Summary of Registrants and Transplants Performed

Type of Organ	No. of Registrants[a] (August 2004)	No. of Transplants Performed (All of 2003)
Kidney	61,766	15,123
Liver	17,857	5,671
Pancreas	1,636	502
Kidney–Pancreas	2,515	871
Intestine	199	116
Heart	3,523	2,057
Heart–Lung	196	29
Lung	3,971	1,085
Total:	91,663	25,454

[a] UNOS allows patients to be listed with more than one transplant center. As a result, the number of registrations may be somewhat greater than the actual number of patients.
  Data is compiled from http://www.unos.org (last accessed August 12, 2004).

1,778 days for blood type B patients. The median waiting time for patients listed for repeat kidney transplants in 1996 was 1,629 days. Generally, patients with panel reactive antibodies (PRAs) of 10–79 percent waited longer (1,631 days for patients registered in 1999) than patients with PRAs under 10 percent (1,107 days for patients registered in 1999; 1,295 days in 2001). Median liver waiting time increased from 43 days for patients registered in 1990 to 767 days for patients registered in 2000; the mean time was 412 days in 2002. Patients with blood type O experienced the longest wait for livers: 1,120 days for patients listed in 1999–2000. Patients are experiencing similarly increasing wait times for other organs. Table 1.2 summarizes the median waiting times for various organ types.[7] The goal of matching organ supply with demand has not been achieved.[8]

Given such circumstances, insofar as commercial markets demonstrate potential to alleviate organ shortages and to decrease the time patients spend on waiting lists, more attention ought to be paid to possible applications. For example, a futures market or a market in cadaver organs might significantly address heart or pancreas needs. Indeed, commercial markets in human organs may be most feasible where need is the greatest: kidney and liver transplants. The transfer of single kidneys from living persons is medically viable: in the United States 6,623 such transplants were performed in 2002 and 6,819 in 2003, with more than 65,966 to date.[9] Perioperative mortality for nephrectomy is very low, approximately 0.03 percent, with other major complications typically occurring in less than 2 percent of cases.[10] The transfer of a liver segment from a living

Table 1.2
Median Waiting Time in Days

Type of Organ	Median Waiting Time (Days)	Years of Waiting List Registration
Kidney	1,144	1999
Liver	412	2002
Pancreas	244	2002
Kidney–Pancreas	275	2002
Heart	141	2002
Heart–Lung	694	2001
Lung	573	1999
Intestine	227	2002

Data is compiled from UNOS, *2003 Annual Report of the U.S. Organ Procurement and Transplantation Network and the Scientific Registry of Transplant Recipients: Transplant Data 1993–2002* (Rockville, MD: HHS/HRS/OSP/DOT, 2003); http://www. optn.org/AR2003 (last accessed August 12, 2004), table 1.6.

donor is likewise medically possible: 355 such transplants were performed in 2002 and 315 in 2003, with 2,392 to date. Provided that healthy donors retain a substantial portion of the liver, its overall regeneration is possible after the donation of a segment.[11] Although some older published reports describe a mortality rate as high as 11 percent for such operations,[12] more recently, most centers with surgeons who have considerable experience in partial hepatectomy report no donor mortalities.[13]

Despite such possibilities, a for-profit commercial market in human organs is often denounced as inappropriately commodifying the human body. Selling human organs for a profit is held to be exploitative and degrading, morally analogous to slavery, as well as incompatible with basic human values, such as human dignity and sanctity of life, and important social goals, such as equality and a spirit of altruism. The human body, it is argued, should not be treated as property.[14] Financial incentives are believed to coerce the poor into selling parts of their bodies and to corrupt the scientific practice of medicine. For example, in 1970 the Committee on Morals and Ethics of the Transplantation Society held that "the sale of organs by donors living or dead is indefensible under any circumstance,"[15] and the World Health Organization's (WHO) "Guiding Principles on Human Organ Transplantation" prohibits giving and receiving money for organs.[16] Moreover, the WHO urges member states to pass legislation forbidding the commercial trafficking of human organs (WHO 1991).[17] In the United States, Title III (Section 301) of the federal National Organ Transplant Act of 1984 (Public Law 98-057) makes it unlawful for any person knowingly to acquire, receive, or otherwise transfer human organs for valuable consideration for use in transplantation.

This study's analysis of the issues at stake, as well as the costs and benefits of a market in human organs, challenges the moral assumptions and conceptual arguments that apparently ground such a "consensus." As this analysis will demonstrate, on balance, prohibition of organ sales fails to sustain central social and medical goals as well as important basic human values.

"GLOBAL CONSENSUS"

The global consensus against for-profit markets in human organs is marked by a view that organs should be understood as gifts, not commodities. Organs are viewed as a social resource to be distributed according to medical necessity and to support public interests, rather than sold for private commercial gain.[18] Organs are to be a "gift of extraordinary magnitude" that transplantation surgeons "hold . . . in trust for society."[19] It is not just that organs are to be gifts, donated in the spirit of altruism and social solidarity; they are to be nationalized and constitute a "national resource to be used for the public good . . . to best serve the public interest."[20] Since the "physicians who select the recipient of a donated organ are making decisions about how a scarce public resource should be used,"[21] organs are to be allocated on the basis of acceptable medical criteria and social goals, rather than patient financial status. These foundational background assumptions, in particular that available organs are a public resource which governments are morally in authority to allocate, colors much of the debate regarding the permissibility of an organ market.[22]

While most laws simply prohibit payment for organs, certain professional statements and moral arguments have been broadly influential. For example, the Transplantation Society,[23] the World Medical Association,[24] the World Health Organization,[25] the Nuffield Council on Bioethics[26] and the U.S. Task Force on Organ Transplantation[27] each condemns the creation of a for-profit market in human organs. This "consensus" is supported by arguments that evaluate the moral and political theoretical parameters as well as the costs and benefits of a market in human organs. Such arguments purport to show that, unlike altruistically motivated donation, (1) offering financial incentives undermines consent, coercing the poor into selling their organs, and (2) that a market in human organs exploits the poor, violates human dignity, and is morally repugnant. Moreover, opponents argue that such a market would lead to (3) greater inequality between the rich and the poor as well as (4) worse health care outcomes than the current system of donation.

Factors That Influence Consent: Commercialism versus Altruism

For consent to organ donation to be morally effective, it must be voluntary and free from coercion. While it is often difficult to insulate patients and family members from institutional and social pressures, it is argued that potential organ donors "should be free of any undue influence and pressure and sufficiently informed to be able to understand and weigh the risks, benefits and consequences of consent."[28] As the U.S. Office of Technology Assessment Report points out, psychological, emotional, and medical needs, as well as a desire to please others, may influence one to donate organs.[29] Family members may agree to donate organs to avoid confrontations or to satisfy personal, family, or social objectives. This is especially the case if the alternative to the proposed procedure is the suffering and death of a loved one. Nevertheless, opponents of an organ market argue that unlike altruistic motivations, the prospect of financial gain, in particular, inappropriately influences a subject's decision to give consent.

Consider the Committee on Morals and Ethics of the Transplantation Society's description of money's coercive potential:

> In a South American country . . . advertisements from desperate individuals have appeared in newspapers offering a kidney or even

an eye . . . for money. In this regard, many of us receive occasional pathetic appeals from people in disadvantaged countries offering to sell a kidney to get money often for care of an ill relative. . . . It does not seem unlikely that a few of the unscrupulous will acquiesce to the profit motive.[30]

Financial gain is considered an influence that overwhelms and subjugates the voluntary consent of impoverished potential donors.[31] The choice to sell a kidney in order perhaps to better the economic status of one's family is considered a decision without merit or scruples.

Numerous professional statements endorse this assessment. The U.S. Task Force recommended that transplanting kidneys from living unrelated donors be prohibited whenever financial gain rather than altruism is the motivating factor. It called for prohibition on federal and state levels.[32] Similarly, the WHO's guiding principles on organ transplantation proscribe advertising for organs with an intent to offer or seek payment.[33] The Transplantation Society simply condemns advertising by transplant surgeons for donors or recipients,[34] and the American Medical Association prohibits the purchasing of organs from living donors for transplantation.[35]

Altruistic donation is believed to support individual freedom by fostering personal choice. As the Transplantation Society argued with regard to living unrelated donors: "altruism on the part of the donor may be a real motivating factor . . . the wish to donate an organ need not be a sign of mental instability."[36] Their guidelines for the distribution and use of organs from cadaver sources and living donors specifically require that donors be altruistically motivated.

It must be established by the patient and transplant team alike that the motives of the donor are altruistic and in the best interests of the recipient and not self-serving or for-profit . . . especially in the exceptional case where the emotionally related donor is not a spouse or a second degree relative, the donor advocate would ensure and document that the donation was one of altruism and not self-serving or for-profit.[37]

Unlike for-profit commercial transfers, altruistic donation purportedly binds persons to their families, friends, and communities.

The market is viewed as corrosive of "gift-of-life" sentiments, which have often characterized organ procurement. After all, altruistic donation has powerful psychological and social repercussions that are of value to society and interpersonal relationships. Altruistic donation is seen as a voluntary expression of important human values as well as of communal commitments. Fox and Swazey encapsulate this view as they lament that many believe that organ transplantation is "analogous to a commercial industry and product and that its nonconformity to a market model is not only curious but possibly subversive."[38] They argue that this position "makes it difficult for us to identify with the way that transplants . . . are now being conceived and interpreted."[39] Rather than parts of living persons "offered in life or death to sustain known or unknown others, that resonate with the symbolic meaning of our relation to our bodies, our selves, and to each other," Fox and Swazey express concern that organs are being considered as mere things—that is, as "just organs."[40] A market in human organs, they argue, would ignore and undermine the gift exchange dimensions of organ donation, with its obligations of giving, receiving, and repaying. It would undermine our willingness to address common problems with collective resolve.[41] The importance of such gifts to individual recipients as well as for community solidarity is believed to be overlooked by commercialization.[42]

Altruistic donation is seen as central to maintaining both public trust and organ availability. The argument is that when organs are donated to the community, they carry "the hopes of the donor's family . . . that the organ will be used to the best possible advantage."[43] As Mary Ellen McNally, coordinator for the New England Organ Bank emphasized, trust that organs are not commodities to be sold underlies public willingness to donate. In one case "the father made perfectly clear . . . that donation was a gift by his son to someone else, and the sale of those organs would diminish the goodness of that gift."[44]

Some have advocated a system of death benefit payments to motivate families of potential organ donors: "Our concerns must focus not on some philosophic imperative such as altruism but on our collective responsibility for maximizing lifesaving organ recovery."[45] Yet others, such as Edmund Pellegrino, have rebutted these proposals as "logically, ethically, and practically flawed."[46] Since such proposals appear to reject the centrality of the gift relationship to organ donation, or to consent to donation, they are criticized as endorsing values that are antithetical to the altruistic, community-oriented culture of donation.[47]

While the purchased organ is conceptualized merely as a commodity, coerced from the seller by poverty, need, and market forces, altruistically donated organs are believed to bind persons to their community and family, as well as to foster "warm satisfaction" in the minds of donors or their bereaved families (in cases of cadaveric donation).[48] While couched in somewhat rhetorical terms, the process of organ donation is regarded as giving something intrinsically valuable back to donors or their families. In short, opponents of organ sales argue that commercialism treats persons as individuals in isolation from family and community, coercing some through the offer of money into parting with their organs. Altruistic donation, in contrast, is held to foster the expression of important personal values as well as family commitments and social solidarity and thus is viewed as consistent with free voluntary consent.[49]

Exploitation, Moral Repugnance, and Human Dignity

The practice of buying organs from living vendors for transplantation arouses in many feelings of gruesome horror. Commercial schemes are viewed as intrinsically exploitative.[50] The historical precedent for such a market, according to Russell Scott, is chattel slavery, in which the human body becomes mere property.[51] At the very least this view does not take seriously the involuntary character of hereditary slavery. Condemnation of a market in human organs is believed to be grounded in basic ethical principles, such as "the dignity of the individual" and "respect for persons."[52] For Paul Ramsey, behind the repugnance lies a real danger that such practices "will only erode still more our apprehension that man is a sacredness in the biological order . . . and our respect for men of flesh who are only to be found within the ambience of bodily existence."[53] According to Leon Kass, there is a general repugnance at owning living nature per se.[54] The concern is that it is precisely because of their general significance and intimate connection with persons that organs ought not to be sold. The body is believed to be part of the basic dignity of the human person; therefore, trade in the body and its parts is held to be deeply morally repugnant and ought to be restricted.

For many the moral repugnance appears straightforward. Indeed, the WHO resolution "Development of Guiding Principles for Human Organ Transplantation" affirms that commerce in human organs is "inconsistent with the most basic human values and contravenes the Universal Declaration of Human Rights. . . ."[55] The WHO resolution "Preventing the Purchase and Sale of Human Organs" similarly asserts that the commercial sale of organs is exploitative and incompatible with human dignity (WHA 42.5). This resolution contends that prohibition is necessary to

> prevent the exploitation of human distress, particularly in children and other vulnerable groups, and to further the recognition of the ethical principles which condemn the buying and selling of organs for purpose of transplantation.[56]

Organ selling purportedly exploits the distress of those in need.

As an example of a commercial venture, consider physician H. Berry Jacobs, founder of International Kidney Exchange Inc. Jacobs asked seventy-five hundred hospitals if they would be willing to participate in his plan to broker human kidneys. He proposed to offer the poor in third-world countries and the United States whatever price would induce them to sell a kidney, and then negotiate acquisition, for a profit, by Americans who could afford to pay for the organs. Jacobs's plan aroused cries of moral indignation in the U.S. Congress. It was denounced by the National Kidney Foundation, the Transplantation Society, and the American Society of Transplantation Surgeons. As the U.S. Task Force summarized the objection: "We are alarmed that . . . certain transplant centers are reportedly brokering kidneys from living unrelated donors. We find this practice to be unethical and to raise serious questions about the exploitation and coercion of people, especially the poor."[57] The contention is that the rich exploit the fact of poverty to encourage the poor into selling their organs, who, given better circumstances, would not have participated in such a transaction.[58]

The potential for exploitation and violation of human dignity, which is perceived to underlie commerce in human organs, is held to trump the possibility of increasing life-sustaining transplants. As the Nuffield Council Report argues, certain uses of human tissue are morally unacceptable because they "fail to respect others or to accord them dignity . . . they injure human beings by treating them as things, as less than human, as objects for use."[59] Morally acceptable uses protect "a central element of the undefined, yet widely endorsed, demand for respect for the human body and for respect for human dignity."[60] Here Caplan, Van Buren, and Tilney note:

> Allowing the sale of the human body reduces people to objects. Offering compensation towards life insurance, cash rebates, estate tax discounts, or payment for funerals contingent upon a favorable decision about the disposition of cadaver remains indicates that medicine and the law are willing to turn the body into a commodity to allow more transplants to be performed. The message conveyed is that it is permissible, even desirable, to treat the body as an object of sale and profit.[61]

This distinction between morally acceptable and unacceptable utilization of human body parts is thus drawn with a judgment regarding whether or not such uses properly respect human dignity.[62]

Edward Keyserlingk argues, in addition, that even though such requirements may make kidney procurement inefficient, this does not provide sufficient reason to override society's commitment to prevent exploitation and to preserve human dignity:

> Assuming and adopting as we do the Kantian injunction that persons should always be treated as autonomous ends and not merely as means to the ends of others, a morally justifiable policy will be one which is likely to provide the largest number of . . . organs . . . without violating the human dignity of potential donors. As for a policy permitting the sale and purchase of human organs, it may well be in some respects the most efficient approach, at least for those in a position to buy and sell, and it can provide direct and full control to buyer and seller; *but because it so badly fails the other tests, it should be rejected.*[63]

Efficient and effective organ procurement and transplantation is not understood as a good worth pursuing at such a price.

Human organs, Keyserlingk continues, have a special status due to their intimate relation with persons. Furthermore, in life the body as an organic whole is a good, since it is the center and means of awareness and vehicle of communication. It is this link between self and body that grounds bodily inviolability. These characteristics, he concludes, make the body and its parts properly the subject of altruism and gift giving rather than commercial sale. To respect these characteristics of persons is to respect human dignity. Organ sales, in contrast, treat the body as a collection of spare parts,[64] independent of the body's intimate relationship to the life of a person. Organ sales thereby violate human dignity.

According to Nancy Scheper-Hughes, cofounder of Organs Watch,

> These people have been reduced to bays of spare parts . . . for doctors to justify this by saying, "Well, the seller is getting something out of it too," is unethical. Turning one person's poverty into an opportunity for someone else is a violation of the most basic standards of human ethics. . . . Doctors should be protectors of the body, and perhaps we should look for better ways of helping the destitute than dismantling them.[65]

Bob Brecher summarizes the objection:

> However much the Turkish peasant who sold a kidney may have needed the money he was paid; however genuinely he may have wished to exercise his autonomy in this enterprising venture . . . however sincere his wish to benefit his family with the proceeds, and however great their need; nevertheless what he did was wrong.[66]

That more patients may suffer and die under current protocols for procurement and distribution than on a for-profit scheme of organ vending is judged as providing insufficient reason to justify the creation of such a market.

Equality and Justice

Building on the assumption that human organs are a common resource to be utilized for the public good with an independent assumption of social egalitarianism, an additional argument levied against commercialization is that equal access to organ transplants is the only distribution consonant with the equality of all candidates. Social justice, it is argued, requires equality of opportunity through redistributing property and forbidding the private purchase and sale of better basic health care. As Childress notes, "the individual's personal and transcendent dignity . . . can be protected and witnessed to by a recognition of his equal right to be saved."[67] The Transplantation Society's statement contends, for example, that allowing the purchase of organs for transplant would lead to inappropriate levels of inequitable health care outcomes between the rich and the poor:

> [If] wealthy individuals from other countries are placed on transplant lists . . . they compete with local patients for scarce cadaver kidneys . . . private hospitals in Europe now perform kidney transplants for foreigners who can afford the substantial fees. . . . The unacceptable consequence of this is that kidneys go only to patients who can pay.[68]

The concern is that a market in human organs will lead to a situation in which the poor sacrifice their bodies for the health of the rich, while the rich gain unequal, and therefore unfair, access to a scarce public medical resource.[69]

This conclusion resonates with that of the President's Commission for the Study of Ethical Problems in Medicine and Biomedical and Behavioral Research (1982), which held that given the circumstance that differences in health status are largely undeserved, and that the distribution of health care needs is uneven and unpredictable, health care has a special status and society possesses a moral obligation to ensure adequate care for everyone: "Equitable access to health care requires that all citizens be able to secure an adequate level of care without excessive burdens."[70] From this viewpoint, society is obligated to sustain the existence of each individual. Moreover, this duty extends not only to providing basic health care but also, if necessary, to organ transplantation.[71]

The U.S. Task Force on Organ Transplantation (1986) similarly concluded that patient financial status should not limit availability of transplantation. They argued that "all transplant procedures recognized as medically effective should be made available through reimbursement mechanisms for the care of patients who have no other source of funds."[72] The task force equated equitable access to transplantation with proscribing organ sales: "implementation of equitable access prohibits any elements of commercialization in the distribution of organs."[73] Insofar as there exists social commitment to provide all with equal access to adequate health care, including organ transplants, equitable access means access regardless of wealth.[74] As the Massachusetts Task Force on Organ Transplantation elaborates this point, rationing human organs based on the ability to pay implicitly sends the message that

> we do not believe in equality and that a price can and should be placed on human life and that it should be paid by the individual whose life is at stake. Neither belief is tolerable in a society in which income is inequitably distributed.[75]

Each assessment stresses equality as a moral constraint on public policy in health care.[76]

Rather than recognizing the guarantee of property rights and free collaboration to be core to human respect and dignity, despite inequalities, opponents of an organ market reflect a vision of social justice that brings into question the good fortunes of those who have more opportunities, wealth, and resources to purchase more extensive health care, such as organ transplantation.[77] In part, the argument concerns which values ought to weigh more in the calculation of the costs and benefits of public health care policy. In part, it is also a debate over which values may be sacrificed for others.[78] Allocation and rationing decisions are inevitable.[79]

For example, one might argue that gains in individual liberty as well as greater organ availability, and thus less total human suffering, compensate at the level of social policy for losses in equal access to expensive health care. However, many assess the value considerations otherwise. As George Annas argues, a market in human organs places a high value on individual rights and a low value on equality and fairness.[80] Similarly, Arthur Caplan maintains that

> Allocating lifesaving organs by the ability of those in need to pay what the market will bear is blatantly unfair to the poor. . . . To argue that the sale of organs as a business is motivated by humanitarian concerns for the well being of those in need simply flies in the face of the fact that selling organs can only increase the cost for those who now receive them for free.[81]

In short, equality of opportunity and of access to organs is appreciated as an essential element of social justice and as trumping important liberty interests. The additional costs of providing more organs to save the lives of more people is considered unjustifiable.

If one assumes that organ donation is a gift to society and that the state has moral political authority to regulate procurement and distribution, it is plausible to raise concerns on grounds of equality that "it seems unfair and even exploitative for society to ask people to donate organs if these organs will be distributed on the basis of the ability to pay."[82] If rich and poor alike donate, but only the rich receive transplants, a significant social class of those who donate will not benefit from transplantation. Thus, opponents conclude, donated organs should be distributed to medically eligible recipients regardless of their ability to pay for the transplant[83]: on these grounds, a for-profit market is argued to lead to unequal health care outcomes and, therefore, is unfair and unjust.[84] Medical suitability and severity of illness are viewed as consisting of more objective data appropriately weighed in allocation of goods and services. They appear to satisfy the requirement that "criteria for organ placement must be objective, medically sound, and publicly stated."[85] However, no one has seemed to notice that the argument as structured is less critical of a market in human organs per se than of (1) selling organs that were donated and (2) charging for health care services that utilize donated organs.

Health Care Outcomes

An additional concern is that a market in human organs would harm the health of donors and recipients. Consider the Transplantation Society's assessment:

> Normal safeguards which protect family donors and recipients are threatened by brokerage arrangements, when otherwise unacceptable donors may become acceptable if the price is right. Similarly, one can argue that less than ideal kidneys could be sold more cheaply than organs of good quality. Even if motivation of both donor and recipient is correct, the sale of organs essentially forces the donor to have an operation. . . . Indeed, as a practical example, it could be argued that the buying and selling of blood for transfusion . . . has led to a less safe and more expensive service.[86]

It is important to note the special health care costs the Transplantation Society identifies: first, that a market in human organs would likely lead to procuring lesser quality organs, second, that this could lead to lower life expectancies for recipients, and third, that vendors would incur inappropriate surgical harms, including possibly death.

Many share the first concern. As Caplan makes the point, medicine cannot morally allow "itself to be used by those who would risk their own health out of greed, desperation or ignorance."[87] Frier and Mavrodes similarly conclude that the profit motive would likely reduce care and caution in the selection of suitable organs.[88] So too Abouna et al. argue that an organ market would lead to inferior medical care with higher complication rates.[89] If profit is the primary objective, they argue, then normal standards of medical screening may not be exerted adequately; for example, R. A. Sells notes that "postoperative deaths from HIV transmission at the time of transplantation have been reported."[90] Moreover, relatives may not be willing to donate genetically well-matched organs, if it is possible instead to purchase the needed organ from another donor.

In fact, the second criticism resonates with general anxiety regarding graft survival. The long-term survival of transplants may be superior when organs are procured from living relatives rather than from unrelated donors.[91] In one 1990 study, the patient survival at one year for transplants utilizing purchased kidneys from unrelated donors was 81.5 percent, compared to 97.8 percent using living related donors.[92] However, other studies rebut this conclusion. One study in India suggested that graft survival from live unrelated donors at one year appeared to be moderately superior to that of live related transplants (84 percent versus 81 percent respectively). They acknowledged, though, that they did not view the difference as statistically significant.[93] For the United States, according to the Organ Procurement and Transplantation Network, the one-year survival data for kidney transplants is 88.1 percent from cadaveric donors and 94.3 percent from living donors. At three years the survival rates were 77.6 percent and 87.5 percent, respectively.[94] If poor transplant results lead to an increased number of transplants per patient, this will be an inefficient and ineffective use of scarce health care resources, presuming that the market does not sufficiently increase the supply of organs to more than compensate for any inefficiencies.

The third criticism identified by the Transplantation Society is often phrased in terms of the Hippocratic injunction first to do no harm, *primum non nocere*.[95] Organ vendors receive operations for which there is no medical indication. "Operations should be performed for therapeutic reasons: a financial reward does not represent a therapeutic indication for surgery."[96] In addition, if the vendor is poor, once his organ is removed and he is discharged from the hospital, there is no protection or guarantee that there will be adequate follow-up. The impecunious vendor can ill afford any future hospitalization for possible complications of the operation.[97] While some have argued that there is no morally relevant difference between selling one's time and selling one's own redundant organs, opponents of commercialization insist that only a minority hold such a view.[98]

Additional criticisms are that legitimating a market in human organs would indirectly[99] lead to a decrease in the number of kidneys available for transplant as well as an unacceptable rise in the financial costs of procuring organs. The first concern is tied to the view that "making organs available only to those who can afford them will only feed preexisting suspicion and paranoia."[100] There are three primary possibilities. First, if organ sales are permissible this may so inflame public response as to turn the public against the organ transplant system. Thus fewer people would be inclined altruistically to donate.[101] In addition, if patients are able to purchase organs, there is less incentive to create and promote local donation programs. Finally, an organ market may also impact living-donor-related transplantation. For example, in Kuwait "several well-matched relatives of potential recipients . . . withdrew their offer of donation after they learned that their relatives [could] go to India and buy a kidney in the market place."[102] If such a decrease in altruism becomes widespread, and if the number of organs available for purchase does not increase to meet the shortfall, there may be fewer organs available.[103]

The Office of Technology Assessment Report identifies two types of additional financial expenses that would be incurred if donors were financially compensated for their organs: the actual cost of compensation and the costs of administering the exchange—that is, additional transaction costs.[104] Transaction costs would likely include advertising for potential vendors, screening for tissue compatibility, and negotiating between patients and vendors, or third parties, over contractual conditions for the transfer of property rights in the organs. Insofar as a market would add significant financial barriers to transplantation, this would further limit the ability of many to gain access to such health care, thereby producing worse health care outcomes than the current system of donation.[105]

In short, it is argued that a market in organs would lead to harms to organ vendors, result in inefficient and ineffective use of scarce health care resources, decrease the number of available organs, raise health care expenses, and procure lower quality organs for transplantation. Such health care costs, if realized, may outweigh the potential benefits of a market in human organs.

PROHIBITION: CONTROVERSIES AND CRITICISMS

While the focus of the debate framing the global consensus has been on the ways in which a market in human organs may undermine consent, exploit the poor, violate human dignity, create greater inequality between rich and poor, and lead to worse health care outcomes than the current system of donation, more analysis is required adequately to evaluate such rhetorically powerful criticisms. Such a consensus, while pervasive, has not proven to be sufficiently justified. Consider the following concerns a nephrologist expressed to the International Transplantation Society at a conference on the permissibility of a market in human organs:

> When I first became aware of commercialization as a possibility in organ transplantation, I, like most everybody here . . . was very opposed to it and thought it a terrible thing. More recently, I am not so sure. I think the issue is much more complex than it appears to be at first and, perhaps, even more complex than its presentation [at this conference].

He questioned the moral grounds as well as the extent of the "consensus" that organ sales are morally illicit:

> I wonder who decided that it was morally wrong. . . . Who is it that sits on these boards and makes these decisions? How many people from the public have been asked if we think it's morally wrong?

Indeed, while apparently possessing evidence that nearly half of the individuals he had polled in the United States did not agree with the assessment of the Transplantation Society's Committee on Morals and Ethics that selling human organs is morally repugnant, he feared professional reprisals if such data was published:

in a survey which I did—that I have never really put together yet for fear of what people would think of it—in which I asked every day Joe Blows what they think about selling their organs . . . somewhere between 40 and 50% of people did not think it was morally wrong.[106]

Similar concerns have been expressed by some surgeons from India. Thiagarajan et al. argue against

those who have allocated to themselves the right to sit in judgment, based on their own environment and prejudices, and to exclude from scientific discussion those observations that come to alternative and controversial, yet acceptable, practices prevailing in other less fortunate areas of the world.[107]

While pointing to the success of their transplantation program in terms of graft survival, lack of donor mortality, return of patients to productive lives, and assistance in resolving the great financial need of donors, Thiagarajan et al. lament that the greatest value lost is professional and academic respectability.

The question that Reddy et al. are faced with is "Do we buy or let die?"[108] Acknowledging that in India money often covertly changes hands even among related living donors and recipients, they rebut the purported moral repugnance that appears to be foundational to the supposed "global consensus." Organ selling is not mere utilitarian spare-parts medicine, they argue; rather, it focuses on basic human values, community connectedness, and fundamental social goals. It conveys essential moral, social, and medical benefits.

To dismiss the idea of paid donors as the ethics of expediency is to deny these patients the right to live. We serve only the corrupt and the unscrupulous if we deny the patient benefit of a transplant that is medically indicated because of our fear that the paid donation process is too complex to be regulated.[109]

Purchasing human organs for transplantation, Reddy, Thiagarajan, and Shunmugasundaram et al. conclude, is in keeping with ethical values, social goals, and fundamental commitments to quality medical care.

The response of the Transplantation Society to such criticisms appealed to the authority of superior information and expertise. Nicholas Tilney stated, for example, "We felt that we had the knowledge and expertise to create these guidelines, knowing some of the facts and innuendoes. . . ."[110] Although they have occasionally revisited the question of paid organ donation over the past two decades,[111] the official position of the Transplantation Society remains unchanged: "organs and tissues should be freely given without commercial consideration or financial profit."[112] The society requires all candidates for membership to sign a policy statement summarizing its views on this and other issues, thereby signifying agreement.

Similarly, in a June 29, 2001, statement, the United Network for Organ Sharing (UNOS) once again condemned the sale of human organs for transplantation, including the brokering of organs for others. It resolved that UNOS members who participate in any such arrangements "shall be considered for status as 'member not in good standing.'"[113]

The criticisms, though, remain largely unaddressed; more careful analysis is required before one should pass judgment against a commercial market in human organs. Before pointing to a global consensus and attempting coercively to impose a particular viewpoint through law and public policy, more voices ought to be heard. Rabbi Moshe D. Tendler urges, for example, that even if altruism remains the gold standard for donation, the shortage of transplantable organs is so acute that donor remuneration may be justified because of the overarching lifesaving considerations.[114] As Johny et al. point out, while the buying and selling of organs is condemned internationally, this doctrine is largely based on sensational press reports concerning the involvement of unscrupulous brokers, as well as the concern to protect desperate recipients and needy poor from exploitation.[115] Insofar as such concerns can be appropriately resolved, legitimate objections to a market in human organs will be diminished.

CHAPTER TWO

Metaphysics, Morality, and Political Theory

The Presuppositions of Proscription Reexamined

INTRODUCTION

Before forming blanket moral judgments whether to condemn or praise, before even considering likely costs and benefits, one must assess what would have to be granted regarding the relationship of persons with their bodies, the ownership of body parts, and the limits of societal and governmental authority for the sale of human organs for transplantation to be morally permissible. Critical assessment of such commercialization must begin with an exploration of the foundational metaphysical, moral, and political theoretical conditions that would need to be granted, if any, for such a market to be established. Utilization of living vendors, for example, is likely to raise rather different moral and political theoretical concerns than a market in cadaver organs. Similarly, because of ways in which the physical brain is experienced as the seat of individual consciousness and personal identity, selling this organ for transplant is likely to pose foundational metaphysical issues that would be unlikely to arise regarding the sale of other body parts, such as blood, sperm, or ova. Perhaps no particular foundational conditions are strictly necessary. Instead, various constellations of understandings of the relationship between persons and their bodies, the ownership of human organs, and the limits of political moral authority may prove sufficient to render a market in organs morally acceptable. Or it may be that certain foundational conditions establish not merely necessary but also sufficient conditions, such that a market could not be rightfully forbidden.

As the analysis proceeds, this chapter will not advance arguments to show that any particular foundational conditions can be established. The justification of a specific moral viewpoint, account of property ownership, ontology of the body, or theory of legitimate political authority is not at issue. Instead, the chapter offers an analytical or geographical portrayal of the presuppositions in which the debate is cast and of the conditions that shift the standard of moral evidence as well as the burden of proof. The general significance of ownership, forbearance, and privacy rights, as well as the closeness of the analogy between dominion/possession/ownership of one's body parts and dominion/possession/ownership of other types of things, for example, will directly impact the relative standard of proof that must be met rightfully to interfere with persons' uses of their own body parts. Other factors, such as the specified body part (e.g., heart, kidney, blood, sperm, or ova) and type of donor (e.g., living or deceased), as well as the grounds and limits of moral political authority, will shift who shoulders the burden of proof: those who would participate in a market for transplantable organs or those who would forbid such consensual human interaction. Such considerations also impact the reasons that are relevant for meeting the appropriate standard of proof.

The result is a multidimensional geography of factors, which in different constellations may be sufficient to render a market in human organs for transplantation permissible, including those constellations of factors that together would establish that such a market could not be rightfully forbidden. This geography will permit systematic and careful assessment of the relative strength of the moral claims individuals put forth to participate in a market in human organs for transplantation and, therefore, of the relative strength of the contraindicating conditions that would be required to defeat the market's moral permissibility.

INITIAL CONSIDERATIONS: ASSESSING STANDARDS OF EVIDENCE AND PLACING THE BURDEN OF PROOF

An initial set of considerations regards standards of moral evidence and the burden of proof. Conceptions of moral permissibility can be located on a continuum beginning with the position that an organ market is intuitively, all things considered, acceptable, ranging to the position that it may not be rightfully forbidden. Intermediary positions describe organ markets as more or less prima facie morally allowable—that is, permissible absent sufficiently significant contraindicating considerations. Among the factors that specify the relative strength of the moral claim to participate freely in such a market are (1) the general significance of ownership rights, (2) whether ownership includes entitlements to exclusive use and alienation, (3) the closeness of the analogy between dominion/possession/ownership of one's body parts and dominion/possession/ownership of other types of things, as well as the force of (4) privacy and (5) forbearance rights (i.e., rights to be left alone and protected from battery). Given different understandings of such foundational concerns, the market will be more or less morally acceptable, thereby increasing or decreasing the burden of proof required to restrict such free human interaction. As foundational conditions supporting organ sales increase in significance, so too will the standard of moral evidence necessary to forbid such transactions.

Whereas an intuitive ceteris paribus judgment may be defeated with sufficient indication of potential harms, the strength of such concerns will turn in part on defensible understandings of reasonable risk. Moreover, such evidence may not rise to the standard necessary to set aside significant forbearance and privacy rights freely to choose to subject oneself to such risks. Here organ vending might appear as simply among the wide range of more or less risk-affirming activities in which individuals are morally free to choose to participate (e.g., hang gliding, rock climbing, motorcycle riding, eating rare meat, working on an oil rig, joining the police force, or pursuing a military career). After all, the same questions regarding appropriate risk are raised anytime a living person is the source of the harvested organ, whether for donation or sale. Relative standard of proof to meet the burden of proof so as to defeat the prima facie permissibility of the market will increase as the significance of such rights and other foundational concerns increase.

This analytic point is similar to the shift in the standard of proof in U.S. law, which increases as the matters at stake become more significant. Standards of proof allocate the risk of error between the plaintiff and defendant by instructing fact finders regarding the degree of confidence for a particular type of adjudication. The selection of a standard of proof indicates, more generally, the value or significance placed on the interests at stake in the litigation.[1] Standards begin with "preponderance of the evidence" for civil cases, which involve loss of property, but not findings of criminal fault, moving to "clear and convincing evidence" for the long-term commitment of persons for psychiatric reasons, or legally to effect the removal of children from the custody of their parents.[2] Since the rights at stake are judged more significant, the proof must be stronger. The test of truth as "beyond a reasonable doubt" is employed in criminal cases, which involve the possibility of loss of freedom and life. These standards are generally understood as the minimum weights of evidence required to support the plaintiff's case to find against the defendant; often thought of as 51 percent ("preponderance of the evidence"), 75 percent ("clear and convincing evidence"), and 95 percent ("beyond a reasonable doubt"). Whereas "preponderance of the evidence" requires the triers of fact to believe that it is more probable than not that the facts are true, and "clear and convincing evidence" requires that they believe that it is highly probable that the facts are true, "beyond a reasonable doubt" requires that they believe the facts to be true of almost certainty. The very strict standard of "beyond a reasonable doubt" is required in criminal cases to satisfy rulings regarding the due process clause of the U.S. Constitution and to protect the important liberty interests of the defendant.[3] As the general significance of the matters at stake increases, so too does the burden of proof to justify interference with the defendant's property, family, or person.[4]

By analogy, insofar as permitting organ sales for transplantation would tend to limit important personal rights and freedoms, imposing net costs on health and restricting individual opportunities, a relatively low standard of moral evidence will be sufficient to forbid the market. However, insofar as forbidding such transactions infringes significant rights and liberties, restricting important opportunities for improving one's life, health, or important personal goals, there will be grounds for significantly increasing the standard of moral evidence required to meet the burden of proof rightfully to proscribe such sales. As the general significance, or strength, of ownership, privacy, liberty, and forbearance rights increases, so too should the standard of proof that must be met rightfully to interfere in one's use of self, body, and property.

As important as the stringency of the standard of proof are considerations regarding the bearer of the burden of proof. Different understandings of property rights, as well as of the authority of the government to intervene in market transfers, will shift the burden of moral justification to the shoulders of either those who would forbid or those who would permit such consensual human activity. For example, the more one can establish universally binding moral content, such as the existence of special goods (e.g., particular understandings of equality or liberty), the more there will exist moral authority to regulate the conduct of persons to promote the creation and maintenance of those goods. Such an account shifts the burden of proof away from institutions that promote or regulate social creation or maintenance of the good, to individuals who would act independently with consenting others. It is presumed that moral authority exists to utilize the time, talent, and property of others to promote the good. Concomitantly, insofar as moral authority is created by and thus limited to the free agreements of persons, the greater will be the burden of proof on those persons and governmental institutions who presume to interfere with free consensual interaction to show that they do so with moral authority.

These two axes, the standard of proof and the bearer of the burden of proof, express the initial complexities of the conceptual geography of conflicting rights and moral concerns underlying a market in human organs. Each axis can be considered as displaying conditions that if granted would make an ever stronger case on behalf of a market in organs. Certain considerations would, by more clearly establishing the plausibility of a market in organs, shift the burden of proof to those who would proscribe such transactions. Moreover, depending on which considerations are established, the standard of moral evidence required to satisfy the burden of proof licitly to proscribe organ sales increases.

PERSONS AND BODY PARTS

Persons are central to the existence of the market. Only persons claim dominion, possession, or ownership over things and self-consciously choose to cooperate with others. Only persons are able to forge agreements to participate in common projects. Roughly speaking, persons are agents that possess sufficient cognitive capacities to understand themselves in a self-conscious, self-reflexive way. As John Locke noted, a person is a "thinking intelligent being, that has reason and reflection, and can consider itself as itself, the same thinking thing in different times and places, which it does only by that consciousness which is inseparable from thinking, and, as it seems to be, essential to it."[5] Such capacities are required for persons to be, in principle, capable of forging agreements to participate in common projects, to choose to convey authority to mutual commitments, and to negotiate and engage in transactions.

Rationality is central to being a person, at least in the limited sense of possessing the capacity to appreciate the relationship between choices and their outcomes or significance. As Kant marked the distinction: "A *person* is a subject whose actions can be *imputed* to him . . . a *thing* is that to which nothing can be imputed. Any object of free choice which itself lacks freedom is therefore called a thing (*res corporalis*)."[6] Here also, Kant noted, persons are not merely agents, but moral agents. To be a person requires the ability, in principle, to appreciate one's actions as praiseworthy or blameworthy. Persons have the capacity to think through their choices and, in principle, to control passionate responses. Persons are morally responsible for the outcomes and significance of their choices. As the agents or causes of actions, persons are able to deliberate and choose, and are thus appropriately the subject of praise or blame. This requires self-consciously seeing oneself as the agent of one's choices and actions. Through reason, deliberation, and choice, persons shape their own characters to a significant extent. Even to protest that one ought to have been treated differently is to construe rational, self-reflexive entities as moral agents.

This account carves out of the phenomenological experienced world the moral and ontological category of persons. Animals and things that do not possess the requisite cognitive capacities cannot be intersubjectively experienced as persons and, therefore, cannot be affirmed as such within the context of general secular morality. Much more would have to be said to establish the moral and ontological status of other beings and things; this account simply points out that whatever their status, such entities and items do not fall into the category of "persons." Indeed, once beings permanently lose the cognitive capacities that sustain personhood, they become beings, if not things, which have the character of being former persons. Without such essential capacities beings cannot, even in principle, participate in self-conscious, self-reflexive moral agency. It is persons for whom there exists the possibility of rational assessment of the costs and benefits of various uses of one's body and property. Only persons can reflect on the relative injustice of a violation of their bodily integrity or of their property. In principle, to possess concern for ownership of or trade in human organs, much less for its moral permissibility or sociopolitical limitations, requires that persons be the sort of beings who are able to express self-conscious, self-reflexive, moral agency.

Persons and Bodily Integrity

The significance of persons, especially regarding individual authority over one's body and one's bodily integrity, has become central to moral and legal reflections on the practice of medicine. Common law understood interest in the integrity of the person to include interest in his body and all the things that are in contact or connected with it. Property expresses the rights of *persons* in and over *things*.[7] The nature of such rights, their character, scope, and form, is drawn from the nature of persons. Under the traditional law of torts, for example, the person includes any part of the body as well as anything attached to it and practically identified with it. Violation of a person includes nonconsensual contact with the individual's "clothing, or with a cane, a paper, or any other object held in his hand."[8] Interest in the integrity of the person includes his body and all the things that are intimately connected with it. The more intimately associated things are with the person, the more they are protected as part of the integrity of the person. Property is an extension of the person and is thereby also protected against unauthorized use or touching; it too is protected against battery.[9]

A person's authority over himself, to freedom of choice regarding the use of his body, is central to understanding personal integrity. Histories of informed consent, for example, often begin with the English case of *Slater v. Baker and Stapleton* (1767),[10] which found two practitioners liable because they failed to acquire consent prior to disuniting and resetting a patient's fracture. Such legal and moral concerns were articulated in the United States in cases such as *Union Pacific R. Co. v. Botsford* (1891). Here the court observed that "[n]o right is held more sacred, or is more carefully guarded by the common law, than the right of every individual to the possession and control of his own person, free from all restraint or interference of others."[11] Similarly, in *Mohr v. Williams* (1905), the court argued that "[t]he free citizen's first and greatest right, which underlies all others—the right to himself— is the subject of universal acquiescence, and this right necessarily forbids a physician or surgeon . . . to violate without permission the bodily integrity of his patient . . . without his consent or knowledge."[12] In these and similar cases, such as *Rolater v. Strain* (1913),[13] a robust understanding of a person's authority over himself, to freedom of choice regarding use of one's body as well as to personal bodily integrity, developed prior to the oft-cited decision of Justice Cardozo in *Schloendorff v. Society of New York Hospital* (1914): "Every human being of adult years and sound mind has a right to determine what shall be done with his own body; and a surgeon who performs an operation without his patient's consent commits an assault, for which he is liable in damages."[14] The moral right to consent and to be left alone has been recognized in a number of court holdings:

> The makers of our Constitution . . . sought to protect Americans in their beliefs, their thoughts, their emotions, and their sensations. They conferred, as against the Government, the right to be left alone—the most comprehensive of rights and the right most valued by civilized men. (*Olmstead v. United States*, 1928, J. Brandeis dissenting)[15]

> Nothing in this utterance suggests that Brandeis thought an individual possessed these rights only as to sensible beliefs, valid thoughts, reasonable emotions, or well-formed sensations. I suggest that he intended to include a great many foolish unreasonable and even absurd ideas which do not conform such as refusing medical treatment even at great risk. (*In re President & Directors of Georgetown College Inc.*, 1964, W. Burger dissenting)[16]

Respect for persons and their individual bodily integrity has become firmly entrenched in much U.S. law. As the court opined, in *Planned Parenthood v. Casey* (1992), the principle at stake is that personal decisions that profoundly affect bodily integrity should be largely beyond the reach of government.[17]

Court decisions regarding forced medical treatment, gathering of evidence in criminal investigations, and abortion give further emphasis to this robust understanding of personal authority over one's body. In *Cruzan v. Director, Missouri Department of Health* (1990), for example, the court noted that "the liberty interest in refusing medical treatment flows from decisions involving the state's invasions into the body. . . . Because our notions of liberty are inextricably entwined with our ideas of physical freedom and self-determination, the Court has often deemed state incursions into the body repugnant to the interests protected by the Due Process Clause."[18]

The court similarly opined in *Schmerber v. California* (1966) that "[t]he integrity of an individual's person is a cherished value in our society";[19] and in *Winston v. Lee* (1985) that "[a] compelled surgical intrusion into an individual's body for evidence . . . implicates expectations of privacy and security of such magnitude that the intrusion may be 'unreasonable' even if likely to produce evidence of a crime."[20]

Concerning abortion, the woman's authority over her body has been held to be of greater significance than the life of the fetus. In *Planned Parenthood v. Casey*

(1992) the court argued that in *Roe v. Wade* the significance of individual control over one's self and body had been correctly applied to a woman's right to choose abortion: "if *Roe* is seen as stating a rule of personal autonomy and bodily integrity, akin to cases recognizing limits on government power to mandate medical treatment or to bar its rejection, this court's post *Roe* decisions accord with *Roe's* view that a state's interest in the protection of life *falls short of justifying* any plenary override of individual liberty claims."[21] Concerns to preserve the unborn living fetus, even in the case of late-term, partial-birth abortion, failed to satisfy the burden of proof necessary to override the significance of individual authority over one's body. Respect for personal authority over one's body, they argued, is of greater significance than preserving life.

Such legal judgments illustrate the central moral concern: as the significance of personal integrity and individual authority regarding the use of one's body increases, so also does the standard of proof that must be met rightly to interfere in one's choices regarding one's body. Increasing too is the significance of claims to be left alone to act in one's own assessment of one's own best interests, thereby also increasing the grounds for placing the burden of proof on those who would interfere with personal use of one's body to show that they do so with moral authority.

The Person: Self and Body

Self and body are often both distinguishable and separable. Sustaining the life of a person requires only that the necessary cognitive capacities for the embodiment and existence of that particular self-conscious, self-reflexively rational moral being endure. Thus, one can distinguish but not separate those parts of the brain necessary to sustain the life of a person. One can distinguish the higher brain as physical tissue from the existence of living persons; however, one cannot separate these parts from the person. Unlike other body parts, the higher brain is a necessary condition for being incarnate in the world. It is the seat of human consciousness, memory, and the cognitive capacities that sustain personhood. Removal of the higher brain demonstrably destroys the necessary conditions for the embodiment and existence of the person. As Puccetti put it, where the brain goes, there too goes the person.[22] Persons are distinguishable from all of their body parts; however, they are only separable from most. This implies that, at least in strictly secular terms, a person's body can be regarded as a collection of things with which the person is more or less intimately associated.

But not all things are created equal. Unlike other types of things that can be protected as part of my personal integrity (e.g., hat, coat, or boots), I experience body parts as "me." Yet one must make distinctions even among body parts. Some parts are necessary for embodiment and existence (e.g., the higher brain);

other parts are necessary for adequate human functioning (e.g., the heart); while still other parts are neither (e.g., the appendix). Some parts are directly experienced (e.g., hands), others are not (e.g., hair).[23] Just like other types of things, body parts that are not essential for embodiment or existence can in principle be replaced at will. What makes such things part of us is experiencing them as such.

Consider a person who requires a cane to walk. When he purchases an improved model, or merely a new cane that suits his fancy, he replaces a thing intimately associated and experienced as part of him. He replaces a thing that is an integral part of his human functioning. Why would the purchase of a new cane disturb anyone? Compare this case to a person with a cybernetic left hand. The hand is experienced much like any human hand would be, with artificial nerves incorporating the extremity into his phenomenological world. If asked, he replies that he does not experience a significant difference in terms of bodily incorporation between his left and right hand. "It is my hand," he says; "I experience it as me." If he decided one day to shop for a new and improved hand, a stronger hand with more sensitive functioning, he would be seeking to replace a thing intimately associated and experienced as part of him. The hand is a body part. Why would the purchase of a new cybernetic hand disturb anyone? The artificial hand is experienced as part of him; it can nonetheless be alienated and replaced.

Similar considerations apply to xenograftic organs. Genetic engineers are attempting to bioengineer pigs to grow internal organs that have sufficiently close DNA for the organs to be transplantable into humans. The hope is that such organs could be harvested and sold to persons in medical need of a transplant.[24] The new organ would replace the defective human part, eventually incorporating into and sustaining the biological life of a person. Is there a significant moral difference between the xenograftic organ and the cybernetic hand? Each is engineered, artificial, and nonhuman in material. Both are things that we can use to replace parts of our bodies at will. Presuming adequate functioning, the organ, much like the hand, will be experienced as me once it is implanted. What ground could one advance as an in-principle objection to a market in fully transplantable xenograftic organs? Given sufficient precautions to prevent interspecies disease transmission, the sale of such organs ought to be no more controversial than the sale of any other animal product.[25] What is the moral difference, if any, between the harvesting and selling of xenograftic organs and human organs?

These fictive cases are constructed to better focus issues concerning the relationship between persons and their body parts. The more the conceptual distance between persons and their body parts is increased, the more body parts become like other objects in the world to be possessed, given away, or sold. A xenograftic organ as fully exchangeable provides no obvious grounds against such sales. Is it its nonhuman, manufactured character that makes its sale seem plausible? The genetically engineered xenograft is living, but not human, tissue. Moreover, the organ is produced or manufactured. Given these considerations, it is possible to re-appreciate the status of those human organs not essential for life or consciousness. Such organs would appear more plausibly to be considered as property rather than as integral to persons. As a consequence, arguments against organ markets that are based on a reluctance to allow persons or their components to be sold would be weakened insofar as those organs are conceptually differentiated from the persons who possess them. The harvesting, selling, and replacing of such parts does not harm the living experiential nature of the person.

Such considerations, in turn, shift the burden of proof. Given certain understandings of body parts the permissibility of an organ market becomes more plausible. Just as one can distinguish between the sale of self and the sale of property intimately connected to oneself, which is not identical with oneself but still experienced within the sphere of the self, one can distinguish between sale of self and sale of most body parts. Body parts are experienced within the sphere of the self, as intimate parts of one's bodily experience. But if they are not necessary for embodiment in this world, persons are able to regard them as things intimately associated with—although not identical to—the self. It is an error to believe that one must justify a market in body parts that are needed for either embodiment/existence or adequate human functioning to justify a market in organs that are neither. It is similarly an error to object to an organ market that trades only in organs that are not necessary for one's embodiment/existence or adequate functioning on grounds that are only concerned with such essential functioning. Equally, it is an error to conflate an argument for an organ market that trades only in organs that are required for neither embodiment/existence nor adequate functioning into a market for all body parts.

Insofar as the self is different from organs that are both separable and distinguishable from the self, then while the self could sell some organs, it could not sell others without destroying the necessary conditions for the possibility of existence. For example, selling one's kidney is different than selling one's brain. While it is caught up in the life of a person, the removal and sale of a redundant kidney will neither undermine individual existence or embodiment as a person nor necessarily adversely impact the conditions for adequate biological functioning. Unlike kidneys, the brain is a necessary condition for the possibility of being incarnate in this world. To sell one's brain is to undermine an essential condition of existence as a person. The burden of proof is on those who oppose an organ market to show that their objections are cogent regarding the applicable part and the character of that part's association with the person.

Potential organ markets include both present and future interests. Unlike present markets that exchange commodities among living vendors and purchasers, an organ futures market would allow persons to contract now for rights to harvest body parts upon death, if any remain usable. An organ futures market would not violate any constraints against killing. The amount of compensation payable to surviving heirs could even be contingent on postmortem viability assessments. Willing organs as part of an inheritance would allow heirs to profit materially through the sale while others profit medically from transplantation. Death defeats any need to sustain the conditions for even essential human functioning, which is why much of the debate regarding harvesting organs has focused on the necessary and sufficient conditions for the death of a person.[26] At death body parts no longer sustain the life of a person; they are things. It is a straightforward error to presume that objections that are telling against harvesting and selling essential organs from living donors are equally cogent against a futures market. Such considerations once again shift the burden of proof to those who oppose an organ market to show that their objections are cogent regarding the characteristics of the particular market.

These reflections disclose the possibility of driving a conceptual wedge between persons and their body parts. Persons, as self-conscious, rational, embodied beings, depend for bodily integrity on some but not all of their organs. Those organs that are necessary conditions for their being embodied in the world possess a unique status. Selling them is tantamount to selling or killing persons. However, such considerations do not meet the burden of proof concerning the sale of organs that are not essential for the continued life of persons. Insofar as the body parts involved can be removed or replaced without a substantial loss in the range of embodied function usual to humans, claims that they should be considered as different from other types of property that can be given away or sold are less plausible. The more body parts are like other replaceable objects (eyeglasses, canes, and artificial limbs), the more it becomes plausible that they should also be open to being bought and sold on the market. A necessary condition for the legitimacy of a market in organs will be that the organs bought and sold are not integral to persons but can be conceived of as outside of the essential core of personal embodiment.

OWNING ONE'S BODY

One must further assess what it would mean to own body parts as property. What does it mean to maintain that a body part is "mine" as a claim regarding ownership rather than as an experiential claim regarding the phenomenology of the lived body? This exploration of ownership will examine both the justification for different senses of ownership—as, for example, in deontological right-making conditions or in certain goods or goals to be realized, as well as different senses of what it is to own an object, such as to have a steward's control over it or absolute dominion. Certain accounts of ownership, of the rights one has over one's property, will be more compatible with the view that one is at liberty to dispose of one's body parts as among the things one owns. The stronger—that is, the less contingent—

such rights are, the more one will be forced to move along the continuum from the mere permissibility of a market toward the position that such a market could not rightfully be forbidden. Intermediary positions differ according to the relative strength/contingency of ownership rights, which in turn help to establish the relative burden of proof that contraindicating considerations must meet to defeat the prima facie permissibility of selling human organs for transplantation.

The range of issues can be situated along three interrelated conceptual grids. First, it is necessary to assess the closeness of the analogy between ownership of body parts and ownership of other types of things. The burden of proof to defeat the prima facie permissibility of an organ market is directly proportional to the closeness of this analogy. Second, certain accounts of ownership are more compatible with an organ market. Rights to exclusivity and to alienation—that is, selling, donating, or abandoning one's property—vary with the ground of ownership. Consider these different foundations:

- Autonomy-based ownership, where persons have rights to exclusive control of their property, and alienation is morally permissible as long as it is freely chosen.
- Benefit-based ownership, where alienation and exclusive use are morally permissible only if they are integral to prudent practices or choices (that is, those that convey benefits to oneself or others).
- Special-consideration-based ownership, where claims to promote special goods (e.g., equality or liberty) may defeat claims to exclusive use, while alienation is illicit if negatively associated with the production of this special good and mandatory if alienation will positively promote such goods.

Third, it is necessary to examine those features of ownership to which one must appeal to grant that body parts may be licitly given away, as in organ donation, while also denying the moral permissibility of a commercial organ market.

Consider the analogies between ownership of one's body parts and ownership of other types of things that would make a market in organs possible. Whether ownership is grounded in individual freedom, social benefit, or special goods, such theories each spell out the acceptable conditions for permissible alienation of property.[27] Although rights to alienate may be limited, a theory of property that held that while one owns the items and has exclusive use, they may never be alienated, would be inadequate. Forbidding alienation, whether through abandonment, donation, or sale, requires sufficiently weighty considerations to defeat the claims of autonomy over one's possessions. Typically, such rights are fairly strong. For example, persons may permissibly sell food and medicine, which are necessary for life, to further goods that the owner holds to be important. If owning body parts is analogous to owning other types of things, then we must look to the general significance of that property to set the standard for justifying interference in the use of it.

Insofar as the relation between persons and their body parts is held to be of greater significance than other types of person-property relationships, interfering with private use of the body must meet a higher burden of proof than interfering with private use of other owned things. As rights to be protected from interference in the use of one's body increase in significance, is it more plausible that the rights to dispose of one's body parts increase, or is it more plausible that they decrease? Absent further considerations, it would appear that rights not to be interfered with, such as privacy and forbearance rights, should increase the significance of claims to utilize one's body as among the items one owns.

How one proceeds further to determine what would support a market in organs depends on numerous and complex considerations. If one may sell oneself, then may one sell one's organs? For example, if one may permissibly join the military, work on oil rigs, climb Mount Everest, or parachute out of airplanes, setting one's life at risk for career advancement, monetary profit, or personal pleasure, does it follow that one can set one's life slightly at risk through the sale of body parts? Even if sales that would necessarily involve a loss of life are ruled out, if the self is different from the organs that are separable and distinguishable from the self, though the self may not sell some organs, it may sell others. Just as one only requires sufficient food and medicine to sustain life, rather than any particular serving of food or dose of medicine, of those body parts that are both distinguishable and separable from the self, one only requires a sufficient set of body parts, rather than any particular parts or replacements, to sustain the biological life that in turn sustains personal life and consciousness. Even replacing one's heart or liver with an adequately functioning equivalent will preserve the existence and embodiment of the person. Indeed, body parts that are distinguishable and separable may be the best example of body parts that can be most easily understood on an analogy with external possessions. Such organs are things that can in principle be exchanged.

Of all the things persons own, these considerations suggest that they have the strongest rights for exclusive use, and thus for alienation, in their body parts, which in turn sets the standard of proof for interference with personal use higher than for other types of property. Yet the significance, or strength, of rights to exclusive use and to alienate one's property will vary with the ground of ownership. Here, more must be said regarding what circumstances might make certain possessions inalienable beyond transfer or sale. Moreover, what conditions would forbid the sale of an organ when it could be given as a gift?

Autonomy-Based Ownership

If ownership is grounded on autonomy-based rights, then alienation through abandonment, donation, or sale would be permissible as long as freely chosen.

Along with association and occupation, economic freedoms are fundamental elements of total freedom.[28] Owners have exclusive use of their property, and among the pursuits to which it may be put is the creation of profit. Things that one owns, including body parts, would then be open to being sold as long as both vendor and purchaser freely agree to the transaction. Particular values or special considerations, such as benefits to others or feelings of moral repugnance, would not easily meet the burden of proof to establish moral authority to forbid sales.

Considerations of benefits to others do not defeat autonomy-based rights. Coercion by need or other external circumstances similarly fails to meet the burden of proof to nullify the agreed-upon transaction. As external conditions are admitted to defeat the claim that a sale or purchase was freely agreed to, they will also destroy the possibility of a market in any product, much less in body parts. Every transaction would be subject to mutually reciprocal claims of external coercion. For example, a poor person who sells a kidney to a rich patient may argue that poverty coerced him into selling. The rich patient may equally argue that kidney failure coerced him into purchasing.[29] The burden of proof to defeat autonomy-based rights is significant. Reasons that would even be relevant to meeting that burden are limited to demonstrating (1) that the individual was coerced, (2) that he was incapable of autonomously consenting to such a contract, or (3) that prior agreements constrained his freedom to consent to the transaction. Defeating the permissibility of the transaction requires demonstrating that one of the parties coerced the other or that circumstances rendered valid consent impossible. In this latter case, the parties are not directly in the relationship of coercer and coerced. Nor are there grounds for holding that the circumstances of the external constraints of nature would render either party incompetent to choose. Other values may be offered peaceably to persuade persons not to enter into certain types of transactions or to motivate different choices, but regarding autonomy-based property rights, freedom in general trumps. Much more would need to be demonstrated to show that valid agreement would not be possible.

Ownership based on individual autonomy is compatible with the view that one is at liberty to dispose of one's body parts as among the things one owns: property rights are actual rather than prima facie and may not be easily overridden or set aside. Such an account of property rights in one's body, if sustained, would be sufficient to establish that a market in human organs could not be rightfully forbidden.

Benefit-Based Ownership

If ownership is benefit based, then exclusive use or alienation is permissible only if integral to prudent individual or social decision making. Rules regarding property would only be justified insofar as they convey benefit to oneself or others, such as maximizing overall benefits while minimizing harms. The nature and extent of property rights will vary according to understandings of prudent individual and social choices. Consider utilitarian property theory: a system of ownership is justified only if it maximizes the good.[30] Or, as with John Rawls, ownership is to be organized such that it maximizes the welfare of the worst-off members of society measured in terms of providing a sufficient material basis for personal independence and self-respect, which are argued to be essential for the development and exercise of citizens' moral powers.[31] As David Hume pointed out, scarcity of resources may cause societal friction and violence as individuals compete for resources. A carefully designed property system ought to promote social stability and peace, minimizing violent competition for the same resources, thereby creating personal and social good.[32] Everyone will be better off because each will be left in the peaceful enjoyment of those items acquired through luck or hard work.

Moreover, private ownership may be a necessary condition for efficient resource usage. Without rights to exclusive use and alienation there is no reasonably assured reward for incurring the costs of developing materials and investing time and labor. For example:

> A farmer plants corn, fertilizes it, and erects scarecrows, but when the corn is ripe his neighbor reaps and sells it. The farmer has no legal remedy against his neighbor's conduct since he owns neither the land he sowed nor the crop. After a few such incidents the cultivation of land will be abandoned and the society will shift to methods of subsistence (such as hunting) that involve less preparatory investment.[33]

Parceling out rights to exclusive use and for-profit alienation cultivates incentives for maximizing the benefits gleaned from available resources.

Here, with respect to benefit-oriented understandings of ownership and their implications for markets in organs, one should note two quite different foci in terms of which to calculate benefits: (1) how best to use the particular organs (e.g., whether a market will lead to better utilization of the available organs), and (2) how best to maximize benefits for persons. The second question will depend on the first. It will always be important, given the benefits of organ transplantation, to examine the first question to address appropriately the second. For example, insofar as regional rather than national distribution would lead to less organ wastage and more donations, it would arguably make the best use of the particular organs, even if patients in more sparsely populated regions experienced greater waiting times. Exclusive use of body parts, on such an account, is contingent on such rights conveying the appropriate benefit, such as efficient use of resources, development of moral powers, or maximization of the good. The distribution and use of internal organs are fixed neither by birth, nor gift, nor sale, but in terms of an a posteriori calculation of benefits.

Such an account of property is in certain ways compatible with an organ market. Insofar as such a market maximizes benefits over harms, it is allowable—indeed, commendable. Confirming rights to exclusive use of one's body parts may efficiently and effectively produce the most beneficial uses of the available organs. Those who would not otherwise donate might be encouraged to sell their internal redundant organs, thereby saving lives and increasing personal wealth. Forbidding such transactions would require defeating the claim that they convey sufficient benefit.[34] The difficulty with the belief that government regulation results in the most beneficial usage of the available organs is that it asserts a claim regarding a particular outcome. It then just assumes that governmental institutionalization of the process, with all of its attendant bureaucracy, will produce this outcome. The assumption is only correct if, in fact, governmental intervention results in reduced economic costs, less organ wastage, and greater transplantation efficiency and effectiveness.[35]

Concerns might be raised about the sale of poor quality or diseased organs. Such concerns are justified only if no adequate system of personal liability or independent methods to monitor quality can be developed. Assuming adequate functioning, a dying patient may prefer transplantation of a diseased or otherwise lower-quality organ to imminent death.

Nevertheless, insofar as property is benefit based, rights to exclusive use and alienation of body parts are straightforwardly defeated by demonstrating that other uses, distributions, or methods of alienation convey greater benefit. Regardless of whether one is calculating across preference satisfaction, wealth, or welfare maximization, the strength of actual ownership rights, and thus the burden of proof to defeat such rights, must be settled by empirical calculation. Depending on the results, alienation of internal organs for redistribution may not simply be permissible but required. If a policy of redistributing working kidneys from those who have two to those with kidney failure would produce sufficient benefits, then this would constitute grounds to redistribute coercively.

While forced redistribution is incompatible with the buying and selling of organs, in itself it commodifies organs as resources to be utilized to maximize benefits. Here, it is important to review the different senses of commodification at stake: commodities are not just items that are bought and sold for money; they may also be resources traded among persons or redistributed through social institutions to produce conditions or social circumstances that are valued, which can be understood in terms of the production of maximum overall benefits, or of the greatest benefit for the greatest number of persons. On such a foundation, persons will only have ownership rights in their own body parts insofar as it is prudent for society to support such rights. The outcome of such empirical calculations may or may not support the view that one is at liberty to dispose of one's body parts as among the things one owns.

Special-Consideration-Based Ownership

Accounts of ownership that focus on special considerations hold that certain goods have a trumping character when one determines the extent of ownership rights to exclusive use and alienation. Consider, for example, the egalitarian argument that to be just, society must be structured so that it promotes fair equality of opportunity—including personal holdings and the private use of property. To justify any private transaction, one must demonstrate that it does not violate the necessary conditions for fair equality of opportunity.[36] For example, if it is claimed that fair equality of opportunity requires substantively equal legal and political liberty, which in turn depends on a sufficient level of economic equality, then insofar as actual distribution of property fails to be adequately equal, there must be further redistribution. Depending on how conditions for fair equality of opportunity are specified, citizens may be entitled to substantively equal material or economic conditions, educational opportunities, or health care. Providing for such positive entitlements requires taxation and redistribution of the time, talent, goods, and resources of other people, defeating claims to have exclusive use of oneself or one's property. Such ownership rights will tend to be much weaker and more contingent than those based on freedom, depending on whether considerations of free choice establish inviolable side constraints as well as on how highly freedom is valued.

Arguments that appeal to the trumping character of equality, or some other special good, attempt to defeat claims of exclusive use of property. The very idea of property is recast in terms of a social benefit to be redistributed. Such theories move the burden of proof away from governmental and other authorities, who would continually interfere with owners' freedoms, placing it on those persons who would freely utilize private property with consenting others. Focus on the special good of equality, for example, supports the creation of a universal single-tier health care system, financed through general taxation and enforced through the prosecution of those who attempt to purchase better basic health care with private funds. It uses the goods and services of some to benefit others. Insofar as property rights are based on the creation of special goods, rights not to participate in the propagation of services that one conscientiously opposes, to utilize private property only in ways that one believes to be morally acceptable, are at best insecure and limited.

Rights to alienation are defeated if exercise of such a right is detrimental to the production or maintenance of this special good. Consider Nozick's "Wilt Chamberlain" case:

> Suppose that Wilt Chamberlain is greatly in demand by basketball teams, being a great gate attraction. . . . He signs the following sort of contract with a team: In each home game, twenty-five cents from the

price of each ticket of admission goes to him. . . . The season starts, and people cheerfully attend his team's games; they buy their tickets, each time dropping a separate twenty-five cents of their admission price into a special box with Chamberlain's name on it. They are excited about seeing him play; it is worth the total admission price to them. Let us suppose that in one season one million persons attend his home games, and Wilt Chamberlain winds up with $250,000, a much larger sum than the average income. . . . Is he entitled to this income?[37]

If the special good that underlies ownership rights is equality, then, in this case, the free alienation of the twenty-five cents per person is illicit—taken as a group, such activity is negatively associated with the production of equality.[38]

Alienation may be mandatory, however, if abandonment, donation, or sale will positively promote the good. Consider egalitarian political theory and its central concern to correct inequalities created by natural and social circumstances. Rawls, for example, rejects a system of natural liberty, which, he argues, improperly allows distribution of property, income, and wealth to be governed by the natural and social lotteries. Such factors, he believes, are arbitrary from a moral point of view. "There is no more reason to permit the distribution of income and wealth to be settled by the distribution of natural assets than by historical and social fortune."[39] Moreover, he argues that we do not deserve our native endowments, talents, and abilities, any more than we deserve our initial starting place in society or having been born into a particular advantaged or disadvantaged family.[40] Egalitarian liberalism, as Rawls interprets it, requires that social institutions, including the family, educational institutions, and health care, be designed to mitigate the influence of social contingencies and natural fortune on distributive shares and fair equality of opportunity.

Insofar as a person's character, native endowments, talents, and family are seen as arbitrary from a moral point of view, so much so are his body's physical characteristics, such as properly functioning eyes, ears, lungs, kidneys, liver, and so forth. Among the most prevalent and pervasive inequalities, which lead inevitably to social and economic inequalities, are those created by the differences in the health status of one's body parts. The aim of health care is to restore individuals so that they return to being fully cooperating members of society.[41] In this view, body parts are simply another natural resource to be distributed so as to promote the favored understanding of the good; in Rawlsian terms, to maximize the welfare of the worst-off members of society. Indeed, such considerations refocus concern away from whether to commodify internal redundant organs to accounts of (1) the fair distribution of body parts (e.g., redistributive justice of natural physical resources) and (2) the fair distribution of economic and social burdens to pay for acquisition, allocation, and transplantation (e.g., redistributive justice of social and economic resources). Such considerations implicitly commit these theories to a market, albeit governmentally controlled, in body parts.

Concerns to promote fair equality of opportunity may entitle persons with organ failure to governmentally supported transplant surgery, including follow-up care and provision of new organs. Even if mechanisms for distribution of internal organs are strictly regulated, noncapitalistic, nonprofit-driven, governmentally financed markets, organs are nonetheless socially traded commodities, utilized for production or maintenance of the special good. These considerations might lead to the blending of egalitarian and liberty-oriented concerns with respect to the development of a state-controlled market in body parts. For example, one might consider matching market-based procurement with a government-based monopoly in distribution. Here the intent would be to increase organ availability, while continuing to distribute organs for transplantation according to a scheme of medical priority. Or, one might imagine circumstances under which the price of body parts in the market would be fixed by the government, and the poor provided with body-part vouchers. Such circumstances would not allow the rich to outbid the poor in the market. There would be the additional virtue of the poor having vouchers at their disposal to act as an incentive to bring individuals to sell organs to those in need. Other regulatory impositions could be fashioned toward the goal of serving other societal interests.

REPUGNANCE: ADJUDICATION AMONG MORAL INTUITIONS

Regardless of the grounds of ownership rights, some insist that the analogy between ownership of body parts and ownership of other things breaks down at the point of for-profit transactions. The contention is that it is precisely because of the general significance and intimate connection with persons that organs ought not to be sold. The body is part of the basic dignity of the human person; therefore, trade in the body and its parts is morally repugnant and ought to be limited.

For example, a report from the Hastings Center asserted:

> The view that the body is intimately tied to our conceptions of personal identity, dignity, and self-worth is reflected in the unique status accorded to the body within our legal tradition as something which cannot and should not be bought or sold. Religious and secular attitudes make it plain just how widespread is the ethical stance maintaining that the body ought to have special moral standing. The powerful desire to accord respect to the dignity, sanctity, and identity of the body, as well as the moral attitudes concerning the desirability of policies and practices which encourage altruism and sharing among the members of society produced an emphatic rejection of the attempt to commercialize organ recovery and make a commodity of the body.[42]

As Paul Ramsey holds, the human body has a sacredness in the biological order. "In terms of our vision of man and his relation to community, there may be little to choose between the blood and soil, organic view of the Nazi and the technological, '(spare parts)' mechanistic analogies of the present day."[43] In each instance, it is an appeal to a moral repugnance apparently felt by some in the case of organ sales.

These vague discomforts and secularized appeals to the "sanctity," "sacredness," and "dignity" of the human body frequently appear as remnants of Christian religious sentiments that cling to the social fabric and moral language of secular society. To some degree they are also due to shifting cultural attitudes regarding the human body and individual freedom, resulting in a new cultural climate that encourages embryo experimentation and third-party assisted reproduction, including the use of donor gametes, embryo wastage, and elective abortion for fetal reduction or simple relief of unwanted children, while still clinging to vague moral repugnance in the case of the sale of human organs for transplantation.[44] Abortion and infanticide are evermore cited as acceptable choices for parents of hemophilic or otherwise disabled newborns,[45] to end lives judged not worth living.[46] Moreover, such practices are perceived and publicly touted as compassionate and just. Each is endorsed in the name of scientific advancement, relief of suffering, reproductive choice, and individual fulfillment.

The contrast between traditional Christian morality and secular ethics, however, is substantial. Contrast Roman Catholic bishop James T. McHugh's diagnosis of this cultural shift, on the one hand, over against Suzanne Poppema's assertion of the goodness of nontherapeutic elective abortion, on the other. McHugh:

> This results from certain violations of the value of human life being justified by public opinion in the name of individual freedom or as a personal choice, thus claiming not only freedom from disapproval or societal regulation but authorization by the state.[47]

Versus Poppema:

> That's precisely what I do. I honor and care for patients who want to end pregnancies. I'm an abortion doctor, and I refuse to mask my work in qualifications or apologies. What I do is right and good and important. Perhaps my story will appall some, but it also may inspire others, particularly the young women who need to know that the struggle between feminism and the patriarchy has not been in vain.[48]

Unfettered access to abortion has become central to arguments for gender equality.[49] Indeed, according to Todd Whitmore, an ethicist at the University of Notre Dame, holding abortion to be an intrinsic moral evil ought to be characterized as a form of oppression.[50] Rather than focused on the beginnings and endings of life, or on the moral status of the embryo, abortion has been fully recast within the guise of human dignity, social justice, and gender power struggles.[51]

Whereas traditionally such practices were understood as directly intending evil, and thereby always illicit, they have become generally sanctioned and nearly universally endorsed by the international bioethical community and encouraged by governmental health care policy. Here one might consider the focus on education as the means to spread AIDS awareness, and thereby to slow transmission. In its 1986 report "Confronting AIDS," the National Academy of Sciences argued that education is the most efficient and effective means to stem the tide of HIV infection.[52] The surgeon general of the United States concurred in his "Report on Acquired Immune Deficiency Syndrome."[53] Yet what information was to be conveyed, who was its audience, and whose moral views and which social values should be incorporated? Education is not neutral. Debate concerned whether to teach abstinence, fidelity within heterosexual marriage, and refraining from drug use or, rather, to utilize graphic images and descriptions of "safe" sex practices (e.g., condom use), the means to avoid infection while injecting narcotics (e.g., cleaning and refusing to share needles), and the means to avoid bearing infected children (e.g., perinatal testing and elective abortion). The Task Force on Pediatric AIDS recommended that an important component of the anticipatory guidance pediatricians provide to young teens should include information about HIV transmission, implications of infection, strategies for prevention (such as abstinence from behaviors that place one at risk), and safer sex options for those electing to be sexually active. Parental permission was seen as desirable but unnecessary.[54]

In contrast, traditional Roman Catholics object to the teaching of condom usage to teenagers, sexual pleasure outside of heterosexual marriage, and the encouraging of HIV-positive women to seek abortions if they become pregnant. Moreover, they object to using public resources (e.g., tax dollars) to endorse such practices. Critics retorted:

> It is unthinkable that religious, educational, and social institutions whose mission is to prepare youth to be good citizens and responsible adults and to be informed in the exercise of their moral agency, would be permitted to deprive them of knowledge essential to that mission and more important, knowledge that might save their lives.[55]

Such criticism, though, misses the point. While public awareness of safe sex practices, abortion, and needle usage may appear to present value neutral medical information, such "instruction" inherently promotes the permissibility of such practices, endorsing particular moral values over others. It is not that religious communities do not understand the utility of such education; rather, they view its message as very effective propaganda in support of values and practices contrary to their deeply held beliefs. Indeed, it combines a particular moral viewpoint with state resources and the powerful endorsement of the medical community to promote social and ethical practices that are contrary to their survival as moral and religious communities.

Similarly, there is a growing endorsement of physician-assisted suicide and euthanasia as the means for reducing human suffering and preserving human dignity. This call ranges from assisted suicide for the terminally ill to promotion of its availability to all who competently request such treatment, and even to both voluntary and nonvoluntary euthanasia for patients in a permanently vegetative state. Even optimal curative and palliative care cannot resolve all loss of personal control and perceived loss of human dignity.[56] Death with dignity is likened to putting an animal out of its misery. Since we would surely aid an animal in pain, the argument proposes, we should extend the same compassion to human beings. Analogous sentiments were expressed by the Ninth Circuit Court with respect to Oregon's Death with Dignity Act: "Those who believe strongly that death must come without physician assistance are free to follow that creed, be they doctors or patients. They are not free to force their views, their religious convictions, or their philosophies on all other members of a democratic society, and to compel those whose values differ from theirs to die painful, protracted, and agonizing deaths."[57] Compassion and love are emphasized as justifying physician-assisted killing in the face of irremediable and severe suffering. Such deaths are presented as alleviating the physical pain and mental anguish of those beyond effective therapy. Adversity can drain a person's life of meaning, and from this perspective the individual appears to have a right to determine when to end his own life.

This view straightforwardly incorporates a purely materialistic calculation of costs and benefits to assess quality of life. It accepts without argument that the focal point of the moral life is autonomous self-determination, where liberty, as the celebration of free individualistic choice, is integral to the good life for persons. Indeed, it fully accepts the axiological assessment that there is no deep meaning to pain, disease, disability, suffering, and death, beyond the firing of synapses, the collapse of human abilities, and the mere end of life. Human life is merely instrumental and meaning is only to be found in the pleasures, beauty, and engagement of this life. Physician-assisted suicide to limit suffering and preserve human freedom is from this perspective simply a commonsense compassionate solution that protects patient "dignity."[58] From such a standpoint, suffering can only be experienced as surd.

Here, one must adjudicate among moral intuitions and distinguish between justified and unjustified moral repugnance. For example, many have deep intuitions regarding the moral repugnance of abortion, contraception, and homosexuality, yet these are practices that society permits. Is such repugnance justified? If so, should such practices be prohibited? In a society that frequently affirms the merits of multiculturalism, abortion on demand (including late-term, partial-birth abortion), embryo experimentation, and, in growing numbers, physician-assisted suicide, there is an obvious irony in the seemingly automatic assumption that rhetorical moral terms such as "sanctity," "sacredness," "dignity," or even "repugnance" should bear any moral weight.

While these and similar moral terms such as "sanctity of life," "respect for life," "human dignity," "best interests of the patient," and "caring" have often been employed to fashion political consensus and settle moral debate, they remain heterogeneous in meaning. Such appeals capture groups of ambiguous and disparate hopes, images, feelings, values, and claims.[59] Moreover, such sentiments often misconstrue and distort their Christian origins.[60] As Torcello and Wear note, for example, capitalistic practices are not in and of themselves objects of Protestant Christian condemnation. Thus, if one were "to condemn the sale of human body parts because it might encourage greed, then all sorts of other activities and professions should be likewise condemned for the same reason."[61] Protestants understand that any number of secular professions can be seen as "callings" from God, even if there exists potential for greed. Commercialization, even of the body and its parts, in itself is not immoral. One might even be called to participate in such a market: "[b]y doing so they not only preserve and enhance altruism, but they create an added means of expressing the grace of God."[62] To assume that an organ market would harm the sanctity of the human body "is to betray a belief that it [the body] is fragile, as well as a hubris regarding man's potential to corrupt what God sanctified."[63] Provided that procurement and transplantation take place in a professional and respectful manner, they argue, financial payment does not in itself threaten such sanctity.

Similarly, both Roman Catholicism and Buddhism hold human life to be sacred. Roman Catholicism draws its traditional view from God, the source of life's sanctity. Human life is sacred and holy because life is a gift from God, who is holy.[64] For Buddhism, in contrast, human life is sacred because all life is inherently sacred. For the devoutly secular, however, the appeal to the sacredness of human life simply assumes the truth of a moral viewpoint that must be proven. Such terms have lost much of their traditional significance. They have become more ethical slogans than moral concerns. Understandings about what it means to care for others, to respect the "sacredness," "sanctity," or "dignity" of life, are contextual. Such rhetorically powerful terms are only adequately understood within a particular moral, religious, or cultural tradition. The terms have no fixed meaning outside of particular content-full moral communities. Outside of particular moral contexts they do not even possess the status of moral nonrigid designators.[65]

If one holds that our natural feelings should be embraced as important, formative elements of morality, then we must have some understanding of the criteria for identifying and ranking the emotions that are to qualify. Do all emotive reactions, by all parties, point to important moral features of a situation? Which emotions should we take as authoritative and how should we quantify them intra- and interpersonally? And if the emotive reactions differ among persons, how can one identify those that, as morally appropriate, ought to guide the formation of public policy versus those that ought to be ignored, if not actively discouraged? Formulating policy utilizing such emotional reactions assimilates and enforces maxims that are very likely merely subjectively contingent; indeed, at times, they may even be pernicious. Regardless, in the case of organ sales, one must determine whether generalized feelings of moral repugnance are justified, prior to presupposing that such intuitions ought to carry any weight in meeting the burden of proof, or lowering the standard of proof, to proscribe organ sales.

Moreover, insofar as such theorists want to allow for morally licit organ donation from living or deceased donors, they must appeal to some special values regarding human organs to support this normative claim. Such values must appeal to "concerns about the inappropriateness of commerce in vital human organs, concerns about justice, a feel for the awesome nature of such gifts, and some uneasiness about shutting families out of the process,"[66] or other similar interests. Yet, not all share such unease. Feelings about the inappropriate nature of commerce in human organs can be countered by equally strong but contrary feelings. Deep intuitions regarding the awesome nature of the "gift" beg the question regarding the meaning, significance, and importance of internal organs.[67] The nature and consequence of the "gift" are no less "awesome" if money changes hands. Those who are concerned about the "dirtiness" of such transactions need not participate. Vigorous searching for donors need not cease merely because of the existence of a for-profit market. Markets in blood, medicine, housing, and food exist side by side with nonprofit charitable counterparts. Moreover, general concerns about shutting out the family must be dealt with regardless of the mechanism for the acquisition of organs.

Finally, all organ procurement and distribution schemes commodify, even donation. That is, on each ground one has specified a market in human organs, albeit a heavily regulated market, with carefully stipulated conditions for bearing the costs and benefits of procurement, distribution, and transplantation. One is arguing not about whether human organs should be commodified but rather about who should receive the resources and who should bear the costs of appropriation and transfer. Insofar as individuals are prohibited from selling their organs, it is a constrained market where donors are required to part with their property without material compensation, while others (including physicians, hospitals, and procurement agencies) benefit financially, and the recipient of the transplant benefits physically. The Office of Technology Assessment considered the following case in their report on the ownership of human tissues and cells:

Suppose, for example, that a market for transplantable kidneys existed. There are three parties to the transaction—the donor, the surgical/hospital team, and the recipient—and they are able to accomplish the transaction at prices agreeable to all. The amount required by the family of the kidney donor to proffer the kidney is $50,000, the amount required by the surgical/hospital team to bring forth its services is $100,000, and the kidney recipient is willing to pay $150,000. Suppose further that a law is passed requiring all transactions in kidneys to be gifts, thereby prohibiting the kidney donor's family from selling the kidney and reaping its economic value of $50,000. Who will now realize this value? The intent of the legislation was that the value of the kidney be transferred as a gift from the kidney donor to the recipient, with the transplant ultimately costing the recipient only $100,000. Yet, because nothing is done to ensure this outcome, a different outcome is possible. Depending on the conditions of the transplantable kidney market, it may be possible for the surgical/hospital team to realize the value entirely by charging the recipient $150,000.[68]

That organs can only be transferred at a price of zero does not thereby reduce the value of such organs to zero. Rather, it straightforwardly transfers the value of the organ from the donor to other parties.

GOVERNMENT, HEALTH CARE POLICY, AND PRIVATE CHOICES

The moral permissibility of establishing a market in human organs for transplantation must also be explored in terms of the nature, force, and limits of societal and governmental authority. The extent of moral political authority will shift the standard as well as the burden of proof regarding the permissibility of establishing an organ market. The foundations of societal moral authority will determine when, how, and to what degree society will possess de jure, rather than merely de facto, authority to forbid, constrain, or regulate markets. This exploration of political concerns will examine the moral foundations for different conceptions of political authority as they might bear on markets in human organs. Attention will be given to the ways in which different foundational accounts of (1) deontological right-making conditions and (2) consequentialist considerations regarding the goods or goals that a society ought morally to realize, as well as (3) understandings of forbearance and privacy rights either establish moral political authority to promote positive welfare entitlements or place limits on legitimate governmental interference into the free choices of persons, protecting negative freedoms. Here one must consider the possibility of securing universally binding moral content. The more one can establish binding moral content, such as the character of special goods or goals, the more there will exist moral authority to regulate the conduct of persons and their interactions to promote those goods.

Certain accounts of the limits of societal and governmental authority, of the strength of persons' rights to forbearance and privacy, will be more or less compatible with the view that the state does not have moral authority to interfere with free interactions among consenting persons. As with rights to ownership, the stronger (i.e., less contingent) forbearance and privacy rights are, the more one will be forced to move along the continuum from the position that organ sales are intuitively, all things considered, acceptable to the position that such transactions cannot be rightfully forbidden. Intermediary positions will differ according to the relative strength or contingency of rights to be left alone, to privacy, and to protection from nonconsensual interference, which in turn will establish the burden of proof that contraindicating considerations must meet to justify state authority to forbid such a market. Here one must note the ways in which the relative significance or strength of persons' forbearance and privacy rights may defeat positive entitlements or claims of others. It may be, for example, that individuals have a right to health care, but that significant forbearance and privacy rights defeat the duty to provide such care. Here also, one must consider the circumstance that even if concerns regarding relations between persons and their bodies, and ownership of body parts, are sufficient to show that a market in human organs should be allowable, analysis of further political theoretical considerations will be required to establish that the moral authority of states is sufficient to meet the standard of proof to forbid such markets.

The conceptual grids that display the geography of political theoretical concerns include the relative strength or contingency of forbearance and privacy rights, as well as the nature and ground of societal and governmental authority. First, the burden of proof to defeat the prima facie allowableness of the market will vary directly with the strength/contingency of individuals' rights to forbearance and privacy that protect persons from nonconsensual interference with peaceable consensual association and interaction with others. Second, certain accounts of the nature and ground of societal and governmental authority will be more compatible with the view that the state does not have moral authority to forbid markets in human organs; others will be more compatible with the view that the state ought actively to create such a market. Such authority can be *freedom based,* where moral authority to interfere in the free interaction of consenting persons is created by and thus limited to the actual agreements forged among persons; *benefit based,* where moral authority is grounded on prudence, such that social institutions are to be arranged, and the interactions of persons organized, so that they maximize benefits while minimizing evils; or *special-consideration based,* where there will exist moral authority to interfere in the free interaction of citizens to promote the moral good or goal to be realized (e.g., equality or liberty).

Freedom-Based Political Authority

If societal and governmental authority is freedom based, there will be different understandings of the legitimate reasons for which the government may forbid, constrain, or regulate markets, depending on whether freedom is an inviolable right-making condition or whether it is simply a highly valued good. If freedom functions as a side constraint, then the moral limits of such authority will be created, rather than discovered, by the free choices of persons.[69] On such an account, forbearance and privacy rights create strong protections from battery (i.e., nonconsensual touching), defining a sphere in which one is morally immune from interference, protecting self-interest and self-preservation in the private use of person, body parts, and other property. Such rights describe side constraints prohibiting nonconsensual interference, which hold against other persons as well as society and state. Unless persons agree, rights as side constraints defeat the claims of others (persons and states) to have positive entitlements to the time, talent, or property of individuals.

On such an account, persons only have rights to their private resources, including body parts, and to those additional resources that they are able peaceably to convince others to donate or sell to them. The moral authority to interfere with such rights (i.e., the standard of proof necessary to meet the burden of proof) is limited to peaceable consent among persons and communities. Under such circumstances the moral authority of the state to enforce general policies regarding the acceptable use of body parts is limited. Morally authorized statutes are confined to the protection of persons' rights to forbearance and privacy, protection of individuals from battery, and those additional policies to which actual persons give consent. Persons, and organizations of persons, may be held responsible for nonconsensual acts against others, including acts of violence and breach of contract, since such actions violate the rights of persons not to be touched or used without permission.

Governmental authority created by the express agreement of those governed is absolutely limited by such agreement. So grounded, the state would have the general character of a limited democracy. It would have no general moral authority to forbid a market in human organs. Strong rights of forbearance and privacy make implausible interventions to forbid persons from freely using personal resources, including their own body parts, with consenting others for fun, beneficence, or profit. Indeed, insofar as strong rights of forbearance and privacy support the absolute dominion of persons over themselves, along with their body parts and other property, where moral authority is created with the free agreement of persons, this account would be sufficient to affirm a market in body parts. Those who disagreed could not be forced to participate. The state would have the moral authority created by agreement to protect persons from coercive transactions, including forced donation and failure responsibly to fulfill contractual agreements. Moral authority, however, would not extend to forbidding the consensual commercialization of human body parts for transplantation.

Benefit-Based Political Authority

If legitimate political authority is benefit based, then societal and governmental policy enactment and enforcement are permissible if prudent. On such an account, state moral authority extends to arranging social institutions, including the market, so that society's infrastructure abounds to social benefit, including the goods of human freedom and liberty. As John Stuart Mill held, the state ought to be organized under the government that "combines the greatest amount of good with the least of evil."[70] Depending on how one understands prudence, this requirement can mean structuring institutions so as to create the greatest benefit for the greatest number, to maximize net social benefit, or to maximize the welfare of the worst-off members of society.

Utilitarianism, for example, provides a defense of the general moral authority of the state to perform useful functions beyond the protection of its citizens from nonconsensual force and fraud. Extensive welfare rights to adequate nutrition, shelter, education, and health care are typically underscored as necessary foundations for citizens to be productive members of society.[71] Rights of forbearance and privacy, including protections from battery, exist only if prudent. Such rights would be contingent upon an a posteriori calculation of the benefits and burdens, on oneself and others, created by rights to be left alone. Even if prudence dictated that forbearance and privacy rights hold against other persons individually, protecting citizens from random rape, murder, and theft, such rights would not necessarily hold against the state without further argument. If prudence requires the state to maximize the welfare of its citizens, then, insofar as its resources allow, the state should provide for the most important needs of its members. This may require taxation, as well as other forms of redistribution, of the personal time, talent, body parts, and other property so as to provide others with welfare, shelter, food, education, organ transplantation, and health care.

It is, however, an empirical question as to whether free markets or socialism, or some intermediary position, will in fact maximize benefits, maximize the condition of the worst off, or create the greatest benefit for the greatest number. For example, it may be that one achieves the best use of scarce resources, such as organs for transplantation, by enforcing strict forbearance and privacy rights—including the liberty to alienate one's body parts in the market. Or, maximizing benefits may require recasting all available redundant organs as public resources for prudent redistribution. As a redundant internal organ, kidneys could be redistributed from those with two healthy kidneys to those in need.

It would be an error, though, to think of the social allocation of public health care resources solely in terms of redistribution from the rich to the poor, utilizing economic criteria. If society is prudently to allocate resources to meet the basic needs of its citizens, this implies redistributing internal redundant organs from those with redundant healthy organs to those with organ failure, regardless of economic status of either donor or recipient. On such health-related issues, redistribution would conceivably flow from the poor to the rich. Organs and other body parts would merely form a pool to be distributed among persons according to the possibility of maximizing prudential benefits. On the other hand, with a free market, persons would control their body parts until they were interested, or provided with sufficient incentive, to sell or donate them. Individuals would have direct economic incentives to cultivate healthy living habits so as to maximize the value of their body parts on the market. The burden of proof, which must be met for a state to forbid organ markets with moral authority on such an account, though, is strictly the result of this empirical calculation. Policy in this matter would be dictated by many considerations, including considerations of equality as well as whether one should first protect the lives of those most likely to contribute to society.

If state moral authority is benefit based, political authority in principle extends to all facets of personal and public life. If intrusion is prudent, it extends to regulation of personal association, private interaction with others, and even to control over utilization of one's body parts. State intrusion to forbid organ sales would in principle be morally authorized. However, if a market would provide for the best use of the particular organs or best maximize benefits for persons, then the state ought to support such a market.

Here one must assess the results of a posteriori calculations regarding the best usage of available organs, as well as the most efficient and effective manner in which to maximize benefits for persons, noting three additional sets of issues: (1) which organs should be understood as "available" for transplantation: organs that persons have voluntarily donated, those that can be harvested with or without consent from deceased persons, or those that are redundantly contained within the bodies of living persons; (2) the benefits and burdens of a market in organs; and (3) the benefits and burdens of forbidding such a market. Here too, one must assess which types of benefits and burdens are to be considered as part of the cost-benefit calculation: preference satisfaction, economic wealth, or welfare maximization in terms of both quality and quantity of life, as well as the appropriate discount rate for the passage of time.

Special Consideration-Based Political Authority

If societal and governmental authority is based on special consideration, its character will vary according to the nature of the good or goal to which special accent is given. Here one may be concerned to distinguish between positive and negative goods, as well as between the goods themselves and the social institutions required to create or to sustain particular outcomes. For example, the importance of realized rights to forbearance and privacy, as well as protection from battery, will differ in relative strength and contingency according to the character of the principles and goods with which they must be balanced.

Consider, for example, concerns to protect individual liberty and the possibility of moral diversity in health care. Suggestions that the market offers significant protection for individual liberty in health care and the preservation of diverse moral commitments is met with considerable skepticism in contemporary bioethics. Market-based financing and distribution of health care, it is typically claimed, fails to protect the most fundamental interests of patients. The forces of the market, it is believed, bring on more harm than benefit.[72] The profit motive is not regarded as leading to the wise use of resources, nor is the market considered a place that rewards responsible, free decision making, while providing tutelage concerning the limitations of the human condition. In short, the market is seen as starkly limiting, rather than enhancing, human liberty and responsible behavior; that is, as restricting rather than preserving the possibility for liberty and moral diversity in health care.

Here, at least four distinct conceptions of liberty compete to frame the foundations of biomedical ethics and moral political authority:

(1) Liberty$_1$ as the entitlement to *realize* one's abilities and choices—that is, to achieve one's own understanding of the good life.

(2) Liberty$_2$ as acting according to an ideal, rather than an actual, account of free choice, informed by rationally discoverable, universal moral norms.

(3) Liberty$_3$ as lived human flourishing—that is, a content-full way of life, fully embedded within a particular cultural or religious context.

(4) Liberty$_4$ as freedom from interference, as expressed in the existence of significant forbearance rights—that is, rights to be left alone and protected from nonconsensual use of oneself and one's private property.

Developing a morally authoritative bioethics will only be possible when the arguments for and the implications of the various conceptions of liberty have been sorted through, and the unsustainable set aside. At stake are starkly different foundational visions of liberty and the limits of moral political authority.

Liberty$_1$ and liberty$_2$ each frame core moral presuppositions of the liberal, social-democratic, universalistic aspirations of Western bioethics. Each supports the imposition of uniform systems of health care and guarantees of equality in the provision of medical services. Whereas the first underscores universal access to comprehensive health care as central to the preservation of the conditions for achieving one's own understanding of the good life, the second judges global establishment of particular biomedical standards, moral principles and precepts, as necessary to preserve individual liberty. While prima facie endorsing liberty and diversity, each privileges a particular, fully secular, concept of morality and human flourishing, prioritizing individual autonomy understood in terms of fair equality of opportunity, self-determinism, and freedom from constraints on the pursuit of self-satisfaction and self-fulfillment.

Such a worldview is at core incompatible with traditional religions and cultures (e.g., Orthodox Judaism, Orthodox Christianity, and traditional Confucianism). Traditional religions and cultures experience morality as part of a living phenomenological world. Here, liberty₃ can be encapsulated, *grosso modo*, as a way of life embodying virtue. Rather than developing action-guiding principles, the focus of the moral life is the development of a particular type of personal character, marked by the cardinal elements of human flourishing. Whereas certain moral positions will be more or less compatible with a virtuous way of life, medical morality and bioethics will not be reducible to the moral principles that generate such choices. A virtuous life is the living experience of true human flourishing. Here the challenge for the establishment of a particular bioethics as the foundation of public policy regarding organ transplantation is that religious and cultural moral diversity runs deep. The national and international political landscape compasses persons from diverse and often fragmented moral communities, with widely varying moral intuitions, premises, evaluations, and commitments. Here one appreciates the significant plurality of fundamentally different, incompatible, and often mutually antagonistic moral visions and moral rationalities, within which complex bioethical issues, such as commercial organ procurement and transplantation, are addressed. Which mode of life or experience of human flourishing should guide bioethical decision making and define the standard of care? Whose bioethics should guide the creation of national law and international treaty?

Whereas the moral vision of Western liberal, social-democratic bioethics offers the hope of a communality binding all persons and the resolutions of biomedical moral controversies through universal moral norms, this hope is chimerical. This cosmopolitan liberal vision offers only the false promise of a global moral consensus, while failing to acknowledge the deep divisions between traditional religious and cultural moral communities and its own posttraditional aspirations. Judging among the rival versions of moral inquiry to guide the establishment of universal bioethical content, therefore, either straightforwardly begs the question of such moral content or arbitrarily embraces a particular moral vision—whether traditionally religious or liberal social-democratic. As a result, the foundations for global bioethics must be found elsewhere. This brings the discussion to consideration of the implications for morally authoritative bioethics grounded in an understanding of liberty₄, freedom from interference, as expressed in the existence of significant forbearance rights. Here, the market creates social space for unencumbered personal interaction, which, while making no judgment regarding the market or its consequences, allows it to exist. In this case, health care—including organ procurement and allocation for transplantation—has no special priority or value. It is simply among the myriad possibilities for expressing oneself in peaceable consensual collaboration with others.

Liberty as the Entitlement to Realize One's Abilities and Choices (Liberty₁)

Whereas all individuals are exposed to the vicissitudes of nature, some will through luck fare better than others, remaining free from disease and major suffering. Others will be born with congenital defects or genetic disorders, confront crippling illness, or through accident or chosen risk become injured or maimed. A focus on preserving the conditions for positive expression of individual liberty espouses a universal vision of autonomy as freedom from constraints on the pursuit of self-satisfaction and individual meaning; each individual is understood as having an equal basic entitlement to achieve his own understanding of the good life, unhampered by the fortunes of nature or social choice. The healthy, talented, and intelligent have natural advantages over those who are sickly, less talented, and less intelligent. Healthy individuals generally spend a less significant portion of their physical resources and personal time on health care, allowing for other opportunities. Moreover, talented and intelligent individuals often hold higher-income, higher-status jobs. These advantages, in turn, are statistically correlated with an increase in the quality and quantity of life.[73] Liberty₁ frames inequalities in the quality and quantity of life as social injustices, because some are less able to realize their positive entitlements to secure their own understanding of the good life; and, in turn, assumes that such injustice ought to be redressed through redistributive state action. As Rawls urges, our natural talents, abilities, and health are to be appreciated as arbitrary from a moral point of view[74] and, indeed, as common assets for the creation of social benefit.[75] Thus, insofar as each do not have an equal chance at realizing their own individual understanding of the good, justice requires state action to mitigate the influences of social contingencies and natural fortune.[76] The free market, he concludes, must be thoroughly constrained within political institutions, which themselves are designed to guarantee fair equality of opportunity and outcome.

Norman Daniels encapsulates this concern as the need to sustain more than the conditions of formal liberty, as freedom from constraint, but to guarantee material liberty, as expressed in fair equality of outcomes.[77] For example, while universal suffrage grants the wealthy and the poor identical voting rights, the wealthy have greater ability to select candidates, as well as to influence public opinion and elected officials. In terms of actual impact on outcomes, political liberty has greater worth for the wealthy.[78] The underlying concern is for equal worth of personal and political liberty, especially concerning the material and social conditions necessary to eliminate natural and social disadvantages so that each may enjoy fair equality of outcomes in terms of the freedom to fulfill their potential, however individualistically defined. Each is understood as possessing an equal basic entitlement to realize one's own understanding of the good life, unhampered by the fortunes of nature and social choice.

Equal worth of liberty, in turn, is dependent on sufficient levels of economic equality as well as personal health and welfare.[79] Preserving personal capacities for forming, revising, and achieving one's own goals and objectives, for defining individual meaning and self-satisfaction, requires removing, as much as possible, the physical, mental, and social handicaps of illness, disease, and disability. Sustaining basic individual liberty$_1$, therefore, straightforwardly requires significant state support and redistribution of resources. Wide-ranging welfare rights to adequate nutrition, shelter, education, and health care are underscored as basic goods necessary to secure successfully individual abilities and choices. Because health care helps guarantee the chance to enjoy the normal range of human opportunities, access to health care as a basic human right, without income-based barriers, is given special status as foundational to preserving liberty and fair equality of opportunity.[80] Here, the state is envisaged as a liberal morally pluralistic democracy, framing economic, institutional, and social structures that guarantee equal access to the basic goods of society (health care, education, and other welfare entitlements), so as to sustain fair equality of opportunity and outcome. Market systems, therefore, are decried as advantaging the wealthier and healthier members of society.[81]

Disadvantages are even greater with regard to organ failure. These concerns suggest that state policies that create positive entitlements for health care, including organ transplants, are justified to the extent that they decrease such inequality. Moreover, it also follows that healthy, well-functioning organs are likewise natural advantages, redistribution of which would help to equalize among persons so that each would be able more equally to share in the benefits and burdens of society. The five-year survival rate of those who receive a kidney transplant is excellent, while life expectancy for donors is not measurably decreased.[82] Redistributing redundant kidneys would be at most a temporary inconvenience for the "donor" that would greatly enhance the recipient's life expectancy, together with his or her social, personal, and political opportunities.

Access to adequate health care, including transplantable organs, without market- or income-based barriers is argued to be essential for eliminating natural and social disadvantages so that each may equally enjoy the liberty to fulfill his or her potential, however individualistically defined: "Because health care is a fundamental good, the moral ideals of justice, equality, and community require that the health care system be universal, comprehensive, and equitable in the sharing of benefits and costs."[83] On such an account of state moral authority to create and enforce health care policy, redistribution to promote the special good or goal to be realized trumps forbearance and privacy rights, which would otherwise protect persons in the private use of their own internal organs and other body parts. Here the state will be perceived as in authority to nationalize organs as a scarce resource to be utilized for public benefits.

Prima facie, such an ethos endorses religious liberty and cultural diversity. Difference in moral, cultural, and religious expression is, after all, the likely outcome of the search for individual meaning and understandings of the good. However, moral and religious viewpoints must not take on an exclusionary character. The status of such diversity may only be affirmed as akin to variations in aesthetic tastes, as differences in individual needs and desires, or predilections and preferences. Toleration, understood in the thick political sense as a willingness to affirm other religions and lifestyles as potentially equally as good as one's own, is central to sustaining this moral vision of a social-democratic, liberal, cosmopolitan polity.[84] Viable political negotiation requires such toleration as a political virtue, since the values realized within national health care systems will not be those that particular persons would choose, but rather the values chosen and ranked in the course of legislative discussion, action, and compromise.[85]

To have a "voice" is not to preserve one's own moral viewpoint, *even for oneself*. It is simply to be one voice among others in the pursuit of politically viable outcomes. Contemporary liberalism thus excludes from public political debate on controversial moral issues the voices of those informed by a thick moral or religious view. As Rawls notes, to secure political agreement public debate must "avoid disputed philosophical, as well as disputed moral and religious questions."[86] As a result, in its very advocacy of tolerance, liberalism is strikingly intolerant of a wide range of traditional moral positions.[87] In *Political Liberalism*'s brief discussion of abortion, for example, Rawls argues that agents who accept the humanity of the fetus can do so only on the basis of a "comprehensive doctrine," which, precisely because it rules out abortion, is "unreasonable" from the standpoint of public reason and thus unacceptable in the public square.[88] While officially endorsing the goods of moral pluralism, this perspective embraces a superficial secular understanding of religion and culture, in which the search for meaning is individualized, all spirituality generic and interchangeable, with all cultures and religions affirmed as equally valuable.[89] To engage in such comprehensive compromise, participants must free themselves from too deep an involvement with any particular values and principles; they must not be burdened with the constraints of traditional religions and cultures; they must "view themselves jointly as authors of the laws to which they are subject."[90] In short, they must be posttraditional. Diversity may only be affirmed as akin to variation in aesthetic taste: at best, the expression of personal or group idiosyncrasy; cultural stops for the secular cosmopolitan tourist.

Real disparity of belief threatens the possibility of reaching significant political agreement for the provision of comprehensive health care or the resolution of controversies, such as organ vending. True believers—that is, those who denounce others as wrong, attempt to convert, or refuse to see central religious or moral beliefs as the appropriate subject of political compromise—are perceived as dangerous and threatening. When traditional constraints collide with the posttraditional individualistic search for self-understanding, one engenders political controversy rather than moral resolution. One can only imagine the discussions of the National Commission for the Protection of Human Subjects in Biomedical and Behavioral Research had the commission when discussing fetal research included the pope of Rome, an atheist feminist, a fundamentalist Baptist, a Maoist communist, a free-market libertarian, the Orthodox Christian patriarch of Antioch, and an advocate of unhindered choice in the matter of abortion.[91] Acknowledging substantive moral diversity requires recognizing the existence of real moral opposition, thereby exposing the aspirations of statewide moral compromise and consensus formation for resolving moral controversies in health care to the significant likelihood of failure.

Consider also its implications for private associations, such as traditional religions, dedicated to developing and sustaining particular understandings of the good in the public space. Sustaining wide-ranging welfare entitlements requires significant taxation and redistribution of the time, talent, goods, and resources of all members of society, defeating individual or group claims to have exclusive use of private property. "Property" is recast as a social benefit to be redistributed as needed to preserve fair equality of opportunity and outcome, thereby ensuring equal worth of liberty. Ownership rights are conveyed insofar as they promote these special goods. The burden of proof is removed from governmental and other authorities, who would continually interfere in private use of one's property, and placed on those who would freely utilize personal property with consenting others. The goods and services of all are simply the means through which to create and finance a universal system of welfare rights. For example, guaranteeing equal access to health care regardless of personal income, social status, or geographical location requires significant redistributive taxpayer financing. Guaranteeing fair equality of outcomes requires state-based, single-tier health care distribution, universal rather than regional or local regulation, and uniform standards of care.

Such systems, however, carry significant financial as well as medical costs. Governmentally financed, single-tier health care predictably lowers the standard of care. Canada, for example, with its single-tier, governmentally financed and regulated health care system, ranks last among developed countries for access to MRI technology, resulting in significant diagnostic degradation (e.g., restricted access to MRI increases the risk of death and disability due to stroke).[92] Those older than sixty-five consume 42.7 percent of Canada's total health care expenditures while only accounting for 12.5 percent of the population. Adjusting for the age of its population, relative to other countries, Canada spends a greater percentage of its GDP on health care than any other industrialized, universal-access country, which the Organisation for Economic Cooperation and Development (OECD) tracks. Yet, Canada ranks tenth among such countries in the percentage of expected disability-free years, seventh in the prevention of death by preventable causes, and sixth in the incidence of breast cancer mortality. Unlike Canada, all six of the countries that experience fewer years of life lost from preventable causes have private alternatives to the public health care system.[93] Since all health care in Canada must be purchased within the governmental system, it is not possible for entrepreneurial physicians or even benevolent charity organizations privately to provide regional centers of medical excellence.

Similarly, even among industrial developed nations, different macro-allocations to health care, and within health care to critical care units, results in significant variation in outcome. When comparing critical care in the United States and Great Britain utilizing the Acute Physiology and Chronic Health Evaluation (APACHE) III scoring system, for example, outcomes of intensive care are qualitatively and quantitatively lower in the United Kingdom than in the United States.[94] As Michael Rie points out, these differential outcomes are not due to measurement problems or definitional difficulties; rather the virtue of such standardized measurements is that they obtain external, objective, third-party critical assessments. Such data allow one to compare outcomes across large populations of ICUs and patients, tracking the quantitative and qualitative vectors of the cost-benefit curve, thereby making possible honest assessment of the benefits and harms of allocating medical and financial resources to critical care.[95]

This cosmopolitan vision of equal worth of liberty and outcome embodies an egalitarianism of envy—a jealous hubris that some might fare better than others—and appears more apt at reducing misery than at creating excellence; more apt to ensure all some access to health care, even at a lower standard of care, than to generate tremendous insight and medical genius.[96] Governmentally sustained mediocrity thus also gives rise to significant losses in private incentive. It is a prioritization of equal worth of liberty over market efficiency, regional centers of excellence, and a higher total standard of care.[97] Here, political creation and enforcement of the privileged conceptions of liberty and equality trump greater availability of high-technology medicine, reduction of suffering, and years of life saved.

State-based health care distribution also gives rise to important moral costs. Significant redistributive taxation to support universal access to health care is hardly compatible with respecting real moral difference. As an example, tradi-tional Roman Catholics consider financing abortion as being complicit with evil. Since the right to abortion is widely endorsed in Western bioethics as cen-tral to gender equality and the equal liberty of women—Rawls, for example, refers to restrictive abortion laws as "cruel and oppressive"[98]—respect for such expression of individual liberty is given priority over deeply held religious objec-tions. Authoritative Catholic teaching forbids obtaining or performing abor-tions, as well as cooperating with or enabling others to obtain abortions.[99] Yet such religious objections are set aside in pursuit of the greater liberty for those whose life plans and personal values affirm abortion as liberating women from patriarchy and enforced pregnancy. (For example, abortion is covered by public expenditure as part of the Canadian health care system.)[100] Given state-based health care, those who object to the provision of particular services, such as abor-tion, find themselves coercively compelled into participating in their purchase.

Rights not to participate in the propagation of services that one conscien-tiously opposes, to utilize private property only in ways that one believes to be morally acceptable, are, at best, insecure and limited. Such losses are not negligi-ble; traditional moral and religious communities are coerced into supporting that which they know to be gravely evil; offering, providing, and financing abortion, physician-assisted suicide, in vitro fertilization, sex reassignment surgery,[101] and so forth. Taxation to support what one understands to be deviant moral visions impoverishes one's own liberty. It is a powerful weapon for suppressing moral dis-agreement and for privileging a particular moral viewpoint.[102]

In summary, liberty$_1$ as the equal entitlement to realize one's abilities and choices creates pro forma space for certain types of idiosyncratic moral differ-ence, akin to aesthetic variation in lifestyle and cultural expression. Substantive moral diversity, however, is ruled out in pursuit of political compromise regard-ing the material, psychological, and social conditions necessary to preserve equal worth of liberty. To forge consensus, different religious, cultural, and moral per-spectives may not appear to have an exclusionary character. Any serious validity claim that is not at the same time presented as a matter of personal idiosyncrasy is seen as endangering social cohesion. Traditional constraints collide with the posttraditional individualistic search for self-understanding, engendering contro-versy rather than compromise. Acknowledging substantive moral diversity requires recognizing the existence of real moral opposition, thereby exposing the aspirations of the liberal cosmopolitan vision and state-based health care to the significant likelihood of failure. Here the state will have a significant role in determining, through powerful legislation and regulatory enforcement, a particu-lar account of bioethics, including organ transplantation; it is legislative moral monism.

Liberty as Ideal, Not Actual, Free Choice (Liberty$_2$)

If liberty is understood as acting in accord with an ideal, rather than actual, account of free choice, informed by universal moral norms, then insofar as particular biomedical standards can be canonically established (such as the immorality of selling human organ for transplantation), they may be legitimately imposed through national law and international treaty. Here, autonomy is not acting in accordance with one's own wishes and desires, but in accord with right reason. Rather than social space for expression of diverse religious and moral beliefs, much of bioethics has sought top-down legislative guidance framed in terms of a rationally discoverable vision of proper conduct, authorizing state authority to constrain and direct citizens, groups, and communities. This is the vision of the universal legislator of Kant's categorical imperative, who derives an understanding of appropriate human choice from a particular account of moral rationality and rational volition. Bioethics as a field of inquiry lays claim to a universal account of proper moral deportment, including the foundations of law and public policy as well as the moral authority for national and international institutions to guarantee uniformity of practice.

Through appeal to core values (e.g., human dignity) and to central principles (e.g., beneficence, justice, and autonomy), bioethics is believed to transcend regional, cultural, and religious differences, binding all nations and peoples. The expectation is that through secular moral reason, bioethics discloses a communality of all persons, justified not in faith but in reason. The hope is to reveal a universally accessible secular basis for human moral community, justifiable without appeal to particular religions or cultures, traditional moral commitments, or insights. Citing objective, rational analysis, freed of the particularities of religious belief and cultural practice, such appeal is held to ground particular, content-full moral conclusions. Thus, much of Western bioethics seeks universal declarations on prenatal diagnosis and selective abortion, physician-assisted suicide, the ethical status of the human genome, the use of animals in research, embryo experimentation, third-party assisted reproduction, the sale of human organs for transplantation, and so forth. Similarly, appeal is often made to the existence of a so-called global moral consensus, which denies the existence of real moral difference, while announcing the secular equivalent of orthodox religious belief.

This compelling moral language—appeals to human dignity, objective reason, global consensus, and the like—rhetorically shifts the burden of proof to those who disagree. Dissenters are thereby made to appear as mean-spirited, idiosyncratic, or superstitious, as acting in "bad faith" or as fundamentalist adherents of irrational dogma. Western bioethics continues to give political and institutional expression to the Enlightenment hope that ethics and thus bioethics should liberate individuals and communities from unjustified customs and constraints—that is, those held to be contrary to the demands of universal moral reason. Choosing other than in accord with "right reason" and the purported "moral consensus"—whether in adherence to traditional religious commitments or to advance diverse secular accounts of the good—is thus characterized as acting under a false consciousness or as the victim of exploitation or social, cultural, or patriarchal despotism. Moral disagreement is to be shunned, if not actively persecuted.

Citing objective, rational analysis, freed of the particularities of religious belief and cultural practice, there is an endorsement of basic rights to prenatal diagnosis and selective abortion, physician-assisted suicide, and animal rights. Similar considerations are mustered in support of legislation prohibiting commercial surrogate motherhood, genetic engineering, and human cloning. There has even been the attempt to assert authority over bioethical professional training and competency assessment.[103] In this fashion, many Western bioethicists have begun elaborating an international bioethics to guide court decisions, public deliberation, clinical decision making, legislative action, and international treaties.[104] Such state-enforced biomedical restrictions are characterized not as limiting legitimate moral diversity or individual liberty but rather as returning individuals, families, and communities to the appropriately objective standards of rationally disclosed morality.

Yet, substantial moral diversity remains. Acrimonious bioethical controversies illustrate that within medicine there exists, as always, foundationally different accounts of the moral life. Indeed, rather than justifying a morality to which no rational being could deny assent, liberal social-democratic bioethics straightforwardly adopts a particular moral content so as to secure specific moral judgments: a content to which reasonable rational dissent is surely possible. To ignore such fundamental differences, while claiming a "global moral consensus" sufficient to establish a particular moral vision through national law and international treaty, engages in what might be termed coercive Western moral colonialism.

The sale of human organs for transplantation is a heuristic example. Regardless of the underlying reasons or likely personal advantages, selling human organs for a profit is held to be exploitative and degrading, morally analogous to slavery, and incompatible with basic human values (such as human dignity), and important social goods (such as equality and a spirit of altruism). The vendors' motives, together with their own judgment of what is in their own best interests, are dismissed as immaterial. Yet, as already explored, many parts of the body, including redundant internal organs, blood, and regenerative tissue, can be removed without destroying oneself or reducing adequate human functioning. While donating such parts as blood, sperm, and bone marrow has become more or less routine, assuming a suitably sterile environment and an appropriately talented surgical staff, even removing redundant internal organs (e.g., a kidney), whether for donation or sale, is less risky than many other occupations. Such medical activities are consistent with personal health, and the practice of saving lives supports the respect of other persons. Those who participate engage in a lifesaving activity, perhaps even heroically, to alleviate unnecessary suffering and death. Dissent to the so-called global moral consensus opposed to the sale of human organs for transplantation appears not merely reasonable but fully rational, if not morally compelling.

Political struggles concern not merely which policies will best achieve desired objectives, but which objectives are themselves desirable—that is, which moral understanding should be established (e.g., prolife or prochoice, individualistic or family-oriented approaches to health care decision making, regional versus global determinations of standards of care). How then should public policy be crafted? Should one simply acquiesce to the personal preferences or deep moral intuitions of academic bioethicists, current biomedical convention, or claims to global moral consensus? Or should one seek moral content to guide public policy through appeal to intuitions, consequences, casuistry, the notion of unbiased choice, game theory, or middle-level principles? All such attempts, as H. Tristram Engelhardt Jr. argues, confront insurmountable obstacles: one must already presuppose a particular morality so as to choose among intuitions, rank consequences, evaluate exemplary cases, or mediate among various principles; otherwise one will be unable to make any rational choice at all. As he points out, even if one merely ranks cardinal moral concerns, such as liberty, equality, justice, and security differently, one affirms different moral visions, divergent understandings of the good life, and varying senses of what it is to act appropriately.[105] In general secular terms, it appears impossible to break through the seemingly interminable bioethical debates to truth.

Given such circumstances, the claims of ideal rational choice theory (e.g., Rawlsian hypothetical contractors) to "global moral consensus," or to rationally discoverable moral truths, are implausible. As already noted, for example, many retain hesitations regarding embryo experimentation and abortion, even though these are practices that society permits and bioethics as a field generally endorses. Even assumptions that "human dignity" and "respect for the human body" possess moral import presuppose particular moral understandings regarding licit uses of the body. Similarly, suggestions that moral guidance is to be found in respect for human vulnerability or social solidarity presume background moral assumptions regarding appropriate expressions of beneficence. Because of divergent understandings of the good life and of what actually counts as doing good, general secular reason cannot comprehend beneficence as the Golden Rule.

Understanding the Golden Rule requires specification of particular moral content. Consider: some argue that social beneficence commands all to participate in the establishment of a totally encompassing welfare state, including universal single-tier governmentally regulated health care, with taxpayer-financed abortions for the impecunious. Those who disagree are to be coerced into participation. Others argue that beneficence requires understanding persons as free to refuse to be complicit in what one sees as evil, with basic welfare needs, such as health care, limited to peaceable consensual interaction, including contractual relationships and acts of private charity. Does "beneficence" command that all accept and participate in embryo experimentation and human cloning, or that all contribute through taxation to its continued development?

Consider also suffering: secular philosophy cannot comprehend pain, disease, disability, suffering, and death as meaningful apart from the loss of the pleasures, beauty, and engagement of this world. Suffering can only be experienced as empty, meaningless torment. As a result, most contemporary bioethical accounts are remarkably thin. Populated with the jargon of duty and obligation, autonomy, virtue, and beneficence, equality and social justice, but bereft of careful analysis of the deep theological or moral significance of health care, they encourage expansion of choice, elimination of suffering, and reduction of death but are unable authoritatively to determine which choices to make, what kinds of suffering to eliminate, or which deaths to postpone. How should one respond to those who suffer with long-term illness and disability: with encouragement toward an end in assisted suicide or toward baptism, rebirth, and redemption? While some see assisted suicide as a justified act of kindness, love, and mercy, which preserves human dignity, others view it as murder. Does "beneficence" require those who abhor the practice either to participate in or to finance assisted suicide?

Whose account of "do unto others what you would have them do to you" (Matthew 7:12) should govern? If others do not share one's convictions regarding beneficence, they may experience one's attempts to act charitably, to do good, as acts of violence. The Golden Rule can be and has been the basis for the coercive imposition of particular concrete understandings of the good life. Without specification of a particular moral framework, the suggestion "to treat others as you would wish to be treated" is at best empty and at worst tyrannical.

The political strategy is evidently to deny or discount the significance of such disagreement, marginalizing those who disagree as nonmainstream or radical, even dismissing alternate views as simply wrong or hopelessly irrational. Yet, outside of an appeal to an all-encompassing moral and metaphysical viewpoint, outside of a particular moral context, moral truth appears deeply ambiguous. Without the presupposition of particular content, morality cannot distinguish among different accounts of the nature of the good life, much less provide definitive guidance on how to proceed when the right and the good conflict. Thus, the imposition of any particular ethical content as the foundation of public policy assumes the veracity of moral claims that have not been established. The inevitably postmodern character of contemporary bioethics is simply the recognition of the foundationally irresolvable character of such moral pluralism in general secular terms. Given such circumstances, the claims of ideal choice theory are implausible. The universalistic aspirations of contemporary bioethics straightforwardly beg the question.

As a result, the so-called consensus regarding the moral impropriety of selling human organs for transplantation is at best coercively imposed. Many might otherwise choose in their own judgment of their own best interests to participate in such a market, whether to benefit others (such as family members) or themselves, or to further other personal, social, or political interests.

Liberty as Lived Human Flourishing (Liberty₃)

The universalistic claims of Western bioethics, as already noted, embody thick understandings of the values of liberty, autonomy, and equality that are incompatible with the often taken-for-granted assumptions of traditional religions and cultures. Drawing on quite different metaphysical and moral assumptions, traditional religions and cultures shape moral conclusions that are often at odds with those that Western bioethicists endorse. Moral understandings, particular accounts of human flourishing, accepted social roles, including appreciation of gender and sexuality, expressed in norms of human form, behavior, and grace, mark the conceptual frameworks that underlie public policy. As the gulf between traditional moral understandings and contemporary bioethical judgments illustrates, there does not even exist a unique canonical account of human nature from which to draw content-full understandings of licit and illicit biomedical conduct. Whereas Western bioethics focuses on the individual and is almost always expressed in discursive terms, within traditional cultures and religions bioethics is part of a living phenomenological world: it is part of a way of life. Liberty is an embodied, living account of full human flourishing.

In much of the foundation of American jurisprudence, persons appear as atomic individuals endowed with a right to determine their own futures.[106] This view of individuals in the practice of informed consent tends to present persons outside of any social context in general and outside of their families in particular.[107] Such individualism does not necessarily exist within traditional cultures and religions. Consider Confucianism. Julia Tao notes, for example, that concerns regarding individualism and individual equality, including equal access to health care, are set aside within traditional Confucian ethics in favor of the family:

> Confucian care ethics rejects universal love. Instead, Confucius himself also urges that a person . . . should start from one's parents and siblings and then extend to other people. . . . There is no requirement to treat

everyone equally with the same impartial treatment. . . . Our obligations are defined by our relationships.[108]

As Tao documents, patients come to health care with their families. Within Confucianism the family offers a natural social structure that provides moral orientation through a community bound in love and a common moral understanding. The family is the central social unit and the presumed locus for appropriate medical decision making.[109]

Similarly, the Western principle of autonomy understood as free individualistic choice is fundamentally incompatible with traditional Confucian understandings of the moral relationships essential to human fulfillment. The practice of free and informed consent for health care in the United States is nested in a cultural affirmation of the moral importance of respecting the choices of individuals. It recognizes as well the difficulty of knowing what it means to choose correctly in a secular, morally pluralistic society. Absent an agreement regarding the requirements of God or the demands of moral rationality, individuals have been identified within rather broad side constraints as the source of authority over themselves and as the best judges of what choices are in their own interest.[110] Thus the surface public morality of the United States gives priority to individuals, who are seen as possessing autonomous authority over themselves. In contrast, as Qiu Ren-Zong notes,

> values seem to be shared by different moral communities or cultures, but their meanings differ among them. Autonomy in Western culture means decisions made by an independent person, but in Confucian culture it means decisions made by a family incorporating the person.[111]

Whereas the family plays a central role in traditional cultures and religions, its place in Western bioethical decision making is ever more marginalized, criticized, and called into question.

In much of Western bioethics the burden of proof is weighed against traditional families and ways of life. As noted, Western health care law and policy is framed in terms of individualistic consent, reflecting the centrality of the individual and ensuring adequate opportunity for persons to free themselves from traditional familial relationships. As Engelhardt argues,

> consider the contrast between those who favor autonomous individualism and those who would give moral priority to family life. Those who regard autonomous individualism as the presumptively appropriate relation among persons would require any deviations to be established by explicit statement and agreement. For example, patients would be presumptively treated as autonomous individuals willing and committed to choosing on their own, unless they explicitly demanded to be regarded

and treated within a traditional family structure. . . . On the other hand, if one considers life within a traditional family structure as the presumptively appropriate relation among persons, the burden of proof shifts. Persons are approached as nested within the thick expectations of traditional family structures, unless they explicitly state that they wish to be regarded and treated as isolated individuals.[112]

Consent in traditional cultures and religions is typically paternalistic and family oriented, where patients may not even know their own diagnosis, much less personally consent to treatment.[113] Western bioethics, on the other hand, seeks legal requirements for patient-oriented confidentiality and informed consent to protect individual autonomous decision making, shielding personal information from spouses, children, parents, and other relatives.[114] Securing equal worth of individual liberty requires liberating morality and personal choice from traditional viewpoints, cultural practices, and religious beliefs. The goal is a secular ethic that begins with the privileged presumption of the sovereignty of the individual—individualistic autonomy and equal worth of liberty. For example, society permits children to speak on their own behalf as soon as they become "sufficiently mature" but does not permit parents to judge for themselves what constitutes "sufficient maturity." Similarly, there is space for women personally to consent, but without women explicitly demanding to be so respected, not for their husbands or eldest sons to consent on their behalf. Securing equal worth of liberty requires liberating morality and personal choice from traditional viewpoints, cultural practices, and religious beliefs.

Those committed to such a goal often perceive ideologically directed state-based civic education of children as crucial for redressing religious assumptions and moral viewpoints that are incompatible with the privileged conceptions of equal worth of liberty and fair equality of opportunity. As Rawls argues,

> a long and historic injustice to women is that they have borne, and continue to bear, a disproportionate share of the task of raising, nurturing, and caring for their children. . . . These injustices bear harshly not only on women, but also on their children and they tend to undermine children's capacity to acquire the political virtues required of future citizens in a viable democratic regime. Mill held that the family in his day was a school for male despotism: it inculcated habits of thought and ways of feeling and conduct incompatible with democracy. If so, the principles of justice enjoining democracy can plainly be invoked to reform it.[115]

State education of children is required to prepare the young "to be fully cooperating members of society and enable them to be self-supporting; it should also encourage the political virtues so that they want to honor the fair terms of social cooperation in their relations with the rest of society."[116] The political virtues include toleration and mutual respect, together with a sense of fairness and civility.[117] Such education teaches children "such things as knowledge of their constitutional and civic rights . . . to insure that their continued membership [in their parent's religion] is not based simply on ignorance of their basic rights or fear of punishment for offenses that do not exist."[118] Accordingly, the family must be subject to significant governmental regulation to ensure proper attitudes and beliefs.

Decisions regarding core curriculum in state education are to be made with the express intention of diffusing a particular societal and civic, fully secular, culture. As Amy Gutmann comments,

> Some kinds of social diversity . . . are anathema to political liberalism. Civic education should educate all children to appreciate the public value of toleration. The basic political principles of liberalism, those necessary to protect every person's basic liberties and opportunities, place substantial limits on social diversity. . . . The limits on racial and gender discrimination, for example, enable many people to pursue ways of life that would otherwise be closed to them by discriminatory practices at the same time as they undermine or at least impede some traditional ways of life.[119]

Since the focal point of the moral life is autonomous self-determination, liberty—as the celebration of free individualistic choice—is integral to the good life for persons.[120] The hope is that through such education the choice to remain in a traditional community or family can be shown to be morally deficient and thereby over time gradually discouraged.[121]

Indeed, Rawls urges that the concern to support equal worth of liberty through fair equality of opportunity tends toward the dissolution of the family. We do not deserve our initial starting place in society or having been born into a particular advantaged or disadvantaged family. "That we deserve the superior character that enables us to make the effort to cultivate our abilities is also problematic; for such character depends in good part upon fortunate family and social circumstances in early life for which we can claim no credit."[122] As long as some form of the family exists, he argues, the principle of fair equality of opportunity can only be imperfectly carried out. The extent to which natural capacities develop and reach fruition depends in large measure on social conditions and class attitudes that influence family structures and environments.[123]

> The consistent application of the principle of fair opportunity requires us to view persons independently from the influences of their social position. But how far should this tendency be carried? It seems that even when fair equality of opportunity (as it has been defined) is satis-

fied, the family will lead to unequal chance between individuals. . . . Is the family to be abolished then? Taken by itself and given a certain primacy, the idea of equal opportunity inclines in this direction.[124]

The liberal cosmopolitan ethos simply presumes the sovereignty of the individual, rather than the family, which in traditional forms is pejoratively caricatured as an institution of repression, injustice, and despotism.

Such an ethos is not morally neutral. Consider, for example, the claim that appropriate procreative autonomy requires sweeping access to prenatal screening technology to detect genetic abnormalities, such as trisomy 21, which causes Down syndrome, coupled with unfettered access to nontherapeutic abortion.[125] Genetics counseling, it is argued, should cover all of the various options, including the appropriateness of abortion.[126] The goal of such counseling is "to empower her (the pregnant woman) to informed and independent decision-making as to which course of action to take at each step in the screening and testing process. . . . It is assumed that the woman's autonomy is best respected if the service empowers her to independent decision-making."[127] The benefits of screening are seen primarily in terms of informed choices regarding selective abortion. In the United States failure to inform pregnant women of the possibility of nontherapeutic abortion has exposed genetic counselors to civil liability under the law of torts.[128] Such suits typically allege malpractice on grounds of either "wrongful life" or "wrongful birth." Civil claims for "wrongful life" involve parental suit on behalf of the child alleging that his nonexistence would have been preferable to his current existence with defects, such that his existence is a wrong done to him as a result of the negligence of the genetic counselor. Under a wrongful birth civil suit, the parents allege emotional and financial harms associated with caring for a defective newborn, whom they would have chosen to abort if they had been informed of the appropriateness of the option. Such legally supported torts require counselors to encourage patients to seek abortions based on quality-of-life judgments, even if in violation of deeply held religious convictions.[129] As Gerhold Becker notes in passing, however, most surveys find that over 90 percent of trisomy 21 diagnosis cases end in abortion.[130] Significantly increased incidence of abortion is the undeniable result of prenatal testing and genetics counseling. Here, authoritative state endorsement gives powerful voice to secular individualistic autonomy.

There is burgeoning evidence, moreover, that the civic education endorsed by the liberal cosmopolitan vision has had a significant impact on traditional religion. In a 1999 survey by the *National Catholic Reporter*, approximately 72 percent of Catholics responded that one could be a good Catholic without following the Vatican's teaching on birth control; 65 percent believed that one could be a good Catholic without following the Vatican's teaching on divorce and remarriage;

and 53 percent responded that one could be a good Catholic without following the Vatican's teaching on abortion. Nearly 50 percent responded that individual choice should be the final arbiter of the morality of abortion, homosexual activity, and sexual relations outside of marriage more generally. Indeed, 23 percent reported that one could be a good Catholic without even believing that Christ rose from the dead, and 38 percent without believing in the Transubstantiation of the Eucharist.[131] Similarly, in one survey of Protestant pastors, 17 percent supported laws in favor of assisted suicide, with over 33 percent of those surveyed who were also associated with the National Council of Churches in favor.[132] Such data represents a striking departure from traditional belief and practice.

The aspirations of many in Western bioethics to articulate a universal medical morality are thus revealed as especially insidious because they are subtly invasive, suggesting that one ought to side with the claims of "rationality," "expertise," and "consensus"—that is, with general secular bioethical "orthodoxy"—over against what one may know in the fullness of a particular moral community to be true, while, at the same time, utilizing national and international legal coercion to eliminate the possibility of moral diversity and liberty in health care. To premise governmental and institutional policy on individualistic understandings of autonomy, or concerns for social justice and individual equality, simply substitutes Western individual-oriented ethical constructs for traditional family-oriented moral commitments without argument. Those who choose to live within thick moral communities confront a governmental and institutional environment that is hostile to traditional understandings of moral goods and important family relationships.[133]

Here, Father Thomas Joseph's reflections on the hostility to the traditional family are also helpful:

> One of the difficulties in attempting to reinvigorate the family is one of its very strengths: families bring within them concrete substantive moral commitments. Substantive commitments divide a society. They ingrain a moral pluralism. In addition, some critics are especially concerned about the family's connection with religious faith because of their commitments to rendering society ever more secular.[134]

The robust, content-full visions of human flourishing available within traditional religions and cultures cannot be captured or recreated within the secular vision of moral theory. Traditional Confucians and Orthodox Christians understand the pursuit of a fully flourishing human life as situated within the thick expectations of family structures rather than in commitments to the pursuit of social justice, equality, fairness, civic duty, or generalized solidarity.[135] From such living moral perspectives, however otherwise different from one another, most of Western bioethics is appreciated as stark and impoverished.[136]

Forbearance Rights and the Freedom to Venture and Fail (Liberty$_4$)

The more general secular reason is unable to disclose a universal, coherent, content-full moral understanding of health care, or to secure the justification for political authority to impose such a vision, without merely assuming the truth of particular moral claims, the more one must seek alternative foundations to construct moral authority for health care policy. Liberty$_4$ understood as freedom from interference, as expressed in the existence of significant forbearance rights, where persons are free to venture with others, open to the possibility that one's choices may lead to success or failure, will support the existence of a free market in health care. Moral authority will not be drawn from assertions of so-called moral consensus, ideal theories of rational action, or deep moral intuitions regarding human rights or repugnance, or cardinal moral concerns, but created through the collaborative agreement of the parties. Collaborators need not agree regarding the background ranking of values or moral principles, cultural or religious assumptions; they need only affirm the particular content of their agreement. All that is needed is the recognition that morally authoritative collaboration can be created through the actual peaceable agreements of persons.

Forbearance rights create strong protections against battery (i.e., nonconsensual touching or use of one's person or property), defining a sphere in which one is morally immune from interference while protecting self-interest and self-preservation in the private use of person and property. Such rights describe side constraints prohibiting nonconsensual interference, which hold against other persons, as well as society and state. Here the market takes on a certain centrality, but not because the market is affirmed as in itself good. Nor is the market or its outcomes in a strict sense valued as such. Rather, the idea of the market is the creation of social space for unencumbered personal interaction. The market and its outcomes are affirmed as the result of respecting the moral authority of persons over themselves and their private property in the exercise of their basic human liberty. Market transactions and contractual relationships draw moral authority from the consent of the participants to be bound by their agreement. The parties to the transactions, themselves, freely convey authority to the enforcement of the specified conditions. General secular moral authority to interfere in the free interaction of consenting persons will not exist, absent its creation through the actual agreements of actual persons. Consequently, health care will not be appreciated as possessing any special priority or value; it will simply be among the many ways in which one may express oneself in peaceable consensual collaboration with others.

Liberty$_4$ grounds significant property rights, where persons have exclusive control of their property, subject only to the constraints of prior agreements and the avoidance of using other persons, together with the property owned by other persons, who do not choose to participate.[137] Alienation, whether through abandonment, donation, exchange, or sale, is morally licit, if freely chosen. Provided that both vendor and purchaser freely agree to the transaction, property may be utilized for fun, beneficence, or profit, including the financing and purchase of health care. Absent actual agreement, forbearance rights act as side constraints, defeating the claims of others, persons and governments, to have any entitlement to the time, talent, or property of individuals. Particular values or special considerations (such as equal positive worth of liberty or equal ability to impact political outcomes, fair equality of opportunity, benefits to others, or judgments of irrational choice or moral repugnance) fail to establish moral authority either to create universal health care systems or to forbid consensual transactions for various types and standards of health care, shaped by varying moral commitments and taken-for-granted background assumptions. As a result, that some find the sale of human organs for transplantation to be morally repugnant, frightening, or inherently exploitative would fail to establish legitimate moral authority to forbid such consensual transactions.

Individuals, families, or communities, including traditional religious communities, would be free to contract for (1) various types of health care (e.g., allopathic, homeopathic, naturopathic, chiropractic, and so forth), with (2) particular standards of care (e.g., regional variations and varying levels of insurance coverage), (3) shaped through divergent moral commitments and (4) framing presuppositions regarding health care practices (e.g., individual versus family or community-oriented consent, or varying concepts of health and disease).[138] Imposition of all-encompassing uniform systems of health care, guarantees of equality in the provision of health care services, and the search for universal health care standards (such as the global prohibition of organ sales) violate such basic human liberty: forbearance rights expressed as peaceable consensual interaction in the market.

The rights of persons will foreclose what many envision to be worthwhile goals. In contrast to liberty₁ as the entitlement to realize one's abilities and goals, or liberty₂ as ideal rational choice, forbearance rights recognize persons as only entitled to their own private resources and those additional resources that they are able peaceably to convince others to donate or sell to them. Basic human rights to health care, much less to the general amelioration of losses due to bad luck, losses in the natural or social lottery, individual choice, disease, ill health, or other misfortunes, do not exist.[139] Seen in this light, financing personal health care choices through coercive taxation clearly forces those with substantive moral or religious commitments, or content-full understandings of the good life, to be complicit in the purchase of health care services that they hold to be at best deviant (e.g., chiropractic or naturopathic), if not evil (e.g., abortion or embryo research). Insofar as freedom is not merely one value among others, or a good that may be valued more or less along with other goods, but rather functions as a side constraint, one may not injure, steal from, tax, defraud, or otherwise coerce unconsenting others, even to produce good consequences. This would violate their status as free and responsible agents. One may not utilize persons, absent actual permission, merely as the means to benefit others.

Morally authorized statutes are confined to the protection of persons' rights to forbearance, protection of individuals from battery, and to those additional policies to which actual persons give actual consent. Persons, and organizations of persons, may be held responsible for nonconsensual acts of violence, fraud, and breach of contract, since such actions violate the rights of persons not to be touched or used without permission.[140] As a consequence, governments, even democratically elected majorities, do not possess moral authority to enforce uniform standards, to finance universal access, or to regulate equal distribution of health care. Governmental authority created by the express agreement of those governed is also limited to the extent of such agreement. So grounded, the state would have no general moral authority to interfere in the medical marketplace. Forbearance rights make implausible interventions to forbid persons from freely using personal resources with consenting others, including the purchase of various types and levels of health care. But note that the market here is not being endorsed as a good in itself, nor are free choice and moral diversity celebrated in themselves as special goods. Instead, the market defines social space and institutional structures for peaceable, consensual, and thus morally authoritative human interaction. Respecting the freedom of persons defaults to protecting liberties of association, contract, conscience, and religion, and thereby to protecting the possibility of substantial moral diversity, including divergent incommensurable instantiations of liberty$_3$ (e.g., Orthodox Christian and traditional Confucian).

Freely chosen, market-based health care financing, procurement, and distribution respects the liberty of persons to pursue their own deep moral commitments. The market creates political space for the free interaction of individuals. It secures the possibility of diversity within particular states as well as for the emergence of a worldwide network of nongeographically based communities with their own particular understandings of moral probity, including bioethics, health care policy, and institutional restrictions. Substantial moral diversity will likely exist, not due to any endorsement of diversity's value—indeed, it may be bitterly regretted—but because moral authority does not exist to foreclose peaceable consensual interaction. We are prohibited from coercively taxing others to create a comprehensive state-based health care system, not because of the simple ascription of positive individual rights but because of the prima facie lack of moral authority to so act.[141] The permission of the parties to collaborate creates, rather than discovers, such moral authority. Unlike liberty$_1$ as the right to realize one's abilities and choices or liberty$_2$ as ideal rational choice, liberty$_4$ understood as freedom from interference actually carves out and protects social space for the possibility of moral diversity in health care, including for those who choose to participate in the commercial sale of human organs for transplantation.

SUMMARY

Assessment of the permissibility of a market in human organs must consider the various factors that directly affect the relative standard of proof that must be met rightfully to interfere with persons and their use of their body parts as well as other property. This will include each of the following considerations. (1) *The significance or strength of ownership rights:* The standard of proof for interfering with persons and their exclusive use of body parts and other property varies directly with the strength of ownership rights. If ownership entails absolute dominion, then rights to exclusive use and alienation will function as side constraints on other persons and social institutions, including governments. Lesser, more conditional ownership will allow other countervailing considerations to overturn claims to exclusive use and at will alienation. (2) *The significance of forbearance and privacy rights:* The standard of proof varies directly with the general strength of such negative rights to be left alone. The stronger and less contingent such rights are, the more they will fix aspects of the external environment, placing constraints on other persons, social organizations, and states. (3) *The closeness of the analogy between dominion/possession/ownership of one's body parts and dominion/possession/ownership of other types of things:* Body parts that are distinguishable and separable may in principle be replaced at will, and may be regarded as things with which persons are the most intimately associated. Indeed, persons utilize their body parts as the embodiment of their will and source of interaction in the intersubjective domain of common experience.[142] Insofar as the general significance of body parts to persons is greater than the significance of other types of things, this suggests that of all the things persons own, they have the strongest rights to the exclusive use, and thus to the alienation of, their own body parts. The standard of proof for rightful interference would thus need to be set higher with regard to uses of the body than for uses of other types of property.

Consider also the various factors that shift who shoulders the burden of proof, as well as which reasons are relevant for meeting an appropriate standard of proof to allow for the restriction of human freedom in entering markets for human organs:

(1) *Not all body parts are created equal:* Some parts are necessary for embodiment/existence (e.g., higher brain), others are necessary for adequate human functioning (e.g., heart, cornea), others are neither (e.g., appendix); some parts are experienced (e.g., hands), while others are not (e.g., hair). Like other types of things that are intimately associated with persons, many body parts, which are not necessary conditions for embodiment/existence, can be replaced at will without thereby harming the liv-

ing experiential nature of the person. Those who object to markets in human body parts will need to provide grounds that focus on the particular body parts at issue. For example, selling one's redundant kidney is not equivalent to selling one's higher brain. Objections that do not meet this condition will fail to be telling at best, or will beg the question outright.

(2) *Not all organs are harvested from living vendors*: Futures markets do not violate any constraints against killing or duties to self. Moreover, death defeats any need to sustain the conditions for either embodiment/existence or adequate human functioning. The burden of proof is on objectors to the market to show that they have not conflated reasons that are telling against utilizing living vendors as if they are equally telling against harvesting and selling organs from deceased donors.

(3) *The ontology of general secular personhood*: The general secular ontology of personhood allows for the possibility of replacing body parts that are distinguishable and separable at will. Replacing such parts is compatible with the full functioning of persons as rational moral agents. Moreover, the secular ontology of personhood is neutral with regard to the origin of the replacement part (e.g., human or mechanical, natural or artificial); it is also neutral with regard to whether money changed hands in the procurement of the part (e.g., charitable donation or for-profit sale). The phenomenological and physical requirements for sustaining particular persons are satisfied with adequate human functioning and minimally sufficient incorporation of the part into the experiential lived world of the person.

(4) *The nature and ground of ownership as well as the nature and ground of moral political authority*: The burden of proof shifts with the nature and ground of ownership and moral political authority. If ownership together with legitimate societal and governmental moral authority are benefit or special-consideration based, authority is founded on the presupposition of canonically binding moral goods, values, or goals. As a consequence, insofar as property is understood as a social benefit to be distributed according to the common good of society, whether "good" is understood as prudently maximizing benefits over burdens or as promoting a particular special value or goal, it will shift the burden of proof to those who would utilize their time, talent, body parts, and other property independently of the concern for the common good. Additionally, state moral authority will in principle extend substantially to all facets of personal and social life. Relevant reasons for meeting the standard of proof vary with the good or goal to be realized. If one is a utilitarian, one will maximize the good; if one is an egalitarian, one will organize social institutions so that they treat all persons equally in the respects relevant to the moral good. An additional consequence, though, is that state moral authority will exist only insofar as such moral content can

be established as canonical rather than merely assumed or intuited. Without such canonical moral content, state authority merely appeals to force.

In contrast, ownership and moral political authority based on freedom begin with persons as the source of moral authority. Insofar as unique canonical moral content cannot be rationally secured, state enforcement of any particular moral content can be appreciated as arbitrary, and as possessing the character of mere force. Avoiding arbitrary appeals to mere force in such circumstances requires moral authority to flow from the agreement of persons. Relevant reasons for meeting the standard of proof will focus only on freedom. If persons act freely with consenting others, then other persons, social organizations, and states do not have general moral authority to interfere. Given this framework the burden of proof shifts away from persons with rights to free association, contract, exclusive use, and alienation of property, to those persons and governments who would presume the right to interfere in the consensual interactions of persons in the market. Access to the market, including markets in body parts, can thus be understood as a basic human right that cannot be rightfully forbidden.

The following considerations would therefore appear to be important in establishing which constellations of factors are necessary or sufficient to render a market in human organs morally acceptable. *First is the special status of separable and distinguishable body parts.* If persons can sell themselves, then they can sell any of their body parts. However, if we eliminate voluntary slavery from consideration, then persons are able to sell some parts but not others. On such an account, a necessary condition for a market in body parts is that the parts being traded are both separable and distinguishable from persons. No other particular conditions appear to be necessary.

Second is the consideration of what policy regarding organ markets will maximize benefits. If an organ market would best utilize the available organ resources, or would best maximize benefits for persons, these factors would be sufficient to render an organ market morally acceptable. Societal and governmental authority would likely extend to the creation and regulation of such a market. Organs would be commodified as resources to produce social benefit. This may entail creating a governmentally controlled market that taxes the body parts of some for prudential transfer to others so as to maximize possible benefits. Who would pay the physical and economic costs of procurement and transplant would depend on a further calculation of possible benefits and burdens, as would considerations as to whether to limit such a market to body parts that are both separable and distinguishable. The possibility of such markets will depend directly on how one conceptualizes prudence (e.g., as maximizing the welfare of the worst off, creating the greatest net benefit, or the greatest benefit for the greatest number) and the results of the empirical benefit/burden calculation, together with an assessment of whether the calculation would range across welfare maximization, preference satisfaction, or wealth maximization, among other possibilities.

Third, one will also need to address the issue of guaranteeing special goods. If ownership and moral authority are based on special considerations, such as social goods, values, or goals, promotion or realization of such goods may require a market in human organs. If the goal to be promoted is free and responsible behavior, then access to such a market should help realize this goal. On the other hand, if the value or goal is equally effective political liberty, this may require transferring the benefits of time, talent, body parts, and other property to those in need of such welfare payments. Sufficient equality of material resources, including adequately functioning body parts, may be a necessary requirement for equal political and social liberty. Equality may be best served by transferring organs from those with redundant internal organs to those in need of such a transplant. On such an account, the argument will focus less on whether to commodify organs than on who pays the physical cost of procurement and who receives the benefit of transplant (e.g., considerations of just distribution of physical resources) and who pays the economic costs of procurement and transplant (e.g., considerations of just distribution of economic resources). It may be that this account of ownership and state moral authority would ground rights of all citizens with sufficient need to receive organ transplants at society's expense.

Finally is the question as to when considerations of liberty will be sufficient. The constellation of factors that define a liberty-based account of ownership and moral political authority are sufficient to render a market in human organs morally acceptable when liberty is an inviolable side constraint or when liberty is understood as freedom from interference, as expressed in the existence of significant forbearance rights. Indeed, if liberty so understood is the sole or primary ground of moral authority or ownership, this would be sufficient to render a market in organs such that it could not be rightfully forbidden.

Each of these ontological, moral, and political theoretical considerations is a factor in determining the analytic geography of the debate regarding markets in human organs. These constellations of factors specify relative burdens of proof, those factors that are relevant for meeting such burdens, as well as on whose shoulders the burden falls. Adjudication among the numerous interrelated factors may require recourse to a theoretical model of balancing appeals.[143] However, before these further arguments can be adequately assessed, the next chapter must consider particular instances of such basic foundational issues, including the geography of benefits and burdens associated with a market in organs: allowing versus forbidding it, as well as possible independent objections to such a market (e.g., considerations of exploitation, sanctity of life, and human dignity).

CHAPTER THREE

A Market in Human Organs

Costs and Benefits, Vices and Virtues

INTRODUCTION

The previous chapter assessed understandings of embodiment, property, and political authority under which a market in human organs would, all things considered, be morally permissible. These necessary and sufficient conditions were assessed by exploring the relationship between persons and their bodies, the senses in which organs can be property, the distinction between justified and unjustified moral repugnance, and the limits of societal or governmental moral authority to interfere in the exchange of body parts. As the chapter demonstrated, given different understandings of these crucial issues a market becomes more or less morally plausible, thereby increasing or decreasing the moral burden of proof that must be met for the permissible creation of public policy, as well as establishing who should bear that burden: proponents or opponents of the market.

But all else may not in every circumstance be equal. In this chapter, the conceptual geography moves to a more subtle arena. The analysis must consider the health costs and benefits of a market, the vices and virtues a market would encourage, thus challenging this ceteris paribus clause and thereby rendering a market more or less morally plausible. Beyond considerations of embodiment, ownership, and morally justified political authority, there are additional moral concerns regarding health care benefits, use of scarce resources, encouragement of free and responsible behavior, liberty, equality, and altruism, which should bear on the moral judgments one may advance regarding a market in organs. There are also special concerns regarding social and personal welfare, as well as human dignity and sanctity of life, often captured under the general rubric of exploitation that are advanced in discussions of the moral permissibility of a market in human organs.

Here, one must attend to counterbalancing interests, which, when gauged against one another, balance, curtail, or defeat arguments against the market. Here also, one must attend to the ways in which normative assessments of costs and benefits vary with theoretical accounts of the consequences and special considerations that are held to be intrinsic or instrumental to the good of persons or society.

Assessing the costs and benefits of a market in human organs requires laying out an analytic geography of underlying values and special moral considerations or goals, as well as assessing the ways in which such factors balance against one another. Such considerations will also bear upon the determination of who shoulders the burden of proof. If a market in human organs supports the realization of significant personal or societal values and goals, the burden of proof will be on those who would forbid the market to provide equally significant counterbalancing considerations, all else being equal. In addition, other concerns, such as human dignity and exploitation, which prima facie might be taken to defeat the allowability of the market, may be better protected with commercialization than through alternative procurement and allocation strategies.

This chapter will not attempt to settle the matter of the permissibility of an organ market. Rather, the focus is on determining under which circumstances a market in human organs advances health benefits, the effective use of scarce resources, as well as other special values and goals, more successfully than alternative organ procurement and allocation strategies.

Unlike the market, most systems of voluntary donation are based on the implicit assumption that organs are a community health care resource, and as such procurement and allocation strategies must take into account community-based moral and health care outcomes. Many contend that a market in human organs would corrupt organ procurement and transplantation protocols, that the possibility for quality medical care and scientific research will be sullied by greed, leading to significant harms to both organ vendors and recipients. Consider Richard Titmuss's claims regarding commercialization of the blood supply. Titmuss argued that the existence of a for-profit market in blood and blood products leads to less blood being available for transfusions, a greater likelihood of distributing blood contaminated with disease, inefficient management of the available supply, and a significant increase in price per pint of blood, while imposing social costs on the poor.[1]

His conclusions, while couched in somewhat rhetorical language, advance important criticisms:

> the commercialization of blood and donor relationships represses the expression of altruism, erodes the sense of community, lowers scientific standards, limits both personal and professional freedoms, sanctions the making of profits in hospitals and clinical laboratories, legalizes hostility between doctor and patient, subjects critical areas of medicine to the laws

of the marketplace, places immense social costs on those least able to bear them—the poor, the sick and the inept—increases the dangers of unethical behaviour in various sectors of medical science and practice, and results in situations in which proportionately more and more blood is supplied by the poor, the unskilled, the unemployed, . . . and other low income groups and categories of exploited human populations of high blood yielders. Redistribution in terms of blood and blood products from the poor to the rich appears to be one of the dominant effects of the American blood banking system.[2]

It is important to note the special moral costs Titmuss identifies: (1) a decrease in altruistic sentiments, (2) an erosion of a sense of community, (3) a lowering of scientific standards, (4) limitations on personal freedoms, (5) limitations on professional freedoms, as well as (6) the legalization of hostility between patients and physicians. In addition, his criticisms presuppose (7) that making a profit from hospital services or (8) from laboratory services is morally suspect, and (9) that the forces of the market bring on more harm than benefit. It is clear that Titmuss does not regard the profit motive as leading to the wise use of resources, nor does he consider the market a place that rewards responsible, free decision making.

This chapter provides an overview of direct and indirect health benefits, efficient and effective usage of scarce resources, free and responsible behavior, liberty, equality, and the maximization of social or personal welfare. The issue of exploitation is then engaged. One must determine whether a market in organs leads to exploitation, or whether policies forbidding organ sales are themselves exploitative. To gauge this issue adequately, one must assess the market over against alternative possible procurement and allocation systems. The chapter then assesses the impact of free choice on personal altruism and community. Here Titmuss's criticisms regarding the impact of markets on a decrease in altruistic sentiments, the erosion of a sense of community, limitations on personal and professional freedom, as well as the legalization of hostility between patients and physicians are brought to bear on procurement and allocation strategies. The criticism that the market lowers scientific standards is then evaluated, along with the virtues and vices of free choice involved in an organ market. Here Titmuss's concerns regarding the making of profits from hospital and laboratory services, as well as the virtues and vices of a for-profit health care market, are addressed. The chapter concludes by reviewing these considerations as well as others in assessing what is at stake in judging the moral allowability of human organ markets.

HEALTH CARE COSTS AND BENEFITS

An initial metric for gauging the acceptability of a market in human body parts is whether it would have better health outcomes—by increasing the quality and quantity of patients' lives, reducing time spent on transplant waiting lists, and avoiding preventable deaths—than alternative procurement and allocation strategies. Alternatively, if the market would lead to inappropriate harms to organ vendors, ineffective and inefficient usage of scarce health care resources, and other more indirect heath care costs, such concerns may outweigh the potential benefits. These considerations can be grouped under the general rubrics of direct and indirect health care costs and benefits.

Direct Health Care Costs and Benefits

Direct health care concerns include whether a market in human body parts would decrease the number of available organs; raise health care costs, thus further exacerbating a constrained health care budget and incurring the health risks of additional rationing; procure only poor quality organs for transplant, contributing to poor health care outcomes for recipients; increase the occurrence of unnecessary surgery, thereby contributing to poor health care outcomes for vendors; or ineffectively utilize the available organ pool, transplanting organs into candidates for whom transplantation will not convey a benefit, or at least not a benefit of sufficient magnitude or duration.

Such concerns affect the balance of considerations with regard to the acceptability of a market in human organs. Significant health costs (because of the availability of fewer organs, the realization of poorer quality outcomes, or the particular surgical harms to vendors, as well as other costs attendant to ineffective and inefficient organ allocation) would tip the burden of proof against a market in organs. Insofar as organ procurement and allocation policies diminish the total number of organs available for transplantation, or otherwise set donors or recipients at considerable jeopardy, such health care costs weigh against the acceptability of the policy. However, if the market is likely to lead to greater organ availability, with organs of good quality and more efficient organ procurement for transplantation, while minimizing potential harms to vendors, such positive health consequences tip the burden of proof against those who would forbid the market.[3] One would need to deny the value of such goods, deny that such goods are produced, or argue that the market engenders or involves costs to significant independent moral considerations, which counterbalance potential health gains, reasonably to prohibit a market in human organs.

Policies that expand the number of living donors would multiply the availability of transplantable body parts, such as kidneys, bone marrow, and liver grafts. If such a policy also engaged families and other third parties (who have authority over the bodies of deceased and dying patients) to make those organs accessible, this would also increase availability of nonredundant organs, such as hearts, from brain-dead and cadaver donors. Expanding the pool of living and cadaver donors would then save lives and reduce suffering. The concern remains that a market in human organs might decrease organ availability.[4] If potential donors sell exclusively to the highest bidder, only the very rich, or those with premier insurance, would be able to purchase needed organ replacements. Other potential recipients would suffer and perhaps die. Terms on waiting lists would extend for the poor, who would then be competing for the diminishing number of donated, or less expensive (perhaps inferior), organs.[5]

Commercial approaches to procurement and allocation are seen as raising numerous issues of social justice. The concern in part is that cash payments will attract primarily poor and low-income segments of the population, including racial minorities, who will disproportionately bear the health care complications of being vendors, as well as being increasingly subjected to exploitation. Once a market exists, family members may be less inclined to donate to a relative in need. Envision, for example, callous individuals chiding a friend or family member: "George, buy your own organ! If you had saved your money, you could have purchased your own replacement kidney for transplant. Why should we give you one?" One might appeal to special moral considerations to respond to such concerns: part of responsible behavior is accepting the consequences of failing to save monetary or physical resources, or of failing to refrain from organ-damaging activities. One might also engage other social or political responses: to blunt such effects, social policy might establish a minimum baseline of welfare or health care benefit packages including organ stamps (i.e., federally supported organ purchase vouchers for the poor). Other market-based responses ought also to be considered, such as the possibility of trading redundant organs (e.g., a segment of healthy liver might be exchanged for a healthy kidney).

Grounds for such health-related concerns, though, are unlikely to be justified. Presuming that the willingness to donate body parts is motivated by actual rather than coerced altruism, those who are willing to donate ought to continue to be willing regardless of the existence of a for-profit market. Though the United States has a market-oriented economy, individual Americans donate over 184 billion dollars annually to charitable and nonprofit organizations.[6] Regardless, most organ donations from living persons are to family members or close friends. The motivations supporting such donations are likely to maintain the same force regardless of the existence of a for-profit market: love, beneficence, loyalty, gratitude, guilt, or avoidance of the shame of failing to donate. These are not donors whose altruism extends to all possible recipients; rather, willingness stems from their relationship with a particular patient. Such transfers are unlikely to change either in general character (i.e., from donation to sale) or in relative number (i.e., become other than driven by the need of a specific friend or relative—e.g., sibling[7] or spouse[8]). Potentially, however, when someone needs a family member to donate a kidney, it may already have been sold.

Also, if organs become perceived as the kind of things that people have to purchase, like cars, they may no longer be considered the kind of good that one can acquire through donation. Note, though, that the motivations that currently support organ donations to family members are also likely to support family pooling of resources to purchase a replacement organ. Indeed, many may find the pooling of financial resources preferable.

Furthermore, the development of such a market provides no reason to stop asking patients or their families to consider donation. Additional strategies designed to increase organ availability, such as required request or directed donation, ought not to be seen as exclusive alternatives to the market. Pursuing multiple parallel strategies may lead to the greatest organ availability. It may be, however, that the goal of increasing organ availability, and thus reducing human suffering, would be more effectively and honestly secured with the existence of an organ market. For example, the concern that an organ market would disproportionately adversely affect health care for the poor, the uninsured, or the underinsured ignores numerous possibilities for influencing the market. Various state incentives could be utilized to avoid the need for direct payments from recipients to donors. Here one might consider allowing donors, or their families, to take tax deductions for the fair market value of the organs. In addition, one might utilize a system of tax credits against income or inheritance taxes owed for the organ's value.[9] These would be governmentally managed systems for the purchase and supply of organs. Both policies would ensure that donors were compensated for the market value of their body parts, while actively encouraging an increase in available organs without raising direct health care costs. Many aspects of such a system could be supported through religious and other charitable organizations. There could, for example, be organ drives supported by particular religious groups or corporations.[10]

Here also, one might consider a system of organ vouchers, which would create certain welfare entitlements. Vouchers might function as straightforward health care entitlements, where the state, or national health insurance, would purchase needed organs utilizing tax dollars for the poor. Alternatively, such vouchers might create a system of entitlements contingent upon personal or family in-kind trade. In an English case, a father, who was not a good tissue match to donate to his son, offered one of his kidneys to the British cadaveric donor pool in exchange for placing his son on the national cadaveric waiting list for a kidney. He offered a cost-neutral option for an in-kind trade.[11] Other market possibilities include the trading of redundant organs (e.g., a barter system in which the families of those in need of transplant trade with each other for the necessary healthy organs). At Johns Hopkins University Hospital, for example, in July 2003, surgeons performed a "triple swap" kidney transplant operation, in which three patients, who were not tissue compatible with their own willing donors, exchanged the donor's kidney for a kidney from another of the three donors. Each donor provided a kidney to one of the three transplant patients.[12] Similarly, a system of incentives, not unlike those utilized to encourage blood donation, could give organ entitlements, or higher priority on the waiting queue, to those families whose member(s) donated organs.[13]

Churches and other charitable organizations could play a significant role in creating health care resources for the poor. One might envision individuals donating rights in organs directly to local churches, which would guarantee high-quality health care for surgery and minimize other risks associated with donation. The organs could then be sold to the rich to raise funds to purchase health care, food, and medicine, or be made available for transplantation to the poor. Imagine a group such as "Mother Teresa's Organs for the Poor" generating resources to provide organs for the impecunious. Such organizations could raise money to provide organs to those who could not otherwise purchase them. One might think of creating "Catholic Kidneys International" to raise funds to purchase specific organs, like kidneys, for the poor, or act as organ brokers for the poor in developing countries to advantage those poor and provide these regions with other important resources. The market creates social and political space to explore additional opportunities and incentives for organ procurement and allocation, without thereby forbidding other types of incentives and opportunities.

Market incentives encourage persons to raise resources to further personal as well as social interests and goals. With the creation of a market in human organs, organ availability need not be limited to acts of altruism. Profits from organ sales would allow for the private pursuit of business and educational opportunities, or to further more public agendas. Given that social and personal advantage is often tied to education and business success, such incentives may be significant. However, even short-term welfare maximization, such as the purchase of housing or health care, may provide some with sufficient incentives to sell redundant internal organs. Commercialization would create opportunities, which some may view as attractive, to secure resources for pursuing their own educational, business, political, and welfare interests. It is likely that utilizing the market as a procurement strategy would encourage individuals, who would not otherwise donate, to sell their organs, which would increase the availability of organs for transplantation.

With regard to minority groups, many argue that there is a disincentive to donate organs because it is perceived as providing a good that primarily benefits the majority establishment.[14] As Arnason points out,

> African-Americans have a higher incidence of renal disease but a very low rate of organ donation. Blacks currently receive three times as many kidneys as they donate; although they receive proportionately fewer kidneys than whites. Blacks also have a smaller rate of graft survival

than whites. The reasons for this pattern include some unique medical predispositions of African-American potential recipients and donors, socioeconomic factors, and mistrust of a predominantly white medical establishment.[15]

Some allege that the use of human lymphocyte antigen (HLA)–based allocation to increase successful grafts actually reduces the chances of African Americans and other minorities to be recipients.[16] Similarly, Cooper-Patrick et al. argue that African Americans and other minorities receive differential and less optimal technical health care.[17] Moreover, according to a 2002 survey, after adjusting for potential confounders, mistrust in hospitals and concerns regarding discrimination were strongly associated with less willingness to donate among African Americans.[18] Such disincentives straightforwardly decrease organ availability for transplantation, increase the length of waiting lists, and thus amplify human suffering and death.

UNOS notes that the need for minority donation is critical: African Americans represent approximately 13 percent of the U.S. population but more than 30 percent of patients waiting for kidney transplant. Similarly, Hispanics and Latino Americans represent approximately 12 percent of the U.S. population but 15 percent of patients waiting for kidney transplant.[19]

Directed donation is often suggested as a means to alleviate and overcome such challenges, because minority families may be more receptive to donation if assured that their loved one's organs will benefit another member of their own minority group. "Seeking ways to enhance the prospect of a black donor's kidney finding its way into the body of a black recipient would certainly remove a *disincentive* for black donors," contends Arnason.[20] Assuming such background conditions, the very directed nature of the market should likewise increase incentives for allowing organ harvesting. Indeed, the market would add further incentives. Individuals and families could pursue either private economic goals or social political agendas. Charging as much as the market is able to bear will transfer financial resources to the particular minority. Selling organs very cheaply to fellow minority members would ensure such patients a higher likelihood of receiving an organ. Either course of action would increase the number of organs available and provide direct health benefits. Unlike donation, sales are empowering and directed in character. Individuals would control their organs as private property to be sold or given at will, provided a willing buyer or recipient can be found. Note also that unlike often proposed systems of routine salvage of organs, which would straightforwardly violate religiously based concerns to maintain the integrity of the deceased body, the market permits but does not require that one sell or donate one's organs.

With the creation of an organ market, one is likely to see an increase in the number of living persons willing to sell organs to recipients who are neither family members nor close friends. Market incentives will likely also lead to the willingness of more families to have the organs of their loved ones harvested upon death. Even if harvested organs only directly benefit members of a particular racial group, such activity will reduce the number of patients on the general waiting lists, thus reducing waiting time for others. Such a policy would thereby incur health benefits for all those in need of a transplant.[21]

The primary health risks for living donors are those associated with the operative procedure for harvesting the organ. For example, perioperative mortality for nephrectomy is approximately 3 deaths for 10,000 donors (0.03 percent), with other major complications occurring in less than 2 percent of cases.[22] Approximations of long-term morbidity risks, such as increased risk of hypertension or proteinuria after living-donor nephrectomy, are more controversial.[23] Other operations, such as harvesting a liver segment, can be somewhat more risky for the donor.[24] Organ failure does not limit itself to the wealthier segments of the population. Yet donation among family members is considered licit, even if those donating are poorer or less healthy than more affluent members of society. Such mortality and morbidity risks exist whenever living donors are utilized, regardless of whether money changes hands.[25] Therefore, presuming that the practice of procurement from living donors will continue, such risks are neutral with regard to the market.

While some may be concerned that individuals will sell poor-quality or diseased organs for private gain, such concerns are only valid if an independent method to monitor the quality of organs is unavailable. In general, the health advantages of transplants from living donors are great. An organ market would allow potential vendors and recipients to "shop" for precise tissue matches. Since vendors can be evaluated with regard to health in advance, the organ can be stored in the donor with few or no concerns about degeneration of tissue. Organs procured from living individuals are more viable than cadaveric organs and are more likely to function well once transplanted. In addition, the transplant can be planned so that both parties are in the same hospital, or in the same operating room, to allow the quick transfer of the organ. This is the same procedure that is utilized for living donative transplants.[26] Greater likelihood of transplant success equates to more efficient and effective use of the available organ pool and other medical resources.

Indirect Health Care Costs and Benefits

Commercialization may lead to other more indirect health care benefits. Such a market, for example, may decrease the long-term financial cost of organ transplantation. While historically organ procurement has not been without significant financial expenditure, the organ itself has typically been donated. In the

United States, for example, average one-year billed charges, including evaluation, procurement, hospital, physician follow-up, and immunosuppressants, ranged from $143,300 to $814,500 in 2002, with no payments to the donor or donor's family. In 2002, U.S. patients, or their insurance companies, paid on average $391,800 for a heart transplant and a year's worth of follow-up care, $313,600 for a liver transplant, $143,300 for a kidney transplant, and $814,500 for an intestine transplant.[27] Surgeons do not generally provide operative services free of charge; hospitals do not provide space, immunosuppressive drugs, and other operative personnel resources without fees. Nor are all organ procurement agencies supported solely through charitable donations. Each of these products and services adds to the high cost of organ transplantation. The concern is that the additional funds expended procuring organs may reduce the overall funds available to purchase other types of health care. Such costs might further stress a single-tier, government-controlled health care system with a fixed global budget for health care expenditures. Within the private insurance market, providers may raise premiums to meet the additional costs.

These potential drawbacks, though, might be blunted in several ways. First, the availability of more organs may lead to reduced overall costs, because timely receipt of a healthy organ may reduce or obviate the need for other types of treatment, such as dialysis.[28] Second, the current costs (in time and money) involved in determining to whom particular organs should be allocated (e.g., setting "match" standards and debating which social and political concerns such as the potential for quality and quantity of life, time spent on waiting lists, and national versus local distribution, ought to play a role in the calculation) could be reallocated to purchasing organs for persons in need.[29] Third, the market would likely reduce the hidden charges generated by current "altruistic" policies. For example, one study, which calculated the financial costs of potential solid organ donors who fail to donate due to medical complications after consent has been obtained, found that additional costs ranged as high as $33,997 per potential donor.[30] Such costs are ultimately passed on to patients' families and third-party payers. Insofar as the market decreased such costs, through an increased number of healthy living vendors, for example, who are less likely to experience these complications, it would liberate resources. Fourth, if private persons sell organs, this may make available more funds to purchase health care or more extensive insurance. That is, in the private sphere, health care is not a zero-sum game: total expenditures are not fixed. Fifth, since an organ market would allow vendors and recipients to seek more precise tissue matches, it would likely lower the long-term financial expenditures associated with transplantation. For example, Schnitzler et al. calculated that follow-up treatment in the three years following transplant was 34 percent less expensive for patients with fully HLA-matched kidneys than for patients with as many as six HLA mismatches.[31]

Selling an organ may not only provide resources for education, training, or starting a business; it could also increase the vendor's overall social and economic prospects, in turn having indirect health benefits. Persons with higher salaries or greater status jobs incur advantages: economic, social, and functional. For example, despite universal single-tier health care coverage, life expectancy in Canada varies according to income and status. In 1971 the difference in life expectancy in Canada between the highest and lowest earning was 6.3 years for men and 2.8 years for women. This deviation had only reduced in 1986 to 5.6 years for men and 1.9 years for women.[32] Consider also the Whitehall II study conducted in Great Britain on civil service workers, which demonstrated an inverse association between employment grade and prevalence of angina, electrocardiogram evidence of ischemia, and symptoms of chronic bronchitis. Morbidity and mortality were each affected by employment grade.[33] The reasons cited to account for these differences include "different attitudes to health," such as "the lower degree of belief among those with lower status jobs that they could take action to prevent a heart attack"; differing "patterns of social activity . . . with clear indication of less, and less satisfactory, social support among those with lower status jobs"; and that the "work environment is perceived differently between grades." The study concluded that "impressive evidence has accumulated that jobs characterized by low control, poor opportunity to learn and develop skills, and high psychological work load are associated with increased risk of cardiovascular disease."[34] Moreover, low job control was closely linked with position in the employment hierarchy. A similar study among Czech men concluded that low job control was related to acute myocardial infarction in middle age.[35] In addition, mortality from heart disease is higher in manual than in nonmanual occupational classes.[36]

Low income has been consistently related to measures of unfavorable birth outcomes. Within lower-income neighborhoods in urban Canada there are higher rates of infant mortality, low birth weight, very low birth weight, prematurity, and small gestational age. According to Wilkins et al., urban Canada experienced a 50 percent decline in infant mortality between 1971 and 1986; however, the ratio of infant mortality rates comparing the poorest neighborhoods with the least poor neighborhoods diminished by only 8 percent.[37] These statistics point to indirect health benefits for children associated with the income level and job status of parents.

Increase in control over one's occupation (i.e., in status as well as salary) leads to economic, social, and functional advantages, which in turn are indirectly associated with increased life expectancy, health, reduced infant morality, and increased advantages for children. Morbidity costs and mortality risks lower with income level and professional status. Measured solely in terms of health care consequences, selling one's internal redundant organs may be a rational strategy to raise one's income, increase one's economic and social prospects, and thereby indirectly to benefit the health of oneself and one's family. Allowing the poor to market their organs will offer opportunities for advantaging their health, as well as empowering them. Even short-term welfare maximization, such as the purchase of housing or health care, may provide some with sufficient incentive to sell redundant internal organs. The market will give them control over their own lives, which, given the foregoing data, is itself statistically related to economic, social, and health advantages.

SPECIAL MORAL COSTS AND BENEFITS: EQUALITY AND LIBERTY

Acceptability of a market in human organs must also be gauged in terms of special moral costs and benefits. Attention must be given to the character of special moral goods and considerations, such as equality and liberty, as well as free and responsible behavior. If commercialization would promote equality and liberty more successfully than alternative procurement and allocation policies, then this would tip the burden of proof against those who would forbid such a market. Alternatively, if the market would inappropriately restrain freedom, increase inequality, or discourage responsible behavior, such moral concerns may outweigh potential benefits.

One might be concerned that the existence of a market in human organs would increase the economic and social gap between the poor (who sell organs) and the rich (who purchase them). Consider, for example, two alternative human organ procurement and allocation policies. On policy A, 100 percent of the patients spend an average of twenty-four months waiting for a suitable organ for transplantation. There is a 5 percent mortality among patients while on the waiting list. On policy B, 50 percent of the patients spend an average of two months on the waiting list, with less than 1 percent mortality while awaiting transplant. The circumstance of the remaining 50 percent of the patients is exactly the same as with policy A. Of these two policies, B may be worse with regard to equality, if measured solely in terms of the possibility of receiving a transplant and the likelihood of dying while awaiting transplant. However, policy B is better with regard to health care outcomes: waiting time for half of the patients is much less, which reduces human suffering; moreover, fewer patients die while awaiting transplant.

As a report on the ownership of human tissue from the U.S. Office of Technology Assessment points out, concerns regarding equality should favor a system of payments to the sources of human tissues.[38] This view incorporates the idea that persons have the right to treat at least some physical parts of their bodies as objects for possession, gift, and trade, such that the sources of human tissues and organs are entitled to the value of any benefits ultimately derived from them.

Legislating that donors may only transfer organs as a gift does not thereby reduce the value of such organs to zero. Rather, it straightforwardly transfers the potentially significant value of the organ from the donor to other parties involved in the transplantation.[39] "If it is possible to determine or estimate the potential value of biological materials, then as information is distributed, patients, or their agents, will come to know the values of tissues and cells they may possess and they will expect recompense."[40] The greater the value of the human tissues or organs to the recipient, the more relevant this view becomes.

One must also weigh the potential of moral harms to equality and liberty, as well as to free and responsible behavior, resulting from forbidding such a market. For example, if one is concerned that the poor will be induced by their poverty to sell their organs, one must also be concerned that removing what the poor may see as an attractive option, so as to assuage feelings of repugnance on the part of the affluent, itself coercively limits the liberty of the poor autonomously to assess available opportunities to better their lives, thereby engendering inequality-related harms. Organ selling may be a means to generate resources for the poor, which can be reinvested in personal and economic development, thereby decreasing inequalities.

Insofar as a disproportionate number of poorer individuals would be exposed to the risks of organ donation, the potential harms of procurement surgery would need to be weighed against the short- and long-term benefits attributed to increased income. As Angeles tan Alora and Josephine Lumitao document, in the Philippines many consider the sale of redundant organs an important means to raise resources to support fledgling businesses and to further family welfare.[41] They argue that in the Philippines the family is the key to understanding and evaluating this problem. Daniel Tiong, for instance, documents the case of Pusakal, a poor inmate who while in prison allegedly sold a kidney to support and benefit his family:

> Given the circumstances, the extreme need of his family appears to outweigh the loss of one kidney. In fact, one could imagine Pusakal giving much more, if the situation demanded it. Subjectively, he senses a greater duty to his family's welfare than to his own well-being. His concern and love lighten the sacrifice he is making. . . . Pusakal recognizes the double burden on Dolor [his wife], who must be homemaker as well as provider, thereby assuming the social roles of both father and mother. Pusakal must protect Dolor, who would have difficulties finding other employment and could get even sicker or die, leaving the children in an even worse situation.
>
> The kidney sale resolves Pusakal's obligation as provider in an extraordinary fortuitous way . . . this one time provision of funds provides

an excellent opportunity for them to survive decently—provided, of course, that they invest the money well and sustain the small business.[42]

Here, the centrality of love and concern for the family provides the central criterion of the moral reasoning underlying the organ sale.

One might also raise concerns that the existence of a market will curtail personal and professional liberty. As was explored in chapter 2, one must first consider how liberty is to be understood. If liberty is freedom from interference, as expressed in the existence of significant forbearance rights, then a market in organs creates social space for unencumbered personal interaction, which while making no specific judgment regarding the market, permits its existence. Alternately, if liberty is appreciated as a right to act on one's abilities, *venturing* with others while open to the possibility that one's free choices may lead to success or failure, this circumstance will entail outcomes that are materially equivalent to freedom from interference. It creates social space for persons to venture freely with others in the market. A third possibility is liberty understood as the entitlement to *realize* one's abilities and goals. In this case, significant state support may be required to ensure outcomes consonant with individual abilities and free choices. As already discussed, this concern is often encapsulated as the need to sustain more than the conditions of formal liberty, as freedom from constraint, but rather to ensure material liberty, as expressed in fair equality of outcomes.[43] At stake in the context of organ procurement and allocation are the ways in which a market in organs, or its prohibition, places limitations on or enhances personal and professional freedom.

Liberty understood either as significant forbearance rights or as freedom to venture with others will support the existence of an organ market. Prohibiting the selling of human organs constrains individual freedoms to use one's body and body parts, fails to respect personal privacy and individual choice regarding lifestyle, and restricts one's ability to venture with others in the creation of contracts from which both parties expect to benefit. Western ideals of freedom from constraint and individual responsibility typically allow for such expressions of liberty. Moreover, insofar as persons are free to venture and fail, the market encourages the development of individual responsibility. It provides tutelage regarding the limits of the human condition and individual ability, as well as the ways in which past agreements can constrain future choices. Agreements formalized as contracts are often a powerful expression of personal freedom.

As Prosser points out, however, since obligations are imposed because of the parties manifesting consent to the agreement, such consent must be autonomous.[44] Here one must assess the possibility for autonomous consent to organ vending. One might argue that actual autonomous consent either may not exist, or may in some fashion be invalidated. For example, organ vendors may be precluded from choosing autonomously because they do not fully comprehend the implications and risks of surgery. While ignorance is not generally held to invalidate all contracts, it is possible that failure to understand significant life-threatening risks associated with donation may be sufficient to raise the standard of proof for consent.

It is unclear, though, that an organ market would fare worse regarding autonomy and consent than other organ procurement strategies.[45] Surgical risks are not a significant concern for harvesting organs from either brain-dead bodies or cadavers. Therefore, concerns that vendors may fail to understand life-threatening risks do not defeat autonomous participation in an organ futures market; nor do such concerns bear on families who sell organs from recently deceased or brain-dead next-of-kin. Moreover, ignorance as a barrier to consent does not respect the distinction between living donors and living vendors. Unpaid donors can be equally ignorant of the risks of surgery or of the potential for serious complications. Insofar as ignorance rules out organ selling, it also rules out organ donation. However, as with donors, not all vendors will be ignorant of the risks, nor will all be irremediably so. Opportunities to receive counseling should ameliorate such concerns.

If the threat of significant harm increases the standard of proof for consent too greatly, this raises the additional concern that other important freedoms will be ruled out as well. Consider, for example, the circumstance where without a job one would starve, or need to take a job that carries substantial risks (e.g., home roofing or oil-platform construction). Would autonomy be impossible in such circumstances? Even if some potential vendors ought to be excluded from selling organs for reasons of irremediable ignorance (e.g., the mentally disabled), blanket prohibitions do not serve the interests of liberty.

Liberty as an entitlement to realize one's abilities and goals supports an organ market insofar as it would more successfully assist persons in fulfilling their talents and choices than a state-mandated system of donation. One might argue that the circumstances of a human organ market are such that forbidding the buying and selling of organs does not limit liberty; or that, on balance, prohibition serves the realization of liberty-based interests more successfully than the market. For example, one might argue that the existence of financial inducements for organ procurement undermines the freedom to donate one's organs. If an organ market is created, while only some will exercise the liberty to sell, the freedom of all to donate will thereby be limited. The private market, Titmuss argued with regard to blood products,

> limits the answers and narrows the choices for all men—whatever freedoms it may bestow, for a time, on some men to live as they like. It is the responsibility of the state, acting sometimes through the processes we

have called "social policy," to reduce or eliminate or control the forces of market coercions which place men in situations in which they have less freedom or little freedom to make moral choices and to behave altruistically if they so will.[46]

Of course this criticism can be turned on its head. Prohibition of an organ market precludes the freedom of all to sell their organs. Given that with a general prohibition on organ vending only some will exercise the liberty to donate, the freedom of all to sell, if they so will, is limited.

Freedoms contingent on realization of significant market-oriented abilities and choices might tip considerations of liberty in favor of the creation of an organ market, even if only a state-sponsored one wherein individuals could take tax deductions or credits for the value of donated organs. If state purchase of organs would realize health-oriented freedoms, this might tip considerations in favor of a government-supported organ market, or allowing patients in need to advertise for organ vendors. Alternately, freedoms contingent on realization of significant community-oriented solidarity or beneficence interests might support blanket prohibition.

Which institutional system would more successfully realize the abilities and choices of persons (the free market, a state-sponsored market, or blanket prohibition) is an empirical question that depends in part on the talents and goals of individuals. Insofar as commercialization of organ procurement and allocation creates social space for unencumbered human interaction, it would not preclude the liberties of the altruistically inclined to realize their need to take care of others. Market-based liberties include, but are not limited to, profit-seeking interests. Unless the state prohibits the practice, an organ market could allow private individuals out of charity to sell organs very cheaply to those in need. Social and political institutions that support the free choices of persons to interact with free and consenting others are formally neutral with regard to the expression of charity.

One possible concern is that the market will intimidate charitably inclined persons who will thereby view themselves as precluded from giving away organs. As with the problem of ignorance, though, such intimidation will not be universal and will not usually be irremediable. One might also be concerned that with the creation of a for-profit market there will no longer exist social institutions for charitable donation of organs. While it is unlikely that the existence of a market would preclude the creation of nonprofit organ acceptance and distribution agencies, even commercial corporations may accept donations to support impecunious care, or simply to cut costs. Commercial markets in food, housing, education, and medicine exist side by side with nonprofit charitable organizations.

Forbidding an organ market straightforwardly limits the liberty of vendors and recipients who are inclined to interact with each other in the profitable exchange of goods and services. It limits personal freedoms of choice, privacy, and association, as well as the freedom of physicians to acquire organs to assist their patients. Those in need of organs for transplant are prohibited from advertising for potential vendors, which straightforwardly also limits patients' freedoms of speech, association, and contract. Prohibition thereby imposes constraints and limits liberties to choose and venture with others. Given that potential recipients are often dying of organ failure, the loss of these freedoms is likely significant. Prohibition will also stifle the realization of market-based abilities and choices, as well as those preferences, which while not directly market based, rely on the availability of private funds. Moreover, prohibition overlooks opportunities for the poor to raise resources to better their prospects, as well as for the state to encourage organ availability, through tax credits and deductions, thereby addressing both income and health inequalities. Even if some consider certain aspects of commercial trade in human organs to be intrinsically unsavory, forbidding such a market may cause worse moral harms to equality and liberty.

EXPLOITATION: ORGAN MARKETS VERSUS OTHER PROCUREMENT AND ALLOCATION STRATEGIES

One must now assess whether and how the market may exploit persons in greatest need, in particular, or whether forbidding the sale of organs is itself exploitative. The core notion is that to exploit someone is to benefit by taking unfair advantage of that person. For example, A may exploit B when A benefits from a transaction that is harmful to B, or from which A receives disproportionate value.[47] In addition, A may exploit B if A benefits from an exchange when B's ability to choose is compromised, even if B's choice is not strictly involuntary.[48] Market exploitation, it is claimed, offers inducements to those who are vulnerable such that intrinsically unattractive options become, all things considered, the best available.

Regarding organ sales, the concern is that financial incentives will tip the balance of interests, inducing the poor into selling their organs to the rich. Consider the case of a twenty-five-year-old Iraqi who, allegedly, was loitering on October 17, 1995, outside of a Baghdad hospital because an elusive Libyan had agreed to purchase one of his kidneys for five hundred dollars, a small fortune in Iraq at that time.[49] Similar reports in Great Britain alleged that in 1989 two Turkish peasants had been paid two thousand pounds each, plus expenses, to travel to London to be live kidney donors in a private hospital.[50] Given conditions of poverty, the poor will have significant financial incentives to undergo the risks of surgery.

Market exploitation can be classified into three types:

(1) *harmful exploitation,* in which purchasers gain from such transactions while organ vendors are, on balance, harmed;

(2) *mutually advantageous exploitation*, in which, though organ vendors benefit from the transaction, it is in a way that remains unfair (e.g., if purchasers benefit substantially more than vendors, or if offering to purchase organs takes unfair advantage of vendors' impoverished circumstances); and

(3) *moralistic exploitation*,[51] in which purchasers and vendors gain from a transaction that, even if freely consented to, is fundamentally immoral. Here, a primary concern is that organ sales improperly commodify human body parts.

Harmful Exploitation

Assessing whether organ sales involve harmful exploitation requires an "all things considered" judgment of the potential for such transactions to cause harm. The question is not whether selling organs has harmful elements, but whether on balance the costs outweigh the benefits. Most uncontroversial beneficial transactions contain negative elements. Individuals may prefer leisure to work, or to receiving expensive medical resources for little or no personal expense; however, such circumstances do not entail either that employment harms workers, or that hospitals that require payment for services rendered harm patients. In each instance, it is presumed that employers and hospitals may permissibly require compensation for the financial or medical benefits one receives, and that the benefits to individuals outweigh the costs. Moreover, adequately to evaluate organ selling as a social practice, the question is not whether any particular individual is harmed, but whether, on balance, the expected value of such exchanges is consistently negative. As Wertheimer points out regarding employment: "If a worker is severely injured on the job, such that employment is a net harm to that worker, we do not say that such employment is harmful as a practice."[52] In short, the issue is not whether an organ market is harmful to any particular individual *ex post*, but whether it can be expected *ex ante* to be harmful as a social practice.[53]

As already noted, the impact on the physical health of organ vendors in terms of long-range mortality and morbidity risks, although crucial to consider, is likely not significant. Indeed, a market in human organs would likely lead to significant positive social and health benefits. Provided redundant internal organs are procured in a suitably sterile environment, by a competent surgeon, selling internal redundant organs is less risky than many other occupations. Regardless, insofar as living donors will continue to be utilized, such harms are neutral with regard to the market.

The additional harms vendors bear are primarily psychological. They will, therefore, be difficult to measure and may differ from person to person.[54] Insofar as organ vendors incur psychological distress (e.g., feelings of violation, embarrassment, or loss of dignity), adequate financial remuneration may compensate. It would, however, be an error to presume that donors are not subject to similar psychological harms. While some argue that compensation itself causes increased psychological harm, the value of the compensation to the organ vendor may out-weigh increased psychological disvalue, thereby obtaining a net benefit.[55] Tit-muss argued in 1971 that the social conditions of blood vending contributed to feelings of duress, stress, and general dissatisfaction among vendors. He con-cluded, moreover, that in states where blood is put up for sale, the fact that oth-ers could sell their blood reduced the satisfaction of donors as well as vendors.[56] *Pace* Titmuss, however, more recent studies have found significant satisfaction among both paid blood vendors[57] and voluntary donors.[58] Organ vendors may experience a deep sense of satisfaction for participating in a lifesaving activity, even, perhaps heroically, at some risk to themselves. It is simply an assumption without adequate argument or evidence that only unpaid altruistically motivated organ donors would experience personal satisfaction.[59] In short, insofar as psy-chological harms can be adequately recompensed, or balanced against psycholog-ical benefits, it is implausible to view organ sales as benefiting recipients at sig-nificant harm to vendors.

Mutually Advantageous Exploitation

Organ sales may also be exploitative if one party benefits a great deal from an exchange that only marginally advantages the other. Marxist accounts of market exploitation, for example, often focus on the ways in which exploiters command significantly more value from an exchange than they bring to the transaction, while for the exploited the reverse is true.[60] Similarly, Joel Feinberg argues that an agreement is exploitative if one of the parties receives excessive profit or dis-proportionate value from the exchange.[61] On such an account, organ vendors are exploited if they receive significantly less value from the transaction than the worth of the transplant to recipients.

The concern is that the poor will be willing to sell organs for relatively little money, because even a small amount will be advantageous. Consider a recent study concluding that impoverished kidney vendors in India are not paid enough to rescue them from poverty.[62] This may be due, in large measure, to the com-paratively small amount of compensation relative to their debt and other desper-ate need. Increasing vendor compensation, however, should rectify this circum-stance. State price controls, for example, could set minimum financial standards for each organ. Minimum price legislation may help prevent exploitation. These considerations also suggest that organ sellers may face a collective action prob-lem. Most individual vendors would not be able to negotiate as attractive an agreement as would be possible if potential vendors negotiated collectively as a group. The goal of escaping poverty is usually better addressed with an increase, rather than decrease, in compensation. Here also one might also raise the concern that prohibition, which forbids persons from realizing any value for their organs, exploits donors.

An offer might be considered coercive if the lure of compensation compromises the voluntariness of the potential vendor's choice. Whereas not all irresistibly attractive offers are coercive, financial gain is often considered an influence that overwhelms and subjugates the voluntary consent of impoverished potential donors.[63] It may even be the case that the purported exploitee stands to gain more utility from a transaction than the purported exploiter. It is because impoverished vendors stand to gain so much from the sale that their bargaining position appears comparatively weak.[64] Marxists have argued that capitalist labor markets are coercive because workers are limited to a choice between unpalatable alternatives, for example, working at low-paying jobs or starving.[65] Others contend that financial offers "may be difficult for a person of little financial means to refuse and would, in that case, be coercive."[66] This account helps to explain why altruistic donation is not regarded as exploitative: it is not that the exchange of value is more fair,[67] but that the motivation underlying the transaction is perceived as more pure.

If poverty is the difficulty, though, one might reduce the financial incentives by lowering the amount paid per organ,[68] or restrict participation in organ markets to those with sufficiently high incomes.[69] Michael Walzer, for example, holds that "what goes on in the market should at least approximate an exchange between equals."[70] While such policies may prima facie appear less exploitative, they have counterintuitive consequences. First, they further restrict options for the poor; second, unlike those better off, the impoverished are prevented from fully utilizing the market for their own advantage.[71] While a poor individual may decide that selling a kidney is more attractive than other options, offers to purchase an organ do not make him worse off if he refuses to sell. Analogously, on the labor market, those who must settle for any unpleasant or more risky occupation, such as ditch digging, oil-platform construction, assembly-line worker, and so on, must make the same type of choice; this does not necessarily mean that they are being coerced. Third, as Margaret Radin notes, it is unclear why engaging in market transactions with the poor constitutes the use of coercive power, while doing so with the middle class or the wealthy is an appropriate expression of personal freedom.[72]

One must also distinguish between coercion and peaceable manipulation. While coercive actions are those that place or threaten to place others into a disadvantaged state without justification, peaceable manipulative actions are those that place or offer to place others into an advantaged state to which they have no prior entitlement.[73] While coercion violates the free choice of persons, peaceable manipulation does not. Indeed, peaceable manipulation undergirds the very process of negotiation through which individuals fashion consensual agreements. As long as offers do not make individual deliberation and voluntary choice among potential costs and benefits impossible, incentives are, in principle, permissible.[74]

As Nozick and others have noted, though, the line between coercion and peaceable manipulation may at times be difficult to draw.[75] What may prima facie appear as peaceable manipulation may under closer scrutiny be shown to be a hidden form of coercion. If, for example, a vendor knowingly exaggerates the quality of a kidney to obtain a higher price, or an employer withholds contractual benefits until an employee agrees to donate, coercion is involved. Each instance is an example of one individual placing another into disadvantaged circumstances through a form of nonconsensual force (e.g., deception or breach of contract).[76]

Opponents of organ sales may argue that such offers, while adding to one's list of options and prima facie enhancing individual freedom, are too good to refuse and in that sense are coercive. If the impoverished individual's status quo is highly unsatisfactory, then an offer to purchase an organ may appear coercive, because it manipulates the victim's preferences, even if it would be rational to accept.[77] The intent of the offer is to elicit behavior that contradicts the individual's normal operative goals, and in that sense attempts to use him as a mere means.[78] Thus, the choice to sell a kidney, even perhaps to belie the economic status of one's family, is typically considered a decision without rational or moral integrity.[79] However, to be coercive, rather than simply peaceably manipulative, requires showing that making such an offer places potential vendors into unjustified disadvantaged circumstances.

One possibility is that the lure of financial gain may motivate a decision that the vendor would have rejected if he had thought carefully about its full effects on his life. The existence of such miscalculation, however, is an empirical question. If the typical organ vendor agrees to sell because he believes that the expected value of so doing is positive, and the resulting value is positive, then there is no miscalculation and no coercion on such grounds. Moreover, the possibility of such miscalculation exists with every commercial transaction; yet, provided they are approached honestly, commercial transactions are not generally speaking coercive. Even if the individual is so interested in money that it would, given the person's values, be irrational to decline the offer, the choice is still plausibly understood as free insofar as he affirms the outcome. Consider the following case. If a rich patient offered an impoverished philosophy graduate student two million dollars to sell a kidney, one might imagine the student thinking: "Wow! I'm very pleased that he offered me two million dollars. I could never rationally refuse such an offer, and I would never want to turn it down in any case. I'm very glad it was made." To develop Harry Frankfurt's suggestion, if the offer moves the student who is being manipulated so that his first-order volitions compel agreement, the action is still plausibly understood as free insofar as his second-order volitions affirm the decision.[80] That is, the second-order willing regarding the types of choices and decisions he ought to make remains free of coercion.[81]

The general difficulty is that the question is not whether the poor are unfree with respect to certain obstacles, but whether financial incentives to purchase redundant internal organs make free choice impossible and thereby coerce potential vendors into complying with the offer. As previously noted, there is no reason to believe that an organ market would fare worse regarding autonomous consent than other organ procurement strategies. Barriers to free choice do not respect the distinction between donating and vending organs. Moreover, it is problematic to describe such offers as coercive, since they do not deprive the potential seller of any preexisting options and rational choice remains possible. While they may be seductive, such offers are not subtle threats.[82] It may be true that the poor generally have fewer options available among which to choose; however, there is a difference between having limited options and being unable to choose rationally in one's best interests among the options available.[83]

Gerald Dworkin has suggested that in certain contexts it is false that being provided with more options leaves one at least as well off as when the individual had a smaller opportunity set.[84] For example, one's bargaining power may be strengthened if one cannot make certain concessions. With regard to an organ market, the concern is that once the floodgates are open, poor individuals may find that others begin demanding their organs as a condition for access to certain goods. Will creditors demand the redundant organs of the poor as collateral for making loans?

Note, though, that such difficulties exist independently of the market. Once transplantation became a medically successful procedure, demand on family members, friends, and even strangers to donate organs became perceived as part of one's obligations. Many may have preferred not to have had to make such a choice; many may have preferred not to have had others attempt to manipulate them into donating. As the U.S. Office of Technology Assessment documented, psychological, emotional, and medical needs as well as a desire to please others may influence one to donate organs, rather than altruism.[85] Family members and friends may agree to donate organs solely to avoid confrontations or to satisfy some personal, family, or social objective.

Paternalistically protecting the poor from a market in human organs only closes a miserable range of options still further. To the dreadful difficulties of poverty are added the moralistic coercions of the state, removing options that the potential vendor may see as the best that they have to improve their lot in life. As Reddy points out, in India organ selling was observed as increasing both self-respect and social status. One saved another's life and enhanced the ability of oneself and one's family to prosper.[86] Janet Radcliffe-Richards concurs: "if some of the unemployed could get a large sum of money and start again, supporting their families instead of living on the dole, would there be anything but a huge increase in their self-respect and the respect of others?"[87] Some may find sale of a redundant organ to be an acceptable, indeed valuable, means to improve one's life circumstances and opportunities. In short, Dworkin's concerns at best support caution; they do not sustain prohibition.

Perhaps such offers are coercive relative to a normative moral baseline. If there exists a moral obligation to provide assistance, then demanding compensation to fulfill one's duty may be coercive. Consider Nozick's example (significantly shortened for clarity):

> *The Drowning Case:* B is drowning. A proposes to rescue B if B agrees to pay him $10,000. Both A and B know that there are no other potential rescuers.[88]

Nozick concludes that this is an example of coercion. While A prima facie offers to improve B's situation relative to the status quo, A actually proposes to make B worse off if B does not pay the $10,000 relative to what B has a right to expect from A.[89] Wertheimer similarly holds that while this case may be properly described as coercive, this is not because B has no acceptable alternative, but because A has an independent moral obligation to save B, either for no compensation or for considerably less.[90] Insofar as there exists a right to be rescued, or a duty to help others in need, which sustains such a moral baseline, the offer is coercive.

It is unclear, however, that this analysis sustains the case against human organ sales. Patients dying of organ failure would not usually be described as having special moral obligations to provide potential organ vendors with financial income without asking for some good or service in return. Indeed, it may be that it is patients with end-stage organ failure who are analogous to Nozick's drowning man. Contrary to the often cited concern that an organ market will exploit the poor, *this analysis suggests that in offering to sell organs, the poor may be exploiting the illness of the rich for personal gain.* Yet, absent prior agreements or special moral obligations, it is unclear why those with healthy organs have a moral obligation to donate. A person's monopoly ownership over his healthy organs is crucially different from monopoly ownership of natural resources. While the second can be secured through a violation of rights, the first cannot. Most significantly, intervening in the commerce of the second can prevent exploitation. In contrast, intervening in the commerce of the first brings about exploitation by forcibly preventing others from paying the owner of the organs as much as it is worth to the owner.[91] In short, adequately to assess claims of coercive offers, one must also inquire as to who is in greater need, and thus in more threat of exploitation: the poor who need financial resources, or the rich who are dying of organ failure.

In general, it is difficult to count a policy as exploitative if, as in the case of legitimizing organ sales, it increases the number of options open to individuals. The Libyan's (or another's) life is saved, and the Iraqi, as well as the Turkish peasants, gain the ability to support their families temporarily while looking for other work. To conclude that such circumstances are exploitative, one must hold that there is something intrinsically wrong or debasing in selling one's organs, so that even if one does this freely, one has been brought to do something morally injurious to oneself.

Moralistic Exploitation: Improper Commodification

An additional possibility is that organ markets are exploitative because they cause moral harm. For example, one might hold that human organs simply should not be exchanged for money. On such an account, a market in human organs is exploitative because it commodifies that which should not be commodified. Insofar as such a view is sustainable, exploitative circumstances do not improve if organs are purchased for significantly more money. According to Michael Walzer, for example, while the proper sphere of money includes "all those objects, commodities, products, services, beyond what is communally provided, that individual men and women find useful or pleasing," certain exchanges ought to be prohibited to set limits on the dominion of wealth.[92] This captures the intuition that while some goods are appropriately distributed through the market, others are not. If organ sales improperly commodify human body parts, it is argued, such transactions should be prohibited.

As Margaret Radin maps the conceptual geography, commodities are marked by (1) objectification (i.e., "ascription of status as a thing in the Kantian sense of something that is manipulable at the will of persons"); (2) fungibility (i.e., as "fully interchangeable with no effect on value to the holder"); (3) commensurability (i.e., that "values of things can be arrayed as a function of one continuous variable"); and (4) money equivalence (i.e., "the continuous variable in terms of which things are ranked is dollar value").[93] Opponents of organ sales must argue that such transactions inappropriately (1) objectify human organs by treating them as objects rather than as parts of subjects or agents; (2) treat human organs as fungible items (i.e., as exchangeable); presume (3) that the value of the organ to the vendor is commensurable to the value of the organ to the purchaser, and (4) that this value can be given a monetary expression. The question, though, is whether organ markets would likely fare better or worse regarding commodification than other strategies of organ procurement and allocation.

An initial challenge for opponents of the market is that organs are in fact manipulable and interchangeable with others of the same kind. This is the very reason that transplantation is medically viable. Whereas one may raise the concern that the market will fail appropriately to weigh and compare economic versus noneconomic values,[94] nonmarket-based strategies for procurement and transplantation face similar difficulties. All treat human organs as exchangeable objects.

One possibility is that organ sales involve an exchange of incommensurable values. Incommensurability represents a concern that the values at stake cannot be relevantly summed and compared.[95] By itself, though, incommensurability will not establish that organ sales are illicit. The permissibility of market transactions does not require that the goods exchanged be precisely commensurable, but rather that the parties transact voluntarily, that deception or other forms of coercion are not employed, and that each is satisfied with the value to be received. This means that what is received in return is worth at least as much to the party as that which was given. As others have noted, one can buy or sell "priceless" Monet paintings without claiming that the aesthetic or historic value of the artwork is "commensurate" with the money that is paid.[96]

Elizabeth Anderson suggests another possibility. There is a kind of exploitation, she argues, that occurs "when one party to a transaction is oriented toward the exchange of 'gift values,' while the other party operates in accordance with the norms of the market exchange of commodities. Gift values, which include love, gratitude, and appreciation of others, cannot be bought or obtained through piecemeal calculations of individual advantage."[97] However, this account oversimplifies: at times one party to an exchange may deliberately sell goods for less than market value as a subtle gift. This suggests that gift values can be brought into play in the market. (This argument will be discussed in greater detail below.) Even if Anderson is correct, however, the difficulty is relevant if and only if such a dichotomy of intentions exists. Persons who negotiate regarding the fair market value of human organs will not likely experience such conceptual dissonance.

One might argue that giving organs a monetary expression is an inappropriate way to value human body parts. Here the concern is that through property discourse and market exchanges, individuals are encouraged to value those goods regarded as "property" solely in economic terms.[98] Ideals that ground how certain things should be valued are typically supported by a conception of human flourishing. Cultivating capacities to appreciate aesthetic and historic values enriches and elevates life. "To fail to value things appropriately is to embody in one's life an inferior conception of human flourishing."[99] For example, in *Moore v. Regents of the University of California*, the question before the court was whether body parts are appropriately conceptualized as property. Justice Arabian argued that treating certain things as commodities may be morally inappropriate:

> Plaintiff has asked us to recognize and enforce a right to sell one's body tissue *for profit*. He entreats us to regard the human vessel—the single most venerated and protected subject in any civilized society—as equal with the basest commercial commodity. He urges us to commingle the sacred with the profane. He asks much.[100]

Arabian concluded that the market norms inherent in property discourse are incompatible with an open discussion and evaluation of nonmarket, nonmonetary, values.[101]

Similarly, Sara Ketchem has argued in the context of commercial surrogacy that use of the market recasts the meaning and nature of women's bodies.

> Sexual or reproductive prostitutes enter the market not so much as agents or subjects, but as commodities or objects. . . . Moreover, once there is a market for women's bodies, all women's bodies will have a price, and the woman who does not sell her body becomes a hoarder of something that is useful to other people and is financially valuable.[102]

It treats women's reproductive capacities as commodities. The analogous claim for organ sales is that once there is a market in human organs, all organs will have a price, and those who do not sell their organs will become hoarders of something that is useful to other people and that is financially valuable.

Such considerations, however, hold equally against systems of donation. As Fox and Swazey point out, as organ transplantation became perceived as the standard of care, organs were recast as mere things.[103] Persons who do not donate parts of themselves, or of their loved ones at death, are seen as withholding life-sustaining medical resources. It is this reconceptualization of persons as sources of scarce medical resources that in large measure has driven the proposals for "required request" laws, as well as "opt out" or "routine salvage" systems of organ procurement. Concerns to avoid recasting persons as collections of spare parts, as well as to encourage noneconomic appreciation of human organs, must be addressed under any system of organ procurement and transplantation.[104]

Perhaps organ selling is exploitative because it involves other types of moral harm. It may be degrading to vendors and thereby violate their human dignity. Consider, for comparison, the example of prostitution:

> In commercial sex, each party now values the other only instrumentally, not intrinsically. And, while both parties are thus prevented from enjoying a shared good, it is worse for the prostitute. The customer merely surrenders a certain amount of cash; the prostitute cedes her body: the prostitute is degraded to the status of a thing.[105]

This degradation, Satz argues, is also objectification—that is, a failure to respect in theory and to make space in practice for the human subject as a person.[106] In transplantation, though, as already noted, donors, surgeons, agencies, and recipients alike objectify organs and treat them as fungible. More generally, we do not treat someone merely as a means if he consents to be so treated. Commodification of human organs is not an obvious violation of the Kantian maxim to treat persons as ends in themselves absent additional arguments showing that even consensual selling of organs is morally injurious. The organ market respects vendors as persons and moral agents. Prohibition, in contrast, may demean the poor by considering them unable to make moral decisions about their own fates.

Such arguments raise additional concerns regarding social exploitation. By forbidding organ sales, are the financially secure and able-bodied exploiting the poor to assuage their own feeling of guilt, so that they can sleep well at night thinking that they have saved the poor from themselves? That is, the rich and able-bodied under this circumstance would be exploiting the poor so as to be able to have the poor not challenge their view of proper moral conduct. But again, some may find the sale of a redundant organ to be an acceptable, indeed valuable, means of improving their life circumstances and opportunities.

Radcliffe-Richards provides a good encapsulation of how the prohibition of a market can in this fashion exploit the poor:

> Prohibition may make things worse for the . . . desperate people who advertise their kidneys, as well as for the sick who will die for lack of them; but at least these people will despair and die quietly, in ways less offensive to the affluent and healthy, and the poor will not force their misery on our attention by engaging in the strikingly repulsive business of selling parts of themselves to repair the deficiencies of the rich.[107]

The rich and able-bodied by forbidding organ sales would be exploiting the poor to support their particular views of moral propriety, improper commodification, or human dignity, denying the poor this opportunity to choose freely on the basis of their own judgments regarding how best to advantage themselves. The outcome is robustly paternalistic.

Some Additional Reflections on Exploitation

In part, language regarding exploitation appears to be parasitic on the distinction between autonomous and heteronomous choices. If one argues that X is exploitative, this often means that persons are being given inducements to act in a way that is heteronomous so that though they are offered a good, to which they had no independent claim, they are required to engage in activities for which there exists independent grounds for holding that it is immoral (e.g., such actions violate human dignity, improperly commodify the human body, and so forth). In that sense, the act involves a heteronomous choice. Therefore, a justified invocation of a view that an offer is exploitative depends on an independent argument to show that the action would illicitly violate the natural good of maintaining the body as a whole, involve a violation of human dignity, improperly commodify the human body, or is justifiably morally repugnant, thereby returning the matter to the arguments addressed elsewhere in this study.

Which is to say that if there are not independent moral grounds to show that the sale of organs is immoral, then the purchase of organs from the poor will be exploitative if and only if either such independent grounds of impropriety can be established or the policy on balance will cause more harm than benefit for the poor. However, assessing this latter condition requires a recognition that allowing the poor to choose on their own view of the good both protects them from being demeaned (by being considered unable to make moral choices about their own future) and helps to educate individuals in their faculties of free and responsible choice.

COMMUNITY, ALTRUISM, AND FREE CHOICE

One might also argue that altruism will be corrupted by the very existence of the market in organs, that philanthropy will be sullied by greed. The concern is that the market would so affect altruistic impulses that it would starkly limit the expression of altruism and thereby lead to far-reaching moral costs to community solidarity and social beneficence. Monetary values, it is argued, ought not to be attached to the presence of a spirit of altruism. At stake are the ways in which individual free choice shapes the character of a community, and which strategy will lead to greater altruism, beneficence, and sense of community: the market or impersonal commitments to civil duty and social solidarity. Titmuss provides in this regard a good summary of the arguments against the market:

> Its role in satisfying the biological need to help—particularly in modern societies—is another unmeasurable element . . . we have used human blood as an indicator; perhaps the most basic and sensitive indicator of social values and human relationships that could be found for a comparative study . . . the extent to which commercialism and profit in blood has been driving out the voluntary donor. Moreover, it is likely that a decline in the spirit of altruism in one sphere of human activities will be accompanied by similar changes in attitudes, motives, and relationships in other spheres.[108]

Weakening of the very moral fabric and social solidarity of a society is argued to be the probable cost of an organ market.

Thomas Murray's defense of the ban on organ vending follows much the same reasoning. He argues that market relationships minimize moral and social dimensions, while gifts are more open-ended, and as such defy such minimization.

Gifts to strangers affirm the solidarity of the community over and above the depersonalizing, alienating forces of mass society and market relations. They signal that self-interest is not the only significant human motivation. And they express the moral belief that it is good to minister to fundamental human needs, needs for food, health and knowledge. These universal needs irrevocably tie us together in a community of needs, with a shared desire to satisfy them, and see them satisfied in others.[109]

These gifts, Murray concludes, serve as a reminder that not all valuable things, such as love, friendship, and fellow feeling, are for sale; that compassion for others reaches beyond impersonal market relationships, large organizations, and impersonal bureaucracies.[110] What we need, he argues, is an alternate interpretation of goods and the principles for distributing goods that "captures more faithfully the complexity of our most deeply held ideas about the meanings of those goods and about distributive justice."[111] If sustainable, such moral costs might tip the scale against the market.

To assess such criticisms adequately, one must consider two interrelated issues. First, one must determine whether current organ procurement practices of donation fare better with regard to encouraging altruism, community beneficence, and personal relationships, as well as staving off the depersonalization of modern society, more successfully than the market. Second, one must assess the ways in which the free choices of individuals, interacting with one another, shape the character of the community.

It is unclear, for example, that "altruism" accurately describes current organ procurement policies. With the documented success of transplantation procedures and the advent of immunosuppressive drugs, such as cyclosporine, that increased long-term survival rates, physicians and the general public quickly changed their view of organ transplantation from an experimental surgical procedure to a medically successful therapy.[112] This shift altered medical social reality to the extent that human organ transplantation has come to be regarded as a treatment to be offered whenever medically indicated. Human organs are construed as a "scarce medical resource." This medical shift, in language, expectation, and practice, placed a greater perceived moral burden on family members and even strangers to make their organs available to others if needed. Moreover, the considerable coercive legal force of the government is brought to bear against the very possibility of selling one's organs, which legislates the necessity of the "donation" and thus calls into question the "altruistic" character of such transactions. Rather than binding potential donors and recipients, as well as their physicians, in the solidarity of shared social values and caring human relationships, dying patients are disinterestedly recast as "sources" of needed medical resources and their grieving families as "access barriers" to be overcome. It may be that it is the current system's blanket prohibition on selling, rather than the market, that reduces organ availability, discourages altruism and social beneficence, and legalizes hostility between physicians and patients.

If it is morally important for organ donation to be an expression of altruism, this requirement will curtail any scheme of presumed consent. It will also weigh against policies of mandatory choice and routine procurement.[113] Routine procurement (organ salvaging) is a social policy that legalizes the taking of organs at death, unless the individual specifically denied permission, while mandatory choice implements the significant force of the state to coerce one into choosing whether or not to "donate."[114] Neither policy is consistent with "gift giving" as a voluntary altruistic expression of beneficence.[115] Consider the structure of such policies for other types of personal property. If the state were to destroy one's house and all of one's stock certificates at death, but did allow their conveyance to others designated as "in need," it would be implausible to describe the deceased as intending an altruistic redistribution, much less as believing that the state is the appropriate mechanism for such redistribution.

Requirements that organ transplant be altruistically motivated, if taken seriously, would also rule out many donations. Persons who stand to be financially supported by a person needing an organ might have other motivations than "kindness" for donating an organ to a relative. Other donations might be premised on reciprocated love, friendship, guilt, or stigma avoidance.[116] Families at times donate out of self-interested desire to see their loved one continue on in another[117] or to perceive something good as coming from their loved one's death. How pure must one's intentions be for organ transfer to be classified as an altruistic act?

Even if it is true that altruism is a necessary building block of beneficent moral communities, social solidarity, and the development of significant personal relationships; even if such altruism reduces the depersonalization of the modern bureaucratic society and ministers to basic human needs—it is unclear why either legislated "altruism" or a depersonalized national bureaucracy for organ procurement and distribution would necessarily possess or foster any of these goods. Indeed, it is often state bureaucratic legislation, rather than the market, which limits altruistic behavior. For example, physicians who accept Medicare patients are generally forbidden to waive the patient's copayment as a matter of kindness, even if such cost is borne solely by the physician.[118] Moreover, such legislation tends to reinforce deceptive practices. Prohibition may lead to the circumstance that altruism alone is insufficient motivation to provide enough organs to meet demand; it may thereby encourage black marketeering, the very opposite of the desired behavior, to purchase needed organs.

Legislated "gift giving" constrains individual altruism in an otherwise commercial setting, where surgeons, nurses, pharmaceutical companies, and hospitals profit, increasing inequality between highly compensated surgeons et al. and the poor who donate organs. This circumstance raises the additional question of who should bear the burden of fostering altruism. On the one hand, those in need of transplants require care and support; on the other hand, so too do the families of the dying, brain-dead, or recently deceased potential organ donors. Rather than being seen as those in need of kindness and sympathy, the specter of organ donation recasts the bereaved family as gatekeepers of a social medical resource. Organ donation inverts those who would otherwise be recipients of beneficence into those who are approached, if not subject to active persuasion, once again to sacrifice.[119] Those who should be recipients of charity are confronted with the additional burden of organ procurement policies.[120] Indeed, studies have found evidence of emotional trauma and posttraumatic stress disorder among families of cadaveric and living donors.[121] The commercial market in organs would allow for altruism for both organ donation and allocation.

Rather than eroding a sense of community, the market may enhance and draw together moral communities, opening significant opportunities for developing personal relationships and for charitably providing for the fundamental needs of others. Expressions of altruism may exist side by side with for-profit markets in human organs. For example, if it is altruism for a parent to give a kidney to a child to save his life, it is similarly altruistic for a parent to sell a kidney to pay for a lifesaving operation.[122] Forbidding a market in human organs restricts persons from joining together with others to pool financial resources to purchase organs for the impecunious. It prevents altruistic donation of organs to nonprofit groups, who could then sell such parts to raise funds to purchase food, shelter, or health care for the poor. A market may open considerable opportunities for the expression of altruistic sentiments, for building a sense of solidarity and community, as well as for charitably providing for the fundamental needs of others. Moreover, instead of encouraging a hostile relationship between physicians and patients, who are potential donors, vendors and physicians would meet on a more equal footing. Indeed, a market in organs would likely be more successful on each of these grounds than current nationalized bureaucratic procedures, or other proposed policies such as presumed consent or routine salvage, in encouraging altruism and community solidarity.

SCIENTIFIC EXCELLENCE AND THE MARKETPLACE

Among the considerations influencing the acceptability of a market in transplantable organs is the concern that market mechanisms will lower scientific standards. The concern is that the market substitutes profit-seeking for truth-seeking behavior. The question, though, is whether the market fares better or worse on such grounds than alternative organ procurement and transplantation policies. At stake is which system will most likely produce high-quality organs and develop innovative transplantation-oriented products. Titmuss, for example, raises the criticism that for-profit markets in medicine create significant conflicts of interest and encourage deceitful behavior among vendors and physicians, thereby leading to a lowering of scientific standards in the search of profit maximization:

> As freedoms are lost in the blood marketplace truth is an accompanying victim. In studying different blood donation, clinical laboratory and medical care systems we were led to ask . . . what particular conditions and arrangements permit and encourage maximum truthfulness on the part of donors—the maximum now demanded by medical science. . . .
>
> [Moreover, the] paid seller of blood is confronted . . . with a personal conflict of interests. To tell the truth about himself, his way of life and his relationships may limit his freedom to sell his blood on the market. Because he desires money and is not seeking in this particular act to affirm a sense of belonging he thinks primarily of his own freedom; he separates his freedom from other people's freedoms. It may be of course that he will not be placed or may not fully realize that he has been placed . . . in such situations of conflicting interests. If so, it can only be because medicine in the person of the doctor has failed to fulfil its scientific basis; it is not seeking to know what is true.[123]

Titmuss's criticisms can be categorized under two general rubrics: whether the market fares worse than government-supported or nonprofit research with regard to (1) fostering conflicts of interest, leading to lower scientific standards, or (2) sustaining the development of high-quality, innovative transplantation medicine.

It is important to recognize, however, that many of the forces that distort data are independent of the market. Political, moral, and other epistemic and nonepistemic background commitments often play roles in surreptitious or unconscious distortion of scientific data so as to acquire research funding, advance one's social standing in the scientific community, or further particular sociopolitical goals. The protection of careers, as well as the furtherance of other goals, may at times take precedence over scientific accuracy.[124] For example, in 1988 Stephen Bruening pleaded guilty in federal court to two counts of filing fake research reports on federally funded research projects. These reports, advocating the use of stimulants rather than tranquilizers, had been relied on nationwide for determining appropriate drug therapy for severely mentally handicapped institutionalized children.[125] Bruening wrote twenty-four of the seventy papers published in this discipline of psychopharmacology between 1979 and 1983, placing him prominently in the field. Under scrutiny, though, it was allegedly unclear how much of his data reflected the results of empirical research. Later research by other scientists demonstrated that use of stimulants heightened self-injury and other behavior-related problems.

In addition, commercial markets are not the only source of profit-seeking behavior. Private nonprofit associations often sponsor research protocols that are expected to yield results supportive of the organization's goals. For example, a recipient of a grant from the American Thoracic Society or the American Lung Association might be hesitant to publish results that confirm health benefits attributable to cigarette smoking. There exists, for example, significant evidence that the nicotine in tobacco smoke assists in the prevention and treatment of active ulcerative colitis,[126] Parkinsonism, and Alzheimer's disease,[127] and it has been linked to the recovery of immune response that had been previously suppressed by immobilization stress.[128] Cigarette smoking has also been shown to heighten short-term and long-term learning ability, to enhance one's ability to reason under stress, and, more generally, to cope with stress.[129] In some quarters the exploration of such areas of benefits might be politically incorrect; indeed, even publicly supporting such research might threaten one's reputation, grant opportunities, and employment.

Moreover, insofar as certain research protocols or scientific theories are seen as supportive of particular political ideologies or sociopolitical movements, this may provide sufficient reason for some to fund, give credence to, or politically back such research. Consider the ways in which HIV/AIDS research has been highly politicized. When AIDS was identified in 1981 the homosexual community was deeply engaged in identity politics—that is, seeking tangible political goals, such as social acceptance, while elaborating an affirmative group identity.[130] Such social and political concerns impacted the structure and goals of HIV/AIDS research. Activists criticized mainstream scientific research as too slow and antigay, and as failing to seek causes that were not associated with HIV transmission through sexual behavior; they demanded further governmentally supported scientific investigation.[131] Public speculation existed regarding whether drug trials for potential therapeutic agents would have been handled differently if the patients had been dying of advanced cancer with no known therapeutic agent.[132] Activists engaged in research established background knowledge about treatments, occasionally conducted their own drug trials, and declared themselves experts to speak on these issues. Moreover, they claimed the expertise to define public health constructs, such as the practices that constituted "safe sex,"[133] challenged the linkage between sexual promiscuity and death, and put forward "sex positive" programs of AIDS prevention, which asserted as a moral community, however diffuse, the rights to sexual pleasure and sexual freedom. Given the impact of such social and political prior commitments on the interpretation and significance of scientific findings, as well as on the structure and goals of science, governmentally supported—rather than market-based—medical research is no guarantee of truth-seeking behavior.[134]

Indeed, the market may fare somewhat better than governmentally controlled research in that the market preserves and expands niches by providing incentives for developing high-quality or innovative products. It is in the interests of profit maximization to produce safer products and procedures as well as to support better access to transplantation. If one is in the business of selling organs, profits would generally be maximized if one provided high-quality organs with low rates of rejection. Given these circumstances, procuring organs from living persons, which usually produce better medical results, will result in higher profits than from cadaveric organs. As noted, organs removed from living persons are more likely to be of significant use to recipients. They have greater vitality and can be screened in advance for defects, diseases, or other negative indicators. In contrast, if organs are only procured from the recently deceased, such as accident victims, one loses both vitality and screening opportunities. A central factor jeopardizing an organ's viability is the time during which it is without oxygen and other nutrients. Damage due to inadequate oxygen, or ischemia, begins immediately when the heart stops pumping.[135] As the Institutes of Medicine Report on organ procurement from non-heart-beating donors points out, such organs have higher discard rates, which leads to increased transplant costs, as well as to the availability of fewer organs. Transplant survivals, though increasingly competitive, are not quite as good as from heart-beating donors.[136] An additional difficulty is rejection by the recipient. Even a well-preserved organ is more likely to be rejected after transplantation if it does not have the same genetic markers as the recipient. Such failures can be fatal. In these areas the market will be advantaged scientifically over a system of donation: commercial sale will likely target living vendors; provide adequate time to screen for organ viability, disease, and potentially deadly immuno-rejections; and have the flexibility to arrange for quick transference of the organ to avoid significant ischemia.

Additional legal safeguards bearing on product liability and tort gear in with market-based organ procurement, transplantation, and research. Consider the Organ Procurement and Transplantation Act of 1984, which prohibited the sale, for "valuable consideration," of human organs for use in human transplantation, punishing violators with a fine of not more than $50,000 or imprisonment of not more than five years, or both. The law prohibits any for-profit commercial harvesting or sale of human organs for transplantation. The act defined "valuable consideration" as excluding "the reasonable payments associated with the removal, transportation, implantation, processing, preservation, quality control, and storage of a human organ or the expenses of travel, housing, and lost wages incurred by the donor."[137] As a result, any transaction with respect to human organ transplantation is classified as the provision of services rather than the sale of goods. The statute thereby directly impacts the grounds on which an individual can base a cause of action for product liability and tort with regard to organ transplantation.

Ordinarily, an individual who alleges an injury caused by a defective product can base cause of action on negligence, breach of warranty, or strict liability.

Negligence can be understood in terms of a duty of the person of ordinary sense to exercise ordinary care and skill. The *Restatement (Second) of Torts* defines negligence as "conduct which falls below the standard established by law for the protection of others against unreasonable risk of harm."[138] Negligence theory requires that the injured party demonstrate that a specific defendant failed "to exercise proper care in designing, testing, manufacturing, or marketing the allegedly defective product and that, as a reasonably foreseeable and proximate result of such negligence, the plaintiff suffered injury."[139] Liability predicated on negligence theory is the standard that applies to providers of services, rather than goods. Negligence is the standard that touches physicians. Courts have generally held that the primary purpose of the physician-patient relationship is the performance or rendition of professional medical services rather than the sale of medical products. Thus, suits against physicians for injury resulting from treatment are typically predicated on professional negligence or malpractice—that is, the failure to exercise the required degree of skill, care, or diligence required by the standard of care in treating the patient.

In contrast, an injured party predicating a cause of action on warranty need only show that the manufacture or seller breached a promise, whether implied or expressed, that the product was both free from defects and fit for the usual purposes for which such a product is typically used.[140]

Strict liability in tort applies even stronger standards to the manufacture or distributor of goods. Liability on the part of the manufacturer or distributor follows the defective product. Strict liability is defined as follows:

Special Liability of Seller of Product for Physical Harm to User or Consumer

(1) One who sells any product in a defective condition unreasonably dangerous to the user or consumer or to his property is subject to liability for physical harm thereby caused to the ultimate user or consumer; or to his property, if
  (a) the seller is engaged in the business of selling such a product, and
  (b) it is expected to and does reach the user or consumer without substantial change in the condition in which it is sold.
(2) The rule stated in Subsection (1) applies although
  (a) the seller has exercised all possible care in the preparation and sale of his product, and
  (b) the user or consumer has not bought the product from or entered into any contractual arrangement with the seller.[141]

To establish a product liability claim under such standards, the injured party need only show that the product causing the injury was defective and unreasonably dangerous when it left the control of the manufacturer or seller, and that as a result of this defect it caused injury.

The circumstance that any transaction with respect to human organ transplantation is classified as the provision of services, rather than the sale of goods, effectively screens out product liability claims predicated on warranty or strict liability. Exposure to liability in this circumstance is limited to the possibility of the physician's negligence or malpractice. With the creation of a market, product liability based on expressed or implied warranty as well as on strict liability becomes applicable. Individual vendors as well as commercial procurement and transplantation corporations could be held strictly liable for defects that cause harms to the transplant recipient. The application of such strict product liability standards is likely to motivate the development of high-quality scientific procurement, screening, and transplantation techniques. Indeed, organ quality may be problematic precisely because of insufficient commercialization, and because of the protection from liability that donation affords those who procure and transplant organs. Given such circumstances, the market may fare better than a system of donation with regard to the search for scientific excellence.

THE MARKET AND PROFIT: THE VIRTUES AND VICES OF FREE CHOICE

One must also attend to the difference in phenomenology between the gift relation and the commercial relation. Gift giving is generally marked by altruism, personal concern for the other, love, and in some cases intimacy. In contrast, love or intimacy rarely marks large-scale commercial relations, which are often anonymous and self-regarding. They are, however, constrained by honesty and agreement. In a commercial relationship, one gets what one contracts or agrees to. One gets what one deserves in terms of what one has agreed to. In a gift relationship, one gets what one does not deserve.

The development of gift giving is core to the enhancement of important areas of character and virtue involved in personal regard and love for others. Gift giving at the very least requires personal concern for identifiable others or identification with the community to which the gift is addressed. Gift giving is tied closely with concerns of compassion and charity, including the root notion of *caritas*, love. As Wuthnow argues, compassion reaffirms that "not all of life depends on efficient, large scale organization and a productive economy. [It helps to] create a space in which to think about our dependence on one another, the needs that can never be fulfilled by bureaucracies and material goods, and the joys that come from attending to those needs."[142] Social policies that encourage gift giving, altruism, or charity express in part the concern that individuals develop a sense of love and concern for others.

In contrast, the success of the market depends on quite other virtues, including the ability to be honest and to keep promises with moral strangers. The market involves a form of willing that binds persons together freely, enabling individuals to pursue their concrete goals with consenting others. It is able to establish bonds among persons and across communities. It is therefore anonymous, transcommunal, and supportive of particular virtues. Private mail services, for example, market the virtues of speed and reliability to patrons who often belong to quite divergent moral communities. As a consequence, if one lives one's entire life within the ambit of the market, one learns only those marks of virtue and character that are beyond particular communities and beyond personal individual relations among moral friends.

The gulf between these perspectives is bridged in two ways. First, to do well in the market, one must often cultivate the virtues of gift giving, kindness, attention, and personal recognition of the other. The goal of customer satisfaction, independently of the goal to maximize profit, is typically necessary to maintain long-term realization of profits. Achieving a long-term successful business generally requires a concurrent commitment to customer satisfaction and to the provision of quality goods and services.[143] Even though vendor and recipient may only meet once in an organ market, reputations are built on relationships with and among surgeons, hospitals, transplant teams, and others who perform specialized services; this will likely provide significant incentives for virtuous tendencies such as quality service, medical follow-up, and ensuring vendor and recipient satisfaction. Even in "spot markets," where vendors and recipients meet only once, necessary third-party involvement provides significant incentives for virtuous behavior. For example, it is in the title company's best interests to effectuate an honest and skillful transfer of real estate. Similarly, surgeons, transplant teams, and hospitals have significant incentives to provide quality services. Given a good reputation, others will be much more likely to utilize their services in the future. Successful organ procurement and transplantation cannot take place without the skilled services of many. Virtue can, therefore, be seen as a profit-maximizing strategy.[144]

Second, small-scale entrepreneurs and tradespeople, such as owners of the neighborhood bar, butcher shop, or bakery, in part enter the market in an anonymous fashion and in part do so as the friend who often offers a free drink, a free slice of sausage, or a free cookie. The pursuit of self-interest frequently requires that one provide benefits to others, outside of disinterested commitments to civic duty or generalized solidarity, to advance their best interests as well as one's own.

Titmuss and others recognize the stark contrast between the personal, loving, community-directed character of the gift relationship and the impersonal businesslike transcommunal character of large-scale markets. They then conclude that if medicine becomes commercial, it will move from being an intimate relationship, or at least from having the character of the mom-and-pop drugstore and bakery shop, to possessing only those points of anonymous regard that characterize large-scale markets. They correctly recognize that patients/customers usually want more. Here one must acknowledge that there are real challenges in moving from small-shop to large-scale medicine.

It is important to recognize, however, that the core concern of this charge is independent of whether the services that are being provided are supported by a capitalist undertaking or a socialist system. In the United States, for example, all organ "gifts" are required by law to be processed through the United Network for Organ Sharing (UNOS), a private corporation that operates the Organ Procurement and Transplantation Network, created under the National Organ Transplant Act of 1984. UNOS manages the national transplant waiting list, matches donors to recipients, monitors every organ match to ensure adherence to UNOS policy, develops policies that utilize the current supply of organs, and, according to UNOS guidelines, supposedly gives all patients a chance at receiving the organ they need—regardless of age, sex, race, lifestyle, financial, or social criteria; moreover, it sets professional standards for efficiency and quality patient care. With 415 member organizations as of January 9, 2004, including 257 transplant centers, 3 consortium members, 59 organ procurement organizations, 153 histocompatibility laboratories, 8 voluntary health organizations, 12 general public members, and 27 medical professional/scientific organizations, the national bureaucracy of UNOS is as impersonal and unconnected from personal relationships and community as any other large-scale corporation.[145] This vast national bureaucracy alienates in the sense of creating a significant distance between donors, on the one hand, and recipients and physicians, on the other.

In contrast, the market's need to satisfy customers may in fact paradoxically lead in the end to a more personal medicine than that available through the state. In Sweden, for example, concerns regarding poor service, long waiting lists and waiting times, as well as impersonal care and little continuity of care, led to reforms in the state health care system in favor of the private market. The success of privately owned and financed drop-in clinics was directly associated with attentiveness to personal needs. As Marilynn Rosenthal reports regarding one such private clinic:

> It is located close to many business offices, in contrast to the public primary health care centers built in the residential neighborhoods. It remains open late, until 7 P.M., and on Saturdays. Its personnel have received special training in consumer relations and it guarantees a shorter wait than the public hospital outpatient clinics. It provides quick, courteous, efficient care in a convenient location.[146]

Here we are back to virtue as a profit-maximizing strategy.

Given this circumstance, reticence regarding the profit motive may involve, first, nostalgia for a past during which medicine functioned more on the model of neighborhood grocery stores, butcher shops, and bakeries. Second, it may reflect a failure to recognize that large-scale government and socialized systems for the provision of health care do not encourage altruism and personal concern for others, even when capitalism or the market are not engaged. Third, there may be a failure to recognize the ways in which virtue is a profit-maximizing strategy, so that the market rewards personal concern and attention to customers/patients. The interests of prospective organ vendors and recipients to have health care choices regarding their body parts respected in a personally attentive manner offer market opportunities that have yet to be adequately explored.

SUMMARY

Assessment of the permissibility of a market in human organs must consider the circumstances in which such a market advances health benefits, the effective use of scarce resources, and other special values and goals more successfully than alternative organ procurement and allocation strategies. The special moral costs of a for-profit market that Titmuss identifies, if sustainable, are significant. If a market in human organs would lead to a decease in altruistic sentiments, an erosion of a sense of community, a lowering of scientific standards, limitations on personal and professional freedoms, as well as increased hostility between patients and physicians, these costs would raise the burden of proof against the creation of such a market. On the other hand, if a market in human organs would support the realization of significant personal or societal values and goals, the burden of proof will be on those who would forbid the market to provide equally significant counterbalancing considerations.

The costs and benefits, as well as the virtues and vices, of a market in human organs that should bear on the moral judgments advanced regarding commercialization include health care costs and benefits; special moral considerations (equality, liberty, exploitation, community, and altruism); and scientific excellence, virtue, and the profit motive. Insofar as the market leads to greater organ availability, with organs of better quality, and more efficient organ procurement for transplantation—while minimizing harms to vendors—such positive health outcomes would tip the burden of proof against prohibition. Similarly, indirect health benefits incurred through increases in income, or resources to support additional education and training, would be advantages weighing in favor of a market in human organs. However, if such benefits are unlikely to be realized, or if they would engender significant costs to other important moral considerations that counterbalance potential health gains, such concerns would weigh against the creation of a market.

The acceptableness of a market in human organs will also depend on the ways in which it promotes or restrains special moral goods and considerations. Insofar as the market promotes equality, liberty, community solidarity, or the free

expression of altruism—while minimizing the possibility for social exploitation—more successfully than alternative procurement and allocation policies,
this would tip the burden of proof against those who would forbid the market. If
the market would inappropriately restrain freedom, increase inequality, and
encourage social exploitation, as well as discourage a sense of social solidarity,
while castigating altruistic impulses, such costs would tip the burden of proof
against the creation of a market. To assess such concerns, though, one must
engage each of the following issues: (1) whether the market would exploit those
persons in greatest need, or whether forbidding the selling of organs is itself
exploitative of those in need; (2) who is in greatest need: the poor who need
financial resources, or the rich who are dying of organ failure; (3) whether the
market enhances and draws together moral communities, opening significant
opportunities for developing personal relationships and for charitably providing
for the needs of others; and (4) whether blanket prohibition on selling recasts
dying patients as "sources" of a needed medical resource and their families as
"access barriers" to be overcome in pursuit of those resources, thereby legalizing
hostility between physicians and patients. The considerations advanced in this
chapter provide significant grounds for concluding that a market in human
organs would fare better regarding each of these concerns than alternative systems of allocation and transplantation.

In determining whether the market substitutes profit-seeking behavior for
truth-seeking or virtuous behavior, procurement and allocation policies must be
evaluated as to whether they more successfully produce high-quality organs and
develop innovative transplantation products and techniques, while encouraging
virtuous behavior. Four general sets of issues frame the assessment of these concerns. (1) It is important to recognize that such concerns are largely independent
of the market. Political, moral, and other nonepistemic background conditions,
such as career development or political goals, often play a significant role in the
surreptitious or unconscious distortion of scientific data to maintain research
funding and social standing in the scientific community, or to further particular
social political goals. (2) Legal safeguards from tort liability, especially product
liability, become applicable with market-based organ procurement, transplantation, and scientific research. Torts predicated on warranty or strict liability are
only possible if the transplanted organ is understood as a good that is being sold
to the recipient. Insofar as transplantation remains only the provision of a professional service, liability is limited to claims of ordinary negligence. Commercializing organ procurement and allocation will, therefore, introduce special legal
safeguards and benefits. (3) The ways in which the market bridges the gulf
between persons and communities includes special moral benefits. To do well in
the market, one must often cultivate virtues of gift giving, kindness, attention,
and personal recognition of the other. Small-scale entrepreneurs in part enter

the market in an anonymous fashion and in part do so as "a friend" who often provides benefits to customers in deeper, more personal ways than commitments to civic duty or generalized solidarity would generate. The market provides incentives for developing high-quality or innovative products and services. In short, virtue can be seen as a market strategy that leads to excellence in both personal relationships and scientific research, thereby maximizing profits.

Each of these underlying background considerations identifies important areas of concern in the analytic geography of the debate regarding the creation of a market in human organs. In considering the moral acceptability of the market, one must assess each factor as well as the ways in which such factors balance one against another. Given different constellations of factors it will be more or less plausible to place the burden of proof on either those who would forbid a market in organs or those who would allow it. It would as well provide a plausible justification of the burden of proof that should be met in evaluating any particular policy.

CHAPTER FOUR

The Body, Its Parts, and the Market

Revisionist Interpretations from the History of Philosophy

INTRODUCTION

The previous chapters had two goals: on the one hand, to assess what understandings of embodiment, body ownership, and political authority would have to be granted for a market in human organs, all things being equal, to be morally permissible; and, on the other hand, to assess the costs and benefits that challenge such a ceteris paribus finding, thereby rendering a market in human organs more or less plausible. The advantages and disadvantages of an organ market were assessed by exploring its costs and benefits in health care, the efficient and effective use of scarce resources, whether such a market would likely lead to increases or decreases in liberty, equality, or altruism, and considering its impact on special moral concerns, such as regard for human dignity, respect for sanctity of life, the exploitation of persons, social solidarity, and the pursuit of scientific excellence. In each case, the analysis indicated that given many constellations of factors, it would be more reasonable to place the burden of proof on those who would forbid a market in organs rather than on those who would permit it.

To extend and deepen this analysis, this chapter turns to the history of philosophy. Contemporary reflection regarding the moral permissibility of the sale of human organs for transplantation usually does not seriously engage arguments from the history of philosophy; indeed, such debate is largely innocent of past moral reflection on the matter. Yet, historically, different foundational understandings of the relationship between person and body have grounded diverse accounts of duties to the body, as well as concerns for the protection of human life and its dignity.

Consider the contrast between the ancient Greeks and traditional Christianity. Greek philosophy often stigmatized bodily sensual life as bestial. The association of the soul with the physical body was seen as distorting the person from his true purpose: contemplation.[1] The body was a burden to bear rather than a blessing to celebrate. Bear in mind Socrates' famous contention that philosophy is the appropriate way for the soul to prepare for the death of the physical body. His contention is predicated on an understanding of the body as distinct from the soul and to be divorced from the soul's more important concerns.[2] Aristotle similarly stigmatized the sensual life of physical pleasures as bestial. While he admits in the *Nicomachean Ethics* that this is the life most individuals seem to prefer, he argues that a truly fulfilled human life cannot be carried out in slavery to one's physical passions.[3] The truly human life, the life of *philanthropia*, is marked by a rational constraint of the passions and taking pleasure only in appropriate things, which are not, for the most part, purely physical pleasures.[4] As Plato and Aristotle illustrate, Greek culture captured a very particular sense of the practice of virtue and right conduct, of human dignity, nobility, and courtesy. It often included a deep sense of alienation from one's body. Rigorous training and domestication of the passions allowed the intellectual life, the life of the person, to flourish. The embodied life was often perceived as an impediment to understanding the true nature of goodness, beauty, appropriate pleasures, justice, and so forth.

For the traditional Christian, however, the goodness of the body as part of God's creation is affirmed. Within Christianity there exists the very real concern to ameliorate the physiological collapse brought on by age, accident, injury, and disease. Even in the fourth century, Saint Basil the Great (AD 329–379) notes that medicine is an important good to be used to relieve sickness and suffering: "Each of the arts is God's gift to us, remedying the deficiencies of nature . . . the medical art was given to us to relieve the sick, in some degree at least."[5] Medical developments, however, did not change the primary undertaking of traditional Christianity. As with all human goods, medicine must be placed within the Christian life and appreciated in terms of man's relationship with God. As a result, the rubric for understanding the relationship between person and body is not ownership but stewardship—that is, the Christian is responsible for proper use of himself, because God will hold him to account for his stewardship.[6] Unlike Plato, traditional Christianity frequently denied that it is the physical body that corrupts the human soul. Saint Cyril of Jerusalem (AD 315–386) writes:

> Do not tell me that the body is the cause of sin. For were the body the cause of sin, why does no corpse sin? Put a sword in the right hand of a man who has just died, and no murder takes place. Let beauty in every guise pass before a youth just dead, and he will not be moved to fornication. Wherefore so? Because the body does not sin of itself, but it is the soul that sins, using the body.[7]

Safeguarding one's body and life are central obligations to oneself, others, and the Creator. Seeking and accepting appropriate medical therapy, including organ donation and transplantation, may be required to fulfill significant duties to oneself and others, such as one's spouse and children.[8]

Insofar as positions for or against a market in human organs presuppose moral intuitions, ontological or political theoretical premises, or understandings of special moral concerns—such as permissible uses of the body and its parts, which have a long history of analysis—attention to that history ought to be rewarding.

This chapter addresses the positions of Thomas Aquinas (1224–1274), John Locke (1632–1704), and Immanuel Kant (1724–1804), which would usually be interpreted as foreclosing a market in human organs, as well as of Robert Nozick (1939–2002), who gives grounds for supporting such a market. On the one hand, Aquinas's principle of totality requires that one preserve the wholeness of the human body; Locke's account of one's duties to support the natural good of individual liberty places constraints on the freedom one has to use one's body; and Kant argues straightforwardly that the categorical imperative rules out selling body parts from living persons. In what follows, the analysis focuses on how these arguments are configured. If certain critical premises are changed in ways that, I will argue, are plausible, then the conclusions come out very different. Prohibiting a market in human organs may depend on a single premise, or a cluster of dubious and allied premises, which when examined cannot hold. In approaching these texts, I will assume the role of a revisionist who takes seriously the core commitments of these authors while at the same time indicating that one can further develop their attitudes about the body in ways that are supportive of the sale of human organs for transplantation while remaining in conformity with the authors' particular core concerns. On the other hand, Nozick views secular morality and the limits of moral political authority as grounded in permission. A market in human organs would thereby be permissible provided parties to such transactions freely consent to participate.

Why these particular philosophers?

Ancient Christianity was one of the central historical sources out of which the West drew its cultural, intellectual, and moral substance. The ancient Christian Church defined Christian belief and culture over against other religions, including the paganism of ancient Greece and Rome. The Roman Catholic Church, while affirming the first seven ecumenical councils,[9] recast such reflections within the framework of Western social, political, and religious institutions.[10] Prior to the Reformation, the Roman Catholic Church was the principal institution that framed the Christian moral vision of Western Europe: from Pope Leo III's crowning of Charles the Great as "romanum gubernans imperium," after the third mass on Christmas, AD 800, to Pope Urban II's announcement of the

First Crusade in AD 1095; from Pope Innocent IV's official inauguration of the Inquisition on AD May 15, 1252, with the bull Ad extirpanda, to the founding of the University of Paris in AD 1208 and the eventual development of natural law moral philosophy. Thus, when Western Christianity explicitly articulated its notions of proper medical deportment, Roman Catholicism offered a significant institutional locus for much of the moral discussion of the first thousand years of Christianity. The morality of Western Christianity became the morality of medicine and of the good physician. Indeed, though diminished in secular authority, the Roman Catholic Church remains a counterweight to the various secular moralities of our time.

Thus, in the West the impact of Roman Catholic and Scholastic thought has been significant. Especially among Western Christianity of the High Middle Ages, as Thomas Aquinas exemplifies, these moral understandings were incorporated in Christian theological doctrine. This defended the ability of persons generally to understand natural law: that there is an objective good for human beings, which reason can articulate, thus justifying the general canons of moral behavior.[11]

Despite considerable secularization following the Renaissance and the Reformation, Western Christian reflection continued to have noteworthy influence. There remained in the West the attempt to fashion rational justification for the general lineaments of Christian culture and moral intuitions as well as its fundamental social structures. Though many recognized the undertakings of modern philosophy and the Enlightenment to be anti-Christian, they were still in great measure attempts to establish the moral commitments of Christianity, albeit without a specifically Christian confession of faith. There was the expectation that one could disclose a communality of all persons, justified not in faith but in reason. For example, Locke reflects Christianity's traditional opposition to suicide. He holds that the duty not to kill oneself is universal and knowable through the natural law construed as the law of reason: "The *state of nature* has a law of nature to govern it, which obliges every one: and reason which is that law, teaches all mankind, who will but consult it."[12] Locke's account of the limited constitutional state, individual rights, and the free market has had a significant impact on the general political theory of the modern liberal state.

For Kant, the Christian community of faith, indeed the Mystical Body of Christ, was restated as the community of reason; the kingdom of grace became the kingdom of reason:

> insofar as we take account only of the rational beings in it, and of their connection according to moral laws under the government of the supreme good, *the kingdom of grace*, distinguishing it from the *kingdom of nature*, in which these rational beings do indeed stand under moral laws. . . . To view ourselves, therefore, as in the world of grace, where all

happiness awaits us, except insofar as we ourselves limit our share in it through being unworthy of happiness, is, from the practical standpoint, a necessary idea of reason.[13]

Prior to Kant and the Enlightenment, God's perspective provided the epistemological gold standard: knowledge of reality as it is in itself. Kant disengaged human knowledge from this cardinal reference point, domesticating scientific, epistemological, and metaphysical investigation within the bounds of possible intersubjective human experience. Following Kant, morality could no longer be understood as a way of life through which one sought salvation. Rather, morality became an account of the grammar of responsible choice and imputable action. It is the framework within which one must think of oneself as an agent who can in principle be praiseworthy or blameworthy. Thus he regarded persons as central to the practice of morality and endorsed the possibility of disclosing through reason canonical moral content that would bind persons as such.

Kant combined precritical, Scholastic, Christian moral views regarding the importance of maintaining the body as a whole with critical arguments concerning the necessary structure for the possibility of morality.[14] Whereas faith in reason made it plausible that rational argument could provide the practical laws of right conduct,[15] Kant continued to incorporate and defend much of Christian moral content, such as the Western Christian principle of totality. He argues, for example, that selling one's body parts, such as teeth or hair, uses oneself merely as a means, rather than respecting oneself as an end, and thus is impermissible.[16] Kant's impact on contemporary bioethics can be seen in arguments that hold that there is something intrinsically wrong or debasing in selling one's organs, so that even if one does this freely, one is being used in a morally inappropriate manner—that one has been brought to do something morally wrong.

The more reason's ability to discover a universal, coherent, content-full moral understanding of organ sales or the justification for political authority to proscribe such sales is brought into doubt, the more one must look for alternative foundations. Here particular attention will be given to the implications of Nozick's *Anarchy, State, and Utopia*. Nozick grounds secular moral authority in permission. Here moral authority is not drawn from claims to religious revelation, so-called moral consensus, or deep moral intuitions regarding consequences, human rights, ethical principles, or views of moral repugnance; rather, it is based on the agreement of the parties to collaborate. It is unnecessary for collaborators to agree on the ranking of values, moral principles, cultural or religious assumptions; they need only affirm the content of their agreement. No value standard or order must be presumed, just the recognition that collaboration is possible through agreement. Market transactions and contractual relationships draw moral authority from the consent of the participants. The parties to the transaction, themselves, freely convey authority to the enforcement of the specified conditions. Given such circumstances, the consent of those who freely choose to participate creates the moral authority of an organ market.

MAJOR THEORIES

Thomas Aquinas: The Principle of Totality and the Selling of Body Parts

Aquinas's arguments regarding the principle of totality reflect a commitment to the coincidence between faith and natural theology. He considers his argument to be binding on all persons as such, even though it is clear that the character of the argument and the content he engages can only be fully appreciated within a set of Western Christian presuppositions. It is important to realize that Aquinas, and later Thomists, do not recognize that theirs is a particular moral rationality. Instead, Western Christian moral reflections are often posited in terms of general discursive rationality: their conclusions are argued to be justifiable through reason alone. Rather than asking, "What do we know to be true in the fullness of Christian faith, practice, and revelation?" the question has been: "What are those principles governing human action to which no rational human being can deny his assent?"[17]

In particular, Aquinas held that it is morally impermissible to remove a part of the body as long as it is healthy and retains its natural disposition.[18] He argued as follows: the life of a human being as a biologically functioning whole is a natural good.[19] Anything that damages this good, endangering or attacking parts of the bodily whole, is prima facie morally impermissible. Therefore, only insofar as one can show that the intervention or removal of the part is in fact intended to preserve the natural good, can the prima facie impermissibility be defeated. Given such an argument, the challenge for organ donation and sales using living donors is the same: cutting away healthy organs from living persons violates the natural good of the wholeness of the body and is, therefore, prima facie morally impermissible.

With the development of blood, tissue, and organ transplantation, as well as arguments pointing to the significant good such activities create, this commitment to rational discourse led contemporary Thomists to reinterpret the principle as implying an obligation to preserve human biological functioning, rather than anatomical wholeness. Human biological life is a natural good: as Finnis argues, "A first basic value, corresponding to the drive for self preservation, is the value of life. The term 'life' here signifies every aspect of the vitality (*vita*, life) which puts a human being in good shape for self determination. Hence, life here includes bodily (including cerebral) health, and freedom from pain that betokens organic malfunctioning or injury."[20] The basic good that must be respected, however, is not the fulfillment of the good of this or that organ, but of the whole human person. That person's bodily health is integral, rather than instrumental, to the fulfillment of this good; a good that ought to be measured in terms of the functional organic whole.[21]

Historical Roots of the Principle of Totality

The historical roots of Aquinas's concern for the natural good of human biological wholeness are found in ancient Christian canons bearing on the preservation of men and women as embodied and gendered beings. Certain heretical sects, such as the Valesians, interpreted Christ's teachings that "if thy right eye offend thee, pluck it out, . . . likewise if thy right hand or foot offend thee, cut it off" (Matt. 18:8–9), as implying that one ought to amputate parts of the body that incite one to sin.[22] Such sects often encouraged castration to avoid sexual sins and to achieve spiritual purity. In response, the church promulgated canons prohibiting the practice of voluntary, nonmedically indicated castration, holding that persons were to master their sinful passions rather than mutilate their bodies as a physical shortcut. Consider canon 1 from the First Council of Nicaea (AD 325):

> If anyone has been operated upon by surgeons for a disease, or has been excised by barbarians, let him remain in the clergy. But if anyone has excised himself when well, he must be dismissed even if he is examined after being in the clergy. And henceforth no such person must be promoted to holy orders. But as is self-evident, though such is the case as regards those who affect the matter and dare to excise themselves, if any persons have been eunuchized by barbarians or their lords, but are otherwise found to be worthy, the Canon admits such persons to the clergy.[23]

Apostolic canons 22, 23, and 24, considered to have arisen from first-century AD moral commitments, tied purposeful self-mutilation to moral and spiritual condemnation. Individuals who castrate themselves are castigated as self-murderers, plotters against their own lives, and enemies of God's creation:

> Let no one who has mutilated himself become a clergyman; for he is a murderer of himself, and an enemy of God's creation. (Apostolic canon 22)[24]

> If anyone who is a clergyman should mutilate himself, let him be deposed from office. For he is a self-murderer. (Apostolic canon 23)[25]

> Any layman who has mutilated himself shall be excommunicated for three years. For he is a plotter against his own life. (Apostolic canon 24)[26]

Castration that results from hatred of being male, or as a physical means to help one control sinful passions, is mutilation that inappropriately rejects the fundamental sexual and gendered nature of God's creation; it thereby constitutes a grave moral evil.

However, as canon 8 of the First and Second Regional Synod, held in Constantinople (AD 861), clarifies, castration for medical reasons, such as to prevent the spread of disease, requires no such intention. It, therefore, can be free of moral and spiritual condemnation:

> The divine and sacred Canon of the Apostles judges those who castrate themselves to be self-murderers; accordingly, if they are priests, it deposes them from office, and if they are not, it excludes them from advancement to holy orders. Hence it makes plain that if one who castrates himself is a self-murderer, he who castrates another is certainly a murderer. One might even deem such a person quite guilty of insulting creation itself. Wherefore the holy Council has been led to decree that if any bishop, or presbyter, or deacon, be proved guilty for castrating anyone, either with his own hand or by giving orders to anyone else to do so, he shall be subjected to the penalty of deposition from office; but if the offender is a layman, he shall be excommunicated: unless it should so happen that owing to the incidence of some affliction he should be forced to operate upon the sufferer by removing his testicles. For precisely as the first Canon of the Council held in Nicaea does not punish those who have been operated upon for a disease, for having the disease, so neither do we condemn priests who order diseased men to be castrated, nor do we blame laymen either, when they perform the operation with their own hands. For we consider this to be a treatment of the disease, but not a malicious design against the creature or an insult to creation. (canon 8, First and Second Regional Synod)[27]

Castration thus could licitly be performed as a necessary means to preserve the health or good of the individual's body.

Aquinas recast these concerns, focused on castration and rejection of one's gendered embodiment, articulating a more general obligation to preserve the wholeness of the body. According to Aquinas, human persons exist as a physical unity, composed of integral parts. Each part exists for and is subordinated to the good of the whole. The body was created as a whole for the natural good of the person. One is obligated to respect the body's integrity and develop its capacities so that it is conducive to moral virtue. Voluntarily maiming or mutilating the body—understood as the removal or functional destruction of parts of the body—violates the natural good of the biological whole, and is therefore prima facie morally impermissible.

As Aquinas argues:

> Since a member is part of the whole human body, it is for the sake of the whole, as the imperfect for the perfect. Hence a member of the human body is to be disposed of according as it is expedient for the body. Now

> a member of the human body is of itself useful to the good of the whole body, yet, accidentally it may happen to be hurtful, as when a decayed member is a source of corruption to the whole body. Accordingly so long as a member is healthy and retains its natural disposition, it cannot be cut off without injury to the whole body. [28]

Insofar as the body is healthy and functioning normally, it is prima facie morally illicit to remove or destroy its parts.

If mutilation is necessary to preserve the health and integrity of the body, however, the prima facie moral impermissibility is defeated:

> If, however, the member be decayed and therefore a source of corruption to the whole body, then it is lawful with the consent of the owner of the member, to cut away the member for the welfare of the whole body, since each one is intrusted with the care of his own welfare. The same applies if it be done with the consent of the person whose business it is to care for the welfare of the person who has a decayed member: otherwise it is altogether unlawful to maim anyone.[29]

Just as the ancient Christian canons permit castration to treat disease, Aquinas concludes that body parts may be removed to preserve the good of the whole, such as the amputation of a gangrenous limb to prevent the spread of disease and decay.

Three general conditions govern the moral licitness of anatomic or functional mutilation. First, the continued presence or functioning of the organ must be causing serious damage or constituting a menace to the body as a whole. Second, the surgical removal in question remediates, or at least measurably lessens, this damage, and there is significant assurance that the operation is efficacious in this regard. Third, the expected positive outcome, in terms of eliminating danger to the whole organism, easing of pain, and so forth, must compensate for the negative effects created by the mutilation and potential harmful side effects of surgery.[30] It need not be that the amputated organ is itself diseased so long as its continued presence or functioning directly or indirectly causes a serious menace for that individual's body. It would be inappropriate, according to contemporary Thomists, to characterize the relationship persons have with their bodies as a form of absolute "ownership." While an owner of a thing may use or destroy it at will, so long as he does not conflict with the rights of others, persons do not own their bodies in such a fashion. "Above all, he must conserve his body and his life, for they do not belong to him, but to God; man may not destroy needlessly his body or any part of his body."[31] Persons possess a stewardship or useful, rather than absolute, dominion over their bodies and its parts. Pius XII emphasized:

> As far as the patient is concerned, he is not absolute master of himself, of his body, or of his soul. He cannot, therefore, freely dispose of himself as he

pleases. Even the motive for which he acts is not by itself either sufficient or determining. The patient is bound by the immanent purposes fixed by nature. He possesses the right to use limited by natural finality, the faculties and powers of his human nature. Because he is the beneficiary, not the proprietor, he does not possess unlimited power to allow acts of destruction or of mutilation of anatomic or functional character.[32]

Maiming the body is, therefore, morally impermissible. But the potential harms of surgery are justified in terms of their effect on preserving the natural good of the biologically functioning whole and the overall well-being of the individual:

> The decisive point rests not in the fact that the organ which is amputated or paralyzed be itself infected, but that its continued presence or functioning cause either directly or indirectly a serious menace for the whole body. It is quite possible that in functioning normally a healthy organ could cause harm to one which is unhealthy, in such a way as to aggravate the evil and the repercussions of this last on the organism as a whole. Or it can happen that the removal of a healthy organ and the paralyzing of its function remove from the evil—cancer, for example— the possibility of extending further, or else change the effect of this evil on the body. If there is no other alternative available, in both cases a surgical operation on the healthy organ is permissible.[33]

More broadly applied, this principle requires that diagnostic and therapeutic procedures be judged in terms of their efficaciousness for producing the good of the particular patient on whom they are used.[34]

As Aquinas articulates the position, the principle of totality is fully consistent with a market in human organs procured from cadaver sources. Taking such organs is not in itself incompatible with respect for the human body; with death obligations to preserve the natural good of the biologically functioning whole, or the well-being of the individual, lose their salience. Once an individual has died, organs removed from the cadaver become much like other types of things. This is why transplanting organs from cadaver sources to living persons does not offer any intrinsic moral problem.[35] Similarly, a futures market, in which one contracts in the present for the sale of organs after one's death, would likewise satisfy the principle of totality. On such grounds, it seems plausible to view certain markets in human organs as consistent with Roman Catholic moral theological concepts of embodiment and God's dominion as well as respecting human dignity.

Applications and Modern Developments of the Principle of Totality

In itself, the principle of totality rules out the procurement of healthy blood, tissue, and organs from living donors. It, therefore, in turn proscribes both donation and selling of healthy organs from living persons. Since the principle requires any removal of a part of the human body to be justified in terms of preserving that person's bodily wholeness, one cannot justify either the donation or sale of body parts in terms of preserving the wholeness of others. As Gerald Kelly argues, the principle of totality is only applicable in cases where there is the subordination of part to whole in the natural body. There exists no such subordination between individuals and society as a whole. "Each person is a distinct entity, with a distinct finality."[36] Persons exist neither for the sake of others nor for the sake of society. Citizens may have certain duties to society, but this is quite different from asserting that they are parts of a quasi-social organism in the same sense as the kidney is part of the body.[37]

Donation or sale of body parts cannot be justified by the fact that the body restores such parts (including blood, skin grafts, and bone marrow). In itself, such reasoning would justify the useless letting of blood or the pointless removal of other regenerating tissues. This would violate the natural good of the biological whole for no reason whatsoever.

Instead, moral appeal must be made to a principle of charity: the donor/seller intends that the body parts be transplanted into another person and thereby wills that other's good. For such an argument to hold, however, it must be structured more or less as follows: (1) Persons are charitable beings and (2) such charity is a good. Moreover, (3) the good of being charitable is often more important than the good of preserving the wholeness of the body. However, (4) directly intending to kill oneself is forbidden (e.g., donating one's heart while still living). Therefore, often charity is sufficient to defeat the prima facie moral impermissibility of removing healthy human body parts, as long as this is not part of an act that intends directly to kill oneself.

For example, Pius XII supports the premises of this argument in his praise of blood donors for their charity, comparing their behavior to the model of Christ:

> Model as He is of all charity, He is your model in a special way . . . to give one's blood for someone unknown to us, perhaps someone ungrateful, who will forget or who will not even want to know the name and countenance of his savior; to donate something of one's own strength only to communicate it to others and give them back what they have lost; to restore one's lost energies only to repeat and renew the same gift and the same sacrifice: it is to this that you are generously dedicated.[38]

Pope John XXIII reiterated this view in 1959:

> Yours is truly, then, an apostolate. But to achieve its perfection it must be rooted and founded in charity, which is love of God and of brother. [39]

The principle of charity, whereby one assumes a cost or burden, intending the good of others, provides sufficient reason to defeat the principle of totality's prima facie moral inappropriateness, and justifies the removal of healthy tissue, blood, and organs.

However, since the principle of totality still holds, it must be reinterpreted as implying an obligation to preserve only a de minimis standard of human biological functioning. One must distinguish between the good of the adequately functioning body and the good of the full integrity of the anatomical whole. The principle of totality must be understood as only strictly requiring the former, not the latter. This reinterpretation of the principle of totality has significant appeal in that transplantation of human tissue, blood, and organs has considerable potential for helping others while still maintaining the adequate biological functioning of the donor.

This change, while departing from Aquinas, plausibly captures the anatomical fact that one must make distinctions even among body parts. As explored in chapter 2, some parts are necessary for embodiment/existence (e.g., the higher brain), other parts are necessary for adequate human functioning (e.g., the heart), while other parts of the body serve little role in effective human biological functioning. For example, the healthy appendix serves no known purpose in the human digestive system. Its removal, even while healthy, does not interfere with the integrity of the body; it neither suppresses nor otherwise harms any organic function of the body. Insofar as there is sufficient reason to subject the patient to the surgical risks—that is, if it is already necessary to open the abdomen to perform another operation—the appendix may be excised prior to closing the incision. The relative unimportance of the appendix, the risk of future appendicitis, and the minimal additional risk to the patient together justify elective appendectomy.[40] Moreover, its incidental removal precludes the possible harms of future surgery, if the appendix were ever to become diseased. As Charles McFadden argues, though, it would not generally be permissible for a person to arrange to have surgery solely for the removal of a healthy appendix. The risks of surgery outweigh the contingent good to be gained given the relatively small possibility that the individual might at some future date have appendicitis, and at that time not have access to medical intervention.[41]

With regard to organ procurement, while persons may not capriciously diminish the integrity of their own bodies, not all of one's organic parts are necessary to preserve adequate biological functioning. Insofar as procurement from living persons is limited to redundant organs (such as a kidney) or regenerating tissue (such as a liver segment), the functional wholeness of the body is maintained. The principle of charity provides sufficient reason to justify the substantial mutilation and the risks of organ procurement surgery, insofar as the organ is to be provided to someone who vitally needs it.[42] Assuming that donating a kidney for transplant does not lessen kidney function, with detriment to one's health generally, it is permissible—even though one accepts a risk to one's health in the event of contracting a kidney disease later.[43] It is morally licit voluntarily to give up an organ, or other body part, which is not needed and assume the risk that the one remaining kidney will continue normally to function.[44] In short, biological function as distinct from simple bodily integrity became the basis for justifying the removal of healthy organs from living donors for transplantation. Provided that functioning is not compromised, one who donates a redundant organ or regenerative tissue is merely accepting a risk to good functioning in the future for the sake of helping another in grave need.

Note, however, that this reinterpretation of the principle of totality is neutral with regard to whether one donates or sells the organ. If one can give away an organ, or regenerative tissue, with sufficient reason, one ought to be able to sell it for sufficient reason. A father, for example, could donate a kidney to his child to save the child's life. The organ is removed for a good purpose consistent with the principle of charity, and the father accepts the risks to his future health as a side effect. Similarly, it seems permissible for a parent to sell a kidney to purchase a life-sustaining operation for one's child. The structure of the action in the second case is the same as in the first. The only difference is that the second has an additional step in the instrumental analysis: obtaining sufficient funds to save the child's life.[45] Moreover, the sale saves the purchaser's, or another's, life directly, which is an act the vendor might well have significant morally compelling reasons to do. Given analogous action analysis, it would seem permissible to sell an organ to obtain life-sustaining food, medicine, or shelter.

It is difficult to understand how giving organs can be permissible but selling organs always impermissible, unless one has some view that accepting payment intrinsically involves a wrong. Selling organs might involve such harm, for example, if done capriciously, without regard for one's welfare. However, as argued in chapter 3, forbidding organ sales may demean the poor and sick, closing off options for improving their lives (i.e., the one sells a kidney to procure funds, the other receives a transplant to regain health).

On the one hand, since the significance of charity must outweigh the principle of totality, this will rule out many donations. Persons who stand to be financially supported by a person needing an organ might have other motivations than "kindness," "love," or "charity" for donating an organ. Other donations might be premised on reciprocated love, friendship, guilt, or stigma concerns for failing to donate.[46]

On the other hand, it is possible charitably to intend the good of another through for-profit market-based transactions. While the virtue of charity is often understood as a benevolent disposition toward others and their welfare, relief of suffering, the bestowal of gifts, and other similar actions, Christian charity has traditionally focused on the love of others for God. "Charity refers to divine love, that is to the love of God for man or the love of man for God. Here, we are considering charity as the virtue by which the creature loves God for His own sake, and others on account of God."[47] Charity, so understood, is consistent with the market. Among examples of charity, John McHugh and Charles Callan include "selling on credit as a favor to a poor customer; a loan granted at a low rate of interest or without interest, help in securing employment, etc."[48] Assisting someone through the market can be a significant act of charity.

Pope Pius XII specifically allowed that for-profit selling of human body parts could be consonant with the principle of charity.

> Moreover, must one, as is often done, refuse on principle all compensation? This question remains unanswered. It cannot be doubted that grave abuses could occur if a payment is demanded. But it would be going too far to declare immoral every acceptance or every demand of payment. The case is similar to blood transfusions. It is commendable for the donor to refuse recompense; it is not necessarily a fault to accept it.[49]

As Pius XII expresses the position, there is nothing intrinsically evil about the for-profit sale of human organs. Removal of a healthy human organ would be permissible even if one accepts or requests monetary compensation, or other valuable consideration, provided that one does not exploit those in need by demanding too great a fee; although, presumably, a poor individual could ask for greater compensation from a rich recipient. One could view this possibility as consonant with the reflections of certain theologians on the priority one should give the poor.[50]

In summary, the principle of totality is fully consistent with a market in human organs procured from cadaver sources as well as with a futures market. With death, body parts are no longer caught up in the life and good of the human person; they are much like other types of things, albeit things that were once parts of a person. Such markets neither degrade human dignity nor depersonalize or dehumanize living human beings. They are fully consistent with the embodied nature of persons and careful stewardship of God's gift to us of our bodies. Moreover, presuming that one sells a healthy organ to a well-matched recipient, the requirement of a sufficient reason for removal of an organ may be satisfied with (1) the expected good to the recipient of the organ of an increase in quality and quantity of life, and (2) the good that the income will provide for the vendor. The vendor may, for example, have morally compelling charitable reasons to sell an organ, such as to purchase medicine, food, or shelter for his family. Insofar as the principle of totality is satisfied in the case of organ donation, it is satisfied in the case of organ vending. As long as one markets only redundant organs, or regenerative tissues, the de minimis standard of adequate biological functioning is satisfied.[51]

Insofar as one's intention in removing the organ is not an attempt to destroy the natural good of biological wholeness but to engage in a market transaction to help others through the market and to assist one's family through the provision of resources otherwise not available, the sale of redundant internal organs is not an example of mutilation that the canons contemplated, nor does the recast principle of totality forbid it. In removing the redundant organ, the natural good of the individual's bodily functional wholeness is not set at risk. It is an instance of an individual cooperating with others in society to provide for the needs of others, as well as for oneself. Given such conditions, it should not be considered a mutilation that offends the Deity or as destroying, or reducing, the natural human good of biological functional wholeness. On such grounds, the organ market may be morally permissible. Indeed, given appropriate circumstances in which the charity of the sale is apparent, it may even be commendable.

John Locke: The Limited State and Natural Duties

There are two primary conceptual foci in Locke's philosophy with which one might forge moral political authority for the state to prohibit a market in human organs: the first considers Locke's contractual account of the derivative and artificial nature of state authority, while the second appreciates the political implications of his natural theology. First, in the state of nature persons are in authority over themselves and their possessions. While political authority, according to Locke, is limited, apparently significant aspects of one's natural liberty are surrendered when one leaves the state of nature for civil society. Here the question is whether one alienates sufficient liberty such that the state has moral authority to forbid the selling of one's own organs. Second, Locke held that persons have moral obligations, such as not to kill oneself, which he secured through a natural theology. In this fashion, Locke limited moral political authority as well as established limits on personal liberty that the state may enforce. Such constraints place in principle limits on the freedom one has to use and dispose of oneself at will. Here the question is whether Locke's natural theological constraints rule out the selling of human organs.

The Limits of Legitimate State Authority

Consider the argument concerning moral political authority. One might argue that within civil society persons cede sufficient liberty over themselves such that it is within the moral authority of the state to forbid the consensual selling of human organs. There are, however, considerable exegetical as well as conceptual difficulties in sustaining such an interpretation. For example, Locke affirms that "every man has a *property* in his own *person*: this no body has any right to but himself. The *labour* of his body, and the *work* of his hands, we may say are properly his."[52] This natural authority of persons over themselves and their property is expressed within the state of nature as a "state of perfect freedom to order their actions, and dispose of their possessions and persons as they think fit, within the bounds of the laws of nature, without asking leave, or depending upon the will of any other man."[53] Such authority includes private legislative rights (e.g., the liberty to act however one believes is necessary for self-preservation) as well as executive rights (e.g., the liberty to punish violators of the natural law);[54] "the execution of the law of nature is, in that state, put into every man's hands, whereby everyone has a right to punish the transgressors of that law to such a degree, as may hinder its violation."[55] Prior to entering civil society, all men are at liberty to preserve person and property, as well as to act in judgment of those who violate these natural goods.

All political authority, according to Locke, is derivative. It must be explained in terms of and grounded on the more basic forms of natural authority that persons have over themselves and their property. States obtain authority only through voluntary alienation of rights by the rightholders (i.e., persons) themselves: "For no government can have a right to obedience from a people who have not fully consented to it"[56]; elsewhere Locke argues that the "only way whereby any one divests himself of his natural liberty, and puts on the *bonds of civil society*, is by agreeing with other men to join and unite into a community for their comfortable, safe, and peaceable living."[57] Only political consent, in which persons surrender those aspects of their natural liberties necessary to form a civil union, binds individuals together in a state.[58]

The reason for forming such a civil society is the effective preservation of our property, life, and liberty.[59] Individuals, therefore, surrender to the political authority only those rights "so far forth as the preservation of himself and the rest of society shall require,"[60] such that the government may achieve these ends.[61] Generally, this includes private legislative and executive rights regarding the natural law, but not extensive authority to create, without consent of the citizens, laws that further limit personal freedom. Basic political authority is limited to the enforcement of the duties and rights of the natural law, securing persons' lives and property holdings:

> For the political society is instituted for no other end, but only to secure every man's possession of the things of this life. . . . Thus the safeguard of men's lives and of the things that belong unto this life is the business of the commonwealth; and the preserving of those things unto their owners is the duty of the magistrate. And therefore the magistrate cannot take away these worldly things from this man or party and give them to that; nor change propriety amongst fellow subjects (no not even by a law), for a cause that has no relation to the end of civil government.[62]

De jure political authority is a fiduciary power that continues only insofar as the state pursues the particular ends for which it has consent, eschewing others for which it does not have consent. In short, while persons must surrender to the society sufficient individual liberty to accomplish the "ends for which they unite into a society,"[63] such "ends" are limited, which in turn constrains the moral authority of the state.

The general character of the Lockean state is a limited constitutional democracy. Such a civil society cannot act arbitrarily over the lives and fortunes of the people.[64] It must rule by established and promulgated laws[65] and cannot take from any person any part of their property without individual consent.[66] Without consent the political authority cannot tax for the maintenance of society,[67] transfer the power of government to any other state or organization,[68] or otherwise enact additional legislation with regard to conduct the natural law does not specifically require or prohibit. With such authorization the political authority can create laws for the good of society as a whole, including those necessary to support effective functioning, such as taxation, as well as national and civil defense: "it is fit every one who enjoys his share of the protection, should pay out of his estate his proportion for the maintenance of it";[69] each "engages his natural force (which he might before employ in the execution of the law of nature, by his own single authority, as he thought fit) to assist the executive power of society."[70]

Insofar as the state asserts more authority than that to which its citizens have consented, they have the natural right forcefully to preserve their lives, liberties, and possessions:

> There remains still *in the people a supreme power to remove or alter the legislative*, when they find the *legislative power given with trust* for the attaining an *end*, being limited by that end, whenever that *end* is manifestly neglected, or opposed, the *trust* must necessarily be *forfeited*, and the power devolve into the hands of those that gave it.[71]

The community retains a "supreme power of saving themselves from the attempts and designs of any body, even of their legislators, whenever they shall be so foolish, or so wicked, as to lay and carry on designs against the liberties and properties of the subject."[72] Indeed,

> should a robber break into my house, and with a dagger at my throat make me seal deeds to convey my estate to him, would this give him any title? Just such a title, by his sword, has an *unjust conqueror*, who forces me into submission. The injury and the crime is equal, whether committed by the wearer of a crown, or some petty villain.[73]

A state or sovereign who asserts and enforces nonconsensual authority is conceptually not much different than a thief[74] or a villain.[75]

Consider the force of such arguments for the morally permissible prohibition of a market in human organs. Procuring and selling internal organs is a consensual transaction involving private property through which both vendor and recipient expect to benefit. For those external to the exchange, the transaction is in Lockean political terms benign: it touches neither their personal security nor their property holdings. Thus, it is implausible that the surrender of the liberty to sell one's redundant internal organs can be understood as necessary to the ends for which persons unite into civil society. Even if it were possible to demonstrate that organ selling is a self-harming, morally repugnant activity, a decision without scruples, general prohibition is inconsistent with Locke's argument's regarding the limits of permissible moral authority of the government. A consistent refrain in his *First Letter on Toleration* is that the magistrate's de jure moral authority does not extend to the prevention of error. An essential aspect of individual liberty is personal responsibility; that is, the right to err, indeed to make costly mistakes that constrain one's future choices. Locke takes care to emphasize that governments do not possess moral authority to regulate self-harming activity—even if such activity is understood as leading to significantly harmful consequences. The right to err compasses individual moral authority to secure one's own ill health, poverty, and damnation.

> [T]he care of souls does not belong to the magistrate. . . . [T]he care . . . of every man's soul belongs unto himself. But what if he neglect the care of his soul? I answer, what if he neglect care of his health, or of his estate, which things are nearlier related to the government of the magistrate than the other? Will the magistrate provide by an express law that such a one shall not become poor or sick? Laws provide, as much as possible, that the goods and health of subjects be not injured by the fraud and violence of others; they do not guard them from the negligence or ill-husbandry of the possessors themselves. No man can be forced to be rich or healthful, whether he will or nor. Nay, God Himself will not save men against their wills.[76]

Persons are in authority over themselves and considered to be the authority of their own best interests. In general, provided that one's actions do not trespass upon the natural forbearance rights of others, or do not violate the terms of one's contractual agreements, the moral authority of the state to interfere in individual choice is limited.

These circumstances imply, as Eric Mack points out, that "Any individual who qualifies as a standard rightholder may subject herself to any medical procedures, i.e., to any form of self-treatment, she chooses; and she may secure for herself any forms of treatment by others that others are freely willing to provide."[77] Self-sovereignty thereby includes individual moral authority over oneself to consensual organ procurement for donation or for-profit sale.

Therefore, unless there are natural theology-based duties that constrain the selling of human organs, absent consent, prohibition of a market in human organs would not appear to be within the derivative authority of the state.

Natural Theological Duties

Locke's natural theology grounds the natural good of individual liberty. It also morally constrains the ways in which persons may use themselves. While such constraints ground limits in principle on the moral authority of the state, they also create natural duties that the state must enforce. One might argue that such restraints also prohibit the procuring and selling of human organs.

For example, Locke holds that persons have natural duties not to commit suicide or to harm others in their "life, health, liberty, or possessions."[78] Such natural theological constraints are grounded not only as correlatives to the rights of persons but also as correlatives to rights that the Deity has in creation:

> . . . for men being all the workmanship of one omnipotent, and infinitely wise maker; all the servants of one sovereign master, sent into the world by his order, and about his business; they are his property, whose workmanship they are, made to last during his, not one another's pleasure.[79]

While such duties constrain the ways one may utilize oneself, they also define a sphere in which persons, vis-à-vis other persons, have natural rights to be left alone. In the state of nature, individuals are at liberty to dispose of their person and possessions; however, they are not at liberty to destroy themselves. While vis-à-vis other persons one has a "right of freedom to his person, which no other man has a power over, but the free disposal of it lies in himself,"[80] with respect to natural theology, one's person and body are not one's own without restriction.[81] The rights of persons over themselves end at the limits of the natural law. Thus "no body has an absolute arbitrary power over himself . . . to destroy his own life." [82] Only God has such absolute dominion.

Locke attempts similarly to ground his argument against slavery. Insofar as one does not have absolute authority over oneself, one cannot transfer such power to another:

> For a man, not having the power of his own life, *cannot* by compact, or his own consent, *enslave himself* to anyone, nor put himself under the absolute, arbitrary power of another, to take away his life, when he pleases. No body can give more power than he has himself; and he that cannot take away his own life, cannot give another power over it.[83]

Just as the rights of God constrain one's liberty to engage in suicide as an exercise of absolute dominion over oneself, they also constrain one's freedom to give others such authority over oneself.[84] Despotic political authority is essentially mass slavery of the citizenry, and is ruled out on similar grounds. Since absolute dominion over life and death belongs only to God, it cannot licitly be ceded to or usurped by other persons or civil institutions.

It is unclear that such natural theological constraints prevent one from selling one's own redundant organs. One might argue that since certain personal freedoms must be infringed (such as rights to commit suicide and to sell oneself into slavery) to support more important liberty-based natural goods, forbidding the sale of organs similarly enhances such goods. However, such an argument is implausible. First, in the case of an organ futures market or of selling organs procured from cadaveric donors more generally, one neither kills oneself nor places oneself in the despotic dominion of another. Therefore, there is no analogy to suicide or slavery, which might justify constraints against such practices on similar natural theology grounds. Second, in the case of living organ vendors, insofar as one only sells redundant internal organs (e.g., a kidney or a liver segment) and the risks of surgery are sufficiently minimized (e.g., a competent surgeon accomplishes the organ removal in a sterile environment), procurement for commercial exchange is not equivalent to suicide. Moreover, the negotiated for-profit transaction gives each party only limited contractual rights, rather than absolute dominion, in the body of the other. Again, there is no analogy to either suicide or slavery. Third, as I argued in chapter 3, it is implausible to construe the prohibition of organ sales as augmenting individual liberty.

Insofar as Locke regards his use of natural theology as a theoretical bar, in principle, against the unlimited authority of the state, it is unlikely that he would have interest in duties to God that forbid the sale of organs. Indeed, Locke specifically denies that the sinfulness of a choice makes it the legitimate concern of others and thus a licit subject of the state's governance. Even eternally damning choices do not necessarily trespass on the legitimate rights of others.

> [O]ne man does not violate the right of another, by his erroneous opinions, and undue manner of worship, nor is his perdition a prejudice to another man's affairs. . . . Every man . . . has the supreme and absolute authority of judging for himself. And the reason is, because nobody else is concerned in it, nor can receive any prejudice from his conduct therein.[85]

Only the actual rights of others are an appropriate subject for the exercise of licit state authority.

> [I]t does not follow that because it is a sin it ought therefore to be punished by the magistrate. For it does not belong unto the magistrate to make use of the sword in punishing everything, indifferently, that he takes to be a sin against God. Covetousness, uncharitableness, idleness,

and many other things are sins, by the consent of all men, which yet no man ever said were to be punished by the magistrate. The reason is because they are not prejudicial to other men's rights, nor do they break the public peace of societies.[86]

Even if some religions find the practice sinful, or if some secular moral viewpoints find it morally repugnant, it is implausible, given Locke's arguments, that governments have legitimate moral authority to forbid a market in human organs utilizing living vendors.

As Locke makes clear, persons have natural liberties to engage in market transactions. Private agreements can transfer property ownership as well as create enforceable duties and rights pertaining to the goods and services of others.

> For it is not every compact that puts an end to the state of nature between men, but only this one of agreeing together mutually to enter into one community, and make one body politic; other promises, and compacts, men may make one with another, and yet still be in the state of nature . . . for truth and keeping of faith belongs to men, as men, and not as members of society.[87]

One's actual rights, duties, and possessions may be expanded or compressed as the result of private contract. Prohibition of a market in human organs would straightforwardly limit the natural liberty of persons to engage in market exchanges. It is plausible to see permissible market transfers as extending to parts of the body, provided that such sales are limited to redundant organs or regenerative tissues, and adequate medical precautions are taken to preserve life.

Insofar as Locke envisions natural theology-based duties as far-reaching and greatly intrusive into individual freedom, moral political authority will also become far-reaching and intrusive. As the number of personal duties under natural theology increase, so too does the moral authority of the state to support and enforce such duties. Given Locke's general commitments to limited government as well as to individual freedom and responsibility, it is unlikely that he would support natural goods, which would in turn justify the moral political authority of the state to prohibit the selling of human organs. In any event, his position does not require such a proscription.[88]

Immanuel Kant: The Categorical Imperative and One's Obligation Not to Use Oneself Merely as a Means

In the *Metaphysics of Morals: The Doctrine of Virtue*, Kant denies the moral permissibility of either donating or selling parts of one's body. He argues, first, that such mutilation constitutes partial self-murder and thus involves the same contradiction in will as suicide; and, second, that it uses oneself merely as a means. The Kantian challenge for these practices is the same: to show that donation or sale of organs can be appropriately universalized, such that it is compatible with the material existence of the moral community both in oneself and in others, and that it supports the respect of moral agents.

An analysis of Kant's arguments may begin with his three formulations of the categorical imperative:

> Act only according to that maxim whereby you can at the same time will that it should become a universal law.[89]

> Act in such a way that you treat humanity, whether in your own person or in the person of another, always at the same time as an end and never simply as a means.[90]

> This is done in the present (third) formulation of the principle, namely, in the idea of the will of every rational being as a will that legislates universal law.[91]

Persons as rational beings are not subjective ends whose existence has worth because we value it, but are beings whose existence embodies reason, which is the ground of the moral law. Their worth is intrinsic rather than instrumental. As he clarifies the second formulation:

> Man, however, is not a thing and hence is not something to be used merely as a means; he must in all his actions always be regarded as an end in himself. Therefore, I cannot dispose of man in my own person by mutilating, damaging, or killing him.[92]

One may not, for example, use one's body to satisfy mere inclination, but only to discharge duties to others or to oneself. "We may treat our body as we please, provided our motives are those of self-preservation. If, for instance, his foot is a hindrance to life, a man might have it amputated. To preserve his person he has the right of disposal over his body."[93] In contrast, removing healthy parts of the body treats the person merely as a means and is likened to partial self-murder.

> Man cannot renounce his personality as long as he is a subject of duty, hence as long as he lives . . . disposing of oneself as a mere means to some discretionary end is debasing humanity in one's own person (*homo noumenon*). . . . To deprive oneself of an integral part or organ (to maim oneself)—for example, to give away or sell a tooth to be transplanted into another's mouth, or to have oneself castrated in order to get an easier livelihood as a singer, and so forth—are ways of partially murdering oneself.[94]

Removing a part of the body, such as an organ, for donation or sale is supposed to involve the same contradiction in will as suicide. It is important to appreciate that in this argument there is no distinction between donating and selling. Either donation or sale of one's healthy body parts, according to Kant, treats one's own person merely as a means.

It is clear that Kant is introducing much of Western Christian morality unexamined into his critical work. For example, he holds that masturbation is equivalent to self-murder.[95] Here he appears similarly to be uncritically adopting the Western Christian principle of totality. Not even those parts that are not necessary to one's biological functioning may be permissibly donated or sold: "cutting one's hair in order to sell it is not altogether free from blame."[96] However, the principle of totality can be understood in a principled fashion for Kant if and only if it can be put within the formulation of the categorical imperative.

The donation or sale of organs violates the categorical imperative only if at least one of three arguments holds: First, that it puts life in danger (and therefore cannot be universalized compatible with Kant's view, which requires taking into account the material existence of the moral community; although this requires some de minimis condition of allowable risk to take account of occupational hazards that people incur in the discharge of their duty). Second, that parts of the body are equivalent to oneself as the subject of morality in one's own person. This premise is necessary for Kant's argument that removing healthy parts of the body involves the same contradiction in will involved in suicide, beyond the considerations of the first argument regarding threat to life. As he argues, "to annihilate the subject of morality in one's own person is to root out the existence of morality itself from the world, as far as one can."[97] Or, third, that donation or sale of organs is not associated with the discharge of a duty (i.e., one ought to donate or sell one's organs not simply to satisfy inclinations but to discharge obligations to others).

Rather than ruling out the donation or sale of organs, the first argument at most requires that adequate precautions be taken during procurement surgery to satisfy the de minimis danger condition of acceptable risk. In such terms, the argument is only telling against the sale of nonredundant organs that are necessary to maintain embodiment/existence or adequate human functioning of the person. Given a sufficiently qualified surgeon, an adequately sterile environment, and so forth, the argument fails. Such use of the self is no more dangerous than many other occupational activities, such as volunteering for the army, which Kant allows as consonant with one's duty.[98]

Kant's position provides no objection to selling organs from cadaveric sources or, more generally, to a futures market. Consider Kant's stark distinction between persons and things. Rational beings are "called persons inasmuch as their nature already marks them out as ends in themselves."[99] Where things have only "a worth for us," persons mark beings "whose existence is an end in itself."[100] "A person is a subject whose actions can be imputed to him. Moral personality is therefore nothing other than the freedom of a rational being under moral laws (whereas psychological personality is merely the capacity of being conscious of one's identity in different conditions of one's existence). . . . A thing is that to which nothing can be imputed."[101] Cadavers no longer have the moral status of persons; on Kantian grounds they are things. They possess only instrumental, rather than intrinsic, value; they are valuable only insofar as actual persons value them. Therefore, they may be used, exchanged, dismantled, and sold as things.

The second argument appears unintelligible on its face. The extension of Kant's argument to the removal of parts of the body as partial self-murder, as being morally equivalent to suicide, only succeeds insofar as particular parts of the body can be identified with oneself as the subject of morality. As I argued in chapter 2, however, not all body parts are necessary for embodiment/existence of the person or adequate human functioning.[102] Therefore, insofar as one only removes parts of the body for donation or sale that are separable from the embodiment/existence or adequate human functioning of the person, one would not destroy the subject of morality in one's own person. Moreover, removing such parts can be universalized as compatible with the material existence of the moral community. Redundant internal organs and regenerative tissues meet such conditions.

The final argument turns on whether one donates/sells one's organs out of obligation or inclination. For example, if persons have a moral duty to be charitable in protecting life, this may include a duty to provide organs. At least, there may be a moral duty to do so if one does not find the transaction morally disrupting. As one is obliged to seek happiness insofar as this aids in the discharge of one's duties, this duty may bind only if not morally burdensome.[103] As a consequence, it may be permissible to sell one's organs for responsible reasons. The presence of payment may outweigh aversive inclinations and responses so that one can act charitably. One ought to be able to donate an organ to a family member to whom one has a duty, or to sell an organ to obtain the material means to satisfy a duty. In principle, Kant should not have an objection to selling organs when the risk to life is de minimis and when it is to discharge a duty, such as to care for one's family.

Moreover, insofar as the argument advanced in chapter 3 regarding the potential health benefits of an organ market is persuasive (i.e., that such a market would likely lead to greater organ availability, with organs of good quality, more efficient organ procurement, and more effective transplantation, while minimizing potential harms to vendors), creation of a market in human organs advantages the health and integrity of persons as ends in themselves. This is not merely a utilitarian point. The end can be categorically willed, since one wills the health and respect of moral agents as such.[104]

While never speaking directly to the concept of a free market in health care, Kant generally endorses private initiative:

For a being endowed with freedom is not satisfied with the pleasure of life's comforts which fall to his lot by the act of another (in this case the government); what matters, rather, is the principle according to which the individual provides such things for himself. [105]

As Klaus Hartman has argued, this affirmation can be seen as plausibly extending to a market in health care, albeit with certain restrictions:

> While duty in Kant could be seen as a non-economic device to ensure performance, commercialism and the market might prove a perfectly satisfactory vehicle to ensure performance without regard to duty. Even medical standards might be assured by the market principle through the competition of physicians in the interest of profit: they might have an interest in tendering service under the aegis of a higher-ranking insurance or medical company. Only ethical questions concerning allocation or distributive justice would remain unanswered.[106]

Kant's support of the market, however, was not unqualified. He argued for some measure of public welfare to care for the impecunious. "The general will of the people has united itself into a society that is to maintain itself perpetually; and for this end it has submitted itself to the internal authority of the state in order to maintain those members of the society who are unable to maintain themselves."[107] It is plausible that such support would include a basic minimum of health care, including, possibly, some organ transplants.

If a market in human organs is limited to redundant organs (e.g., a single kidney) and regenerative tissue (e.g., a liver segment), the Kantian elements for morally permissible action are present. First, the vendor does not will to destroy himself, and the procurement and selling of such organs is not incompatible with the health of moral agents. Second, the practice can be universalized at the level of individual and social risks. The increased personal risks associated with procurement surgery and having sold a redundant organ are lower than those associated with many other aspects of day-to-day life. Third, selling an organ is a plausible manner in which to discharge a duty of charity, or to gain the material means to discharge such a duty. Fourth, the practice of saving others supports the respect of moral agents. Since persons are always to be treated as ends in themselves, it is plausible that Kant could endorse the moral permissibility of organ selling as helping others to maintain that personhood. It would support the special dignity of persons as central to morality. Fifth, given his support of basic welfare rights, plausibly extended to include a basic package of health care, Kant could have supported the state purchase of organs for the impecunious.

Robert Nozick: The Moral Authority of Consent

As the discussions of Aquinas, Locke, and Kant illustrate, a significant difficulty for resolving moral controversies such as the permissibility of a market in human

organs is that all do not appeal to the same background assumptions to guide resolution. Given different presuppositions regarding the nature of the right and the
good, the character of virtue, and the consequences endorsed or eschewed,
rational argument will support disparate conclusions. Even if one appeals to natural law, one must specify how to interpret and rank findings about nature. For
example, the permissibility of procuring healthy organs from living persons
depends on whether one assumes, with Aquinas, that the life of a human being as
a biological anatomical whole is a natural good that must be unconditionally
supported, or whether it is a good to be pursued, balanced with the pursuit of
other goods. According to contemporary Thomists, it is morally sufficient to preserve the natural good of the human body as an adequately functioning whole,
while also donating an organ in response to the principle of charity. To follow
the view of Aquinas's text, organs may only be removed if diseased, or would
otherwise constitute a direct or indirect threat to the body, so as to preserve the
good of the whole. In contrast, contemporary Thomists consider other factors,
such as charitably intending the good of others, to be sufficient to justify the
removal of healthy organs. Such background moral assumptions in turn bear on
one's assessment of the permissibility of a market in human organs.

Similarly, following Locke, background assumptions concerning (1) the
extent of the personal liberty one surrenders to political authority and (2) the character of natural law duties will lead one to conclude for or against the moral authority of the state to prohibit a market in human organs. For example, as individuals
cede a greater amount of freedom to the government, it becomes more plausible
that political institutions have moral authority to prohibit the selling of human
organs. Additionally, insofar as individuals surrender the legislation and enforcement of the natural law to civil society, as the requirements of natural theology
increase so too does the moral authority of the state to enforce such duties. If selling human organs significantly infringes natural goods, there may exist moral
authority for the state to forbid such activity. In contrast, if one appeals to the natural good of individual liberty, the benefits of market freedoms, respect for the
authority of persons over themselves, and the limited reasons for which persons
form civil society, it will be much less plausible within a Lockean framework that
the state possesses moral authority permissibly to forbid such a market.

More generally, just as Aquinas and Locke each engage a particular content-
full morality with specific presuppositions regarding natural goods, duties, liberties, virtues, and consequences, which when defended in a rational framework
give their arguments force, much of contemporary bioethics has sought top-down
guidance framed in terms of a rationally discoverable vision of proper conduct,
which authorizes state authority to constrain and direct citizens, groups, and
communities. As noted in chapter 2, this is the vision of Kant's universal legislator, who derives from a particular account of moral rationality and rational voli-

tion an understanding of appropriate human choice. Bioethics as a field of inquiry lays claim to a universal account of proper moral deportment, which thereby provides morally justifiable foundations for law and public policy—as well as, it is claimed, the legitimate authority for national and international institutions to guarantee uniformity of practice.

Consequently, bioethics has come to have a socialist, liberal, statist character, seeking protection of equality in the provision of health care and individual choice freed from the influence of traditional family and community power structures. Claiming the existence of "global moral consensus," bioethics seeks universal declarations on the ethical status of the human genome, the use of animals in research, embryo experimentation, third-party assisted reproduction, human organ sales for transplantation, and so forth. In short, bioethicists claim for themselves moral expertise with authority to guide court decisions, public deliberation, clinical decision, and legislative action.

As chapter 2 explored, however, in general secular terms, it is impossible to break through the seemingly interminable bioethical debates to univocal truth. All such attempts confront insurmountable obstacles: one must already presuppose a particular morality so as to choose among intuitions, rank consequences, evaluate exemplary cases, or mediate among various principles; otherwise one will be unable to make any rational choice at all. Even if one merely ranks cardinal moral concerns—such as liberty, equality, justice, and security—differently, one affirms different moral visions, divergent understandings of the good life, and varying senses of what it means to act appropriately. The price of particular content—that is, the adoption of content-full moral commitments—is the sacrifice of rationally attainable universality.

Claims to "global moral consensus," or to rationally discoverable moral truths, are implausible. Where reason can demonstrate that one must fulfill one's moral obligations to preserve oneself from blameworthiness, it can provide no necessary content with which to determine the nature or extent of such obligations. Here Hegel's account of why determinative moral content requires the specification of a particular context is illustrative of the challenges: "Since action for itself requires a particular content and a determinate end, whereas duty in the abstract contains nothing of the kind, the question arises: *what is duty?* For this definition [*Bestimmung*], all that is available so far is this: to do *right,* and to promote *welfare,* one's own welfare and welfare in its universal determination, the welfare of others."[108] Nothing in particular follows from the general notions of duty, the right, and so forth. Even to sort useful information from noise, one must already possess a moral sense, standards of evidence, and inference. That is, one must first specify a particular moral context within which to make decisions. Removing or ignoring the theological and cultural particularities that mark religious and moral differences thereby eliminates any context for understanding and assessing the content and veracity of moral claims. Without particular content, morality cannot distinguish among different accounts of the nature of the good life, much less provide definitive guidance on how to proceed when the right and the good conflict.

If one could through reason secure a particular moral content, there would in principle be a unique canonical rational morality to provide the terminus ad quem for the reasoned search for proper moral deportment and the justification of its enforcement.[109] The difficulty is that outside of an appeal to an all-encompassing moral and metaphysical viewpoint, such as those to which Aquinas, Locke, and Kant appeal, outside of a particular moral context, moral truth appears deeply ambiguous. The inevitably postmodern character of contemporary bioethics is simply the recognition of the foundationally irresolvable character of this moral pluralism in general secular terms. Given such circumstances, the claims of ideal choice theory, whether Kantian categorical imperative or Rawlsian hypothetical contractors, and so forth, are implausible. These intractable and sustained conflicts regarding the nature of the right and the good, appropriate choice among intuitions, ranking of consequences or cardinal moral concerns, and choosing among alternative evaluations of exemplary cases—much less how to reason by analogy from exemplary cases to new situations—demonstrate that the imposition of any particular moral content as the foundation of public policy simply assumes the truth of a particular morality.

The more general secular reason is unable to disclose a universal, coherent, content-full moral understanding of health care, or universal canonical moral justification for political authority to impose such a vision, the more one must seek alterative foundations. One possibility, which Nozick endorses in *Anarchy, State, and Utopia*, is to ground secular moral authority in freedom as permission—that is, freedom as a side constraint. Resolution of moral controversies regarding organ sales in such a framework will turn on whether the parties to the transaction have given consent. Freedom as a side constraint, as expressed in the existence of significant forbearance rights (where persons are free to venture with others, open to the possibility that one's choices may lead to success or failure), will support the existence of a free market in human organs. Moral authority is not being drawn from claims to "moral consensus" or ideal theories of rational action, or discovered through deep moral intuitions regarding consequences, human rights, or cardinal moral concerns, but rather is created from the actual agreement of the actual parties to collaborate. Collaborators need not agree regarding the background ranking of values or moral principles, cultural or religious assumptions—indeed, they may be deep moral strangers to each other. They need only affirm the content of their actual agreement, with the recognition that collaboration is possible through voluntary choice and peaceable agreement. Agreement or permission is the ground of the moral justification of such collaboration.

Nozick's account of legitimate moral authority distinguishes between the secular rights of persons and what may be virtuous, good, or proper to do. This contrast derives from his distinction between freedom as a side constraint and freedom as one value among others. For Nozick, one may not use other persons without their consent, even to achieve a significant good. Even if using some would be a good thing to do (e.g., in the sense that it would save lives or otherwise benefit the common good), no one has a right to do it. This appeal to the moral inviolability of persons is a variation on the Kantian insight that if one is obligated to respect persons as ends in themselves, one is obligated to respect their freedom. Freedom is not merely one value among others or a good that may be valued more or less along with other goods, but rather is a side constraint that captures a general secular moral obligation to respect the separateness of persons. Thus, one may not injure, steal from, defraud, or otherwise coerce unconsenting others—even to produce good consequences—without using them merely as a means to one's own ends. This would violate their status as free and responsible agents. Such an argument provides significant force to forbearance rights as well as rights to be protected from nonconsensual touching or use of one's person or property. It does not, however, create any content-full duties to others aside from those to which persons freely agree. One needs the actual consent of actual persons before using them to respect individuals as free persons.

Here the market is central for understanding morally authoritative human interaction. Market transactions and contractual relationships, including those that engage in commerce in human organs for transplantation, draw moral authority from the consent of the participants to be bound by their agreement. The parties to the transactions, themselves, freely convey authority to the enforcement of the specified conditions. Actual agreements among actual persons, therefore, limit the moral authority of others to interfere with the free interaction of consenting persons. Forbearance rights define a sphere in which one is morally immune from interference, protecting self-interest and self-preservation in the private use of person and property. Such rights describe side constraints prohibiting nonconsensual interference, which hold against other persons, as well as society and the state.

Nozick encapsulates this position as treating persons as individuals with separate lives, where one may not be sacrificed to achieve another's particular understanding of the good:

> Why not . . . hold that some persons have to bear some costs that benefit other persons more, for the sake of the overall social good? But there is no *social entity* with a good that undergoes some sacrifice for its own good. There are only individual people. . . . Using one of these people for the benefit of others, uses him and benefits the others. Nothing more. . . . Talk of an overall social good covers this up.[110] (original emphasis)

This is the case whether one seeks beneficently the good of others or paternalistically the good of individuals themselves. As Nozick argues:

> A line (or hyper-plane) circumscribes an area in moral space around an individual. . . . Voluntary consent opens the border for crossings. . . . My nonpaternalistic position holds that someone may choose (or permit another) to do to himself *anything*, unless he has acquired an obligation to some third party not to do or allow it.[111]

Respecting the freedom of persons constrains one to allow individuals to choose freely in their own best interests, even if they choose in ways one considers unwise.[112]

Moral political authority is derivative of the permission of persons. Thus, as already noted, the rights of persons will foreclose what many envision to be worthwhile goals. As Nozick argues, "the rights possessed by the state are already possessed by each individual in a state of nature . . . the state has no special rights."[113] Rather, governmental institutions may legitimately exercise only those rights that persons freely transfer to them. Persons consent to political authority and thus convey moral authority to social structures. Insofar as persons consent to transfer protection of particular rights to state institutions, such governmental authority gains moral legitimacy. Governments, even democratically elected majorities, do not possess moral authority to enforce uniform standards, to finance universal access, to regulate equal distribution of health care, or to forbid the consensual sale of human organs for transplantation. Morally authorized statutes are confined to the protection of persons' rights to forbearance, protection of individuals from battery, and to those additional policies to which actual persons give actual consent.

Persons, and organizations of persons, may be held responsible for nonconsensual acts of violence, fraud, and breach of contract, since such actions violate the rights of persons not to be touched or used without permission.[114] Forbearance rights make implausible interventions to forbid persons from freely using personal resources with consenting others, including the purchase of various types and levels of health care. The express agreement of those governed creates and thus also limits governmental authority to the extent of such agreement. So grounded, the state would have the general character of a starkly limited democracy. It would have no general moral authority to interfere in the medical marketplace generally, much less to interfere in the consensual choices of persons freely to participate in a commercial market for human organs.

Note, though, that the market is not being endorsed as a good in itself, nor are free choice and moral diversity celebrated in themselves as special goods. Rather, the market defines social space for peaceable consensual human interaction in all aspects of life. Here morality exists as the marketplace of ideas, moral visions, and understandings within which each peaceably pursues his own ends without necessarily sharing a common moral vision or understanding of justice. Respecting the freedom of persons defaults to protecting liberties of association, contract, conscience, and religion, and thereby to protecting the possibility of substantial moral diversity. Freely chosen, market-based health care financing, procurement, and distribution respects the liberty of persons to pursue their own deep moral commitments.

Consider Nozick's argument that individuals already own things prior to any particular society. There is no particular a priori distribution of wealth and resources that represents just allocation; provided that the history of acquisition and transfer has been without coercion, the final disposition of property is just. "There is no *central* distribution, no person or group entitled to control all the resources, jointly deciding how they are to be doled out."[115] The principles of justice are those of just acquisition, just transfer, and retribution for past injustice in acquisition and transfer. Persons receive resources from others who give to them in exchange for something or as a gift. "There is no more a distributing or distribution of shares than there is a distributing of mates in a society in which persons choose whom they shall marry."[116] Diverse individuals control varying resources, and new distributions arise out of the exchanges and actions of persons.[117] So, absent actual permission, it would be unjust to remove a kidney for transplantation from an individual with two healthy kidneys, even if another person would thereby significantly benefit.

Nozick captures this circumstance in terms of a distinction between freedom-based justice and goals-based justice. Goals-based justice is concerned with the achievement of the good of individuals in society. Freedom-based justice, in contrast, relates to permissible institutional moral authority and the distribution of goods made in accord with the actual consent of actual persons. Permission sets constraints on the permissible pursuit of beneficence, including the philanthropic use of human organs.[118] Morally permissible strategies to eliminate the disparity between organ availability and patients, who could benefit from transplantation, do not include compulsory redistribution, presumed consent, or coercive donation. Particular acts of kindness, such as donation of one's redundant kidney, or all of one's organs at death, are premised on the permission of individual persons who wish to make their organs available. Proponents of compulsory redistribution schemes, presumed consent, or governmental control over organ allocation should instead attempt to persuade people to donate organs voluntarily—according to an account of just distribution of organs—and to ignore those who offer organs for sale. Absent actual agreement, however, it would violate moral constraints to compel people who are entitled to their organs to donate against their will, to control to whom they may freely donate, or coercively to prohibit those who are inclined to buy and sell organs from doing so.

Nozick's account has special force with regard to ownership, distribution, and transfer of human organs. Human organs are not social resources that are grown, harvested, and distributed independently of actual persons. Rather, they come into existence already part of and owned by individuals.[119] On a goals-based account of distributive justice, one only has entitlement to things, including one's organs, insofar as such title is consistent with the promotion of the particular social goals or goods at stake.[120] In contrast, on Nozick's freedom-based justice, human organs are preeminent examples of "things [that] come into the world already attached to people having entitlement to them."[121] If one really owns things, such as one's internal organs, there will be forbearance-rights-based limits on distributive justice as well as on moral political authority to regulate one's use of such property. One may not claim title to the bodies of others without prior permission. The needs of others to organ transplantation will not erase the rights of some to utilize their organs as they see fit: to possess and enjoy or to transfer through donation or sale. On such an account, the permission of those who choose to participate settles the controversy regarding the moral authority of a market in human organs.

SUMMARY

While Aquinas, Locke, and Kant each argue for positions that, if taken at face value, would foreclose a market in human organs, on closer examination their standpoints do not unequivocally preclude the selling of redundant internal organs. If certain critical premises are reexamined in ways that are plausible, then these philosophers' arguments can support the permissibility of organ sales. It is important to note, however, that while these divergent moral accounts would in particular circumstances endorse the same conclusion regarding the permissibility of organ sales, they will not agree in all instances. Each presupposes quite different moral frameworks and background metaphysical assumptions, including assumptions regarding persons and the relationship of persons with their bodies. Moreover, the significance or theoretical force of the conclusion is in each case different.

For example, while the recast principle of totality and Nozickian libertarianism both allow one to utilize market institutions to create beneficence-based goods, they differ regarding when such appeal is morally acceptable as well as concerning the significance of charity. The reinterpreted principle of totality requires that one maintain the biological functional integrity of the donor when procuring organs or other body parts and tissues for donation or sale. While one can through charity take burdens upon oneself, and seek to help others through the market, one cannot seek directly to kill oneself. Nozick requires no such restrictions. Moreover, Thomists recognize the importance of charity as a good in its own right. For Nozick, the market merely creates social space for persons to

express philanthropy should they wish; the market neither endorses such beneficence as a good, independent of the ways in which persons value it, nor does the
market value beneficence-based transactions more than other types of for-profit
ventures. Philanthropy is an instance of persons cooperating with others in society to provide for themselves as well as for the needs of others.

Similarly, if one assumes with Locke that moral political authority is derivative of the consent of persons, then (as Nozick is aware) morally permissible social
prohibition of an organ market will depend on the ends for which persons form a
polity and whether they freely alienate sufficient liberty over themselves to societal institutions to authorize such proscription. Locke makes clear that individuals
have natural liberties to engage in market transactions. However, Locke also limits the authority persons have over themselves through natural-law-based duties.
Nozick's account fully endorses freedom as a side constraint, as defining a sphere
in which persons, vis-à-vis others, including political institutions, are morally
inviolable. Absent natural-law constraints that would forbid the selling of human
organs, Locke would likely agree with Nozick that only consent will create the
moral authority to prohibit a human organ market. Absent prior agreements, the
permission of those who freely choose to participate is sufficient morally to
authorize the creation of such a market. Locke's constraint against suicide would
likely limit sales from living vendors to redundant organs and regenerative tissues.
In this, his conclusion would resonate with that of the recast principle of totality.
However, while contemporary Thomists require an appeal to the good of others to
justify the removal of the healthy organ, Locke would likely embrace the natural
good of individuals having the freedom and responsibility to make such choices
over their lives. The significance of the conclusion thus varies from the importance of charity to the structure of individual liberty.

While Nozick argues that the rights of persons forbid, in principle, coercing
some beneficently to seek the good of others, he acknowledges that persons may
consent to philanthropy contracts, in which one agrees to protect the life and
health of others. Such agreement can create obligations to sell body parts. Past
agreements can constrain future choices. As the examination of Kant illustrated,
selling an organ is a plausible way, which would otherwise not be available,
directly to discharge a moral obligation or to raise funds to satisfy one's duties.
For Kant, insofar as the vendor does not will to destroy himself, the procurement
and sale of the organ is not incompatible with the health of the individual as a
moral agent, and the action is undertaken out of duty rather than inclination,
selling healthy human organs should be compatible with the categorical imperative. Nozick requires no such special conditions to be met morally to justify organ
sales. If the parties to the transfer give permission, the sale is permissible.

The context in which the moral decision to sell one's organs is made shapes
the significance of one's choices and actions. The recast arguments of Aquinas,

Locke, and Kant lead to conclusions similar to Nozick's position regarding the permissibility of selling redundant organs and regenerative tissues. However, each engages quite different premises and moral constraints and presumes a different moral theoretical context, including (1) the nature of liberty and responsibility, (2) the significance of acts of beneficence, (3) the moral importance of granting permission, (4) the ways in which seller intent shapes the permissibility of actions, and (5) the limits of moral political authority.

CHAPTER FIVE

Prohibition

More Harm Than Benefit?

ASPIRING TO AN INTERNATIONAL BIOETHICS

As a field of inquiry, Western bioethics aspires to an international political stage. Bioethicists almost inevitably lay claim to a universal account of morality, and professional moral deportment, including the purported foundations of law and public policy, as well as the moral authority for national law and international treaty to guide and hopefully guarantee uniformity of practice. Its claims are framed as assertions or discoveries of universal truths—for example, that there exists a global consensus that selling human organs for transplantation is a violation of basic human dignity, exploitative, and morally impermissible. Bioethics rarely pays adequate attention to the significant challenges that religious, cultural, and secular moral diversity presents to the crafting of political and institutional policy. Compassing persons from disparate and more or less intact moral communities with often widely varying moral intuitions and narratives, taken-for-granted moral norms, evaluations, and commitments, as well as diverse understandings of the common good, the national and international landscape is indeed complex and fragmented. One need only consider the acrimonious bioethical debates concerning abortion, human embryo research, health care allocation, stem cell research, euthanasia, and the marketing of human organs for transplantation to note that this fragmentation is often significant. Policy must be created to span a diverse set of individuals, cultures, and communities.

Yet such policy is never neutral. It inculcates and promotes the social and moral acceptance of certain practices, endorsing particular moral values over others. Political struggles regarding the structure and content of what will become the prevailing medical, moral, and social ethos are substantial. As chapter 2 illustrated, the various religious and secular moral viewpoints do not typically share a mutual understanding of the good life, much less of the meaning and significance of birth, suffering, and death. They differ regarding standards of evidence and rules of inference and generally do not share sufficient moral premises to resolve moral controversies through sound rational argument. Moreover, as believers of different religions, and followers of various secular "philosophies of life," persons do not usually agree on those individuals or institutions who are in authority to resolve moral controversies. For example, there exists a significant range of opinion regarding whether very low weight premature neonates should be sustained regardless of expense, likelihood of survival, or quality of life.[1] Similar questions arise regarding treatment of patients in a permanently vegetative state.[2] Should they be sustained, and if so, for what length of time, and using what methods (e.g., artificial nutrition and hydration)? Consider also: Is assisting in the suicide of a patient with terminal cancer an act of love and compassion or of murder? Which acts or omissions preserve human dignity?[3] Is the use of human embryos for research a positive good or is it equivalent to murder?[4] Should persons be understood as in authority over themselves to utilize their body parts for beneficence and profit? In short, we often meet as moral strangers.

Medical clinical encounters, as well as attempts to frame society-wide medical policy, are encumbered by these divisions.[5] Health care policy is fashioned out of the characteristics of the particular cultural and moral traditions of the underlying community. However, in contemporary morally pluralistic society there is no single moral tradition that binds all in a common normative or evaluative understanding. Policy must be created to span a diverse set of individuals and communities. Framing health care policy involves fashioning agreements that engender a common (and usually artificial) medical, social, and moral reality. Here, the crucial challenge is that given varying ontological, epistemological, and axiological presuppositions, different moral positions and political objectives will appear as not merely morally permissible but socially obligatory. Such fundamental conflicts define what have come to be referred to as the culture wars.[6]

FALSE CLAIMS TO MORAL CONSENSUS

As has been explored in this volume, much of contemporary bioethics advances philosophical arguments concerning the character of the moral world and its significance for medicine as if there were an uncontroversial common moral reality to which all appeal. Contemporary bioethics inevitably holds that a common moral foundation exists upon which a single content-full moral perspective can be erected. Bioethics has breathed new life into the Enlightenment hope of disclosing a single content-full morality binding on all persons as such. This effort is reflected in the significant recent attempts to capture and legislate a thick secular morality, including the proscription on the sale of human organs for transplantation.

Such unjustified assertions, however, cannot heal the fragmented character of moral reality. Within Western Europe, for example, there are substantial communities of socialists, Christian democrats, and liberals with a significant cleft between Christian and non-Christian moral and metaphysical understandings, including commitments to both family and society. In the United States and Canada, divisions are often even more substantial among Protestants, Roman Catholics, Mormons, and Orthodox Christians;[7] Orthodox, Conservative, Reform, and Secular Jews,[8] Buddhists, Muslims, Hindus, and so forth,[9] and yuppie cosmopolitan atheist secularists. Moreover, there are significant distinctions between the moral assessments of Western bioethicists working within industrial first-world medicine versus those in the developing world[10] or Asia.[11]

As Kazumasa Hoshino observes regarding the differences that characterize the United States and Western Europe versus Japan, such disputes are often substantial: "There are many subtle and overt racial, national, social, cultural, and religious differences among divergent societies, such as Japan and the United States. Such differences may explain the difficulties that the Japanese and other cultures have in accepting many Western principles of bioethics."[12] As he notes, Western bioethical reflections have, for better or worse, been imported into Japan, altering traditional Japanese understandings.[13] Yet, unlike the West, Japan remains in large measure a traditional society, with shared, non-Western, understandings of value and strong ties to culture, community, and family. The Japanese moral perspective draws on cultural and religious understandings that are often at odds with the conclusions that Western bioethicists endorse. In sum, moral understandings, accounts of human flourishing, and accepted social roles (such as the meaning of gender and appropriate expressions of sexuality) embodied in often taken-for-granted norms of human form and permissible behavior denote the conceptual frameworks that underlie moral decision making and thereby impact on public policy.

As this study has explored, such fundamental moral understandings are essential for critically assessing the possible metaphysical, moral, and political theoretical foundations of a market in human organs. The study has examined the metaphysical and moral conditions that would need to be met to legitimate the selling of human organs for transplantation. It has considered what it means to own internal organs, the circumstances in which governments have moral authority to regulate how persons dispose of their own body parts, and the probable advantages of a market in human organs. It has evaluated not only the likely moral and other benefits of such a market, but also the probable disadvantages of its prohibition. In so doing, the study has explored the arguments and assumptions cited in support of the supposed moral "consensus" that frames the nearly global prohibition on selling human organs for transplantation: that unlike altruistically motivated donation, offering financial incentives under-mines consent, coercing the poor into selling their organs, and that a market in human organs exploits the poor, violates human dignity, and is deeply morally repugnant. Moreover, opponents argue that such a market would lead to greater inequality and injustice between the rich and the poor as well as worse health care outcomes than the current system of donation.

The results of this study suggest that there are significant grounds for suspi-cion that such a "consensus," while pervasive, fails either to be universal or suffi-ciently justified. For example, it does not adequately consider basic foundational concerns regarding those factors that shift who shoulders the burden of proof as well as which reasons are relevant for meeting that burden. These include physi-ological and phenomenological distinctions among body parts (i.e., not all parts are necessary for embodiment or continued existence or even for adequate human functioning, nor are all parts experienced as part of oneself); the ontology of personhood (i.e., replacing body parts that are distinguishable and separable from the existence and embodiment of persons is compatible with the full con-tinued functioning of persons as rational moral agents); and the closeness of the analogy between ownership of one's body and ownership of other types of things (e.g., it is implausible simply to presuppose without significant further argument that human organs are a social or governmental, rather than private, resource). Moreover, the "consensus" tends to gloss over distinctions between future and present markets and the fact that many organs are harvested from cadaveric sources (i.e., former persons, who cannot be physically harmed by procurement) and that certain organs are more central to the existence of persons (e.g., the higher brain versus a redundant kidney). Often disregarded, as well, are the ways in which the burden of proof shifts with assumptions regarding the nature and ground of morally justified political authority.

The preceding chapters have argued that the global "consensus" appears in many areas to be not only unfounded but also misguided. While opponents argue that consent to organ sales is not fully voluntary, it is unlikely that barriers to autonomous consent respect the distinction between altruistic donation and commercial sale. It may be true that for consent to organ donation to be morally effective it must be informed and free of coercion; however, concerns to provide adequate information regarding the risks of surgery or of the potential for serious complications apply to both donation and sale. Such concerns can be amelio-rated in each case in the light of further analysis. Moreover, offers to purchase organs cannot easily be understood as coercing the poor into selling. Such offers do not situate potential vendors in unjustified disadvantaged circumstances, nor do they deprive vendors of any preexisting options. Regardless of whether organs are donated or sold, it is impossible fully to insulate patients and family members from external social and institutional pressures. In either circumstance, incentives are strongest if the medical or financial resources are needed to avoid the suffering and death of a loved one. While offers to purchase organs may be seductive, they are not necessarily coercive. Indeed, they propose to advantage vendors in ways to which they have no prior entitlement. Moreover, autonomous rational choice among the available options remains possible.

Provided that physical and psychological harms are adequately compensated, vendors and recipients each benefit from the exchange. If moral harms, such as the objectification of persons as mere collections of spare parts, are minimized, it is implausible to understand the market as necessarily exploitative. The market increases the number of options open to impoverished individuals to improve their prospects while saving the lives of patients who are desperately ill. In contrast, prohibition appears to exploit the poor and sick to support particular views of moral propriety and human dignity, denying those impoverished and ill an important opportunity freely to choose how best to advantage themselves.

All systems of organ procurement and allocation objectify and commodify human body parts, even donation. Incentives and policies to increase organ availability, whether through donation or sale, evoke an industry designed to procure, allocate, and transplant human organs. This industry, whether for-profit or nonprofit, recasts organs as a scarce medical resource and "product" of exchange. In each case, one has specified a market for human organs, albeit a heavily regulated market, with carefully stipulated conditions regarding who bears the costs and benefits of procurement, distribution, and transplantation. It is inadequate to criticize commercial markets as improperly commodifying human organs without also addressing this critique to systems of donation. In short, while at times couched in terms of improper commodification, the debate is less about commodification than about who should receive the medical resources and who should bear the costs of appropriation and transfer.

As the exploration of Kant's position demonstrated, selling organs is consistent with many influential conceptions of human dignity: vendors do not will to destroy themselves, and selling an organ is a plausible manner in which to discharge a duty of charity. Moreover, organ selling is less risky than many other occupations. It is consistent with the health of persons, and the practice of saving others supports the respect and dignity of moral agents. Those who sell redundant internal organs participate in a livesaving activity, heroically, at some risk to themselves, which is intended to alleviate suffering and to foster human dignity. Indeed, as the analysis of Aquinas's principle of totality suggested, insofar as one's intention in removing the organ is not to destroy the natural good of the body, then the sale of internal redundant organs can be consistent with the good of bodily functional wholeness.[14] Those who sell organs engage in transactions that can help others through the market and through the provision of resources otherwise not available. Selling an organ enables an individual to cooperate with others in society to provide for the needs of others, as well as for oneself. While prohibition is robustly paternalistic, demeaning the poor and sick by considering them unable to make moral decisions about their own fates, the market respects the dignity of vendors and patients as persons and rational moral agents able to make choices about their own lives.

On balance, concern with issues of equality and liberty favors a system of payments to those who supply organs and other human tissues. While opponents claim that a market will lead to a situation in which the poor will sacrifice their bodies for the health of the rich, while the rich gain unequal (and therefore unfair) access to a scarce medical resource, prohibition forcibly prevents those worse off—that is, the poor and the sick—from bettering their own situations. Insofar as a commercial market leads to an increase in the number of available organs for transplant, all potential recipients, whether rich or poor, stand a better chance of receiving transplants.

This view also incorporates the idea that persons have the right to treat at least some physical parts of their bodies in some respects as objects of possession, gift, and trade, such that it is plausible to understand the sources of human organs as entitled to the value of the benefits ultimately derived from their use. Legislating that donors may only transfer organs as a gift does not thereby reduce the value of such organs to zero. Rather it utilizes state coercive force to transfer the value of the organs from donors and their families to other parties—nothing more. Increasing vendor compensation reduces this strikingly unequal allocation of costs and benefits.

Organ selling may be a means to generate resources for the poor that can be reinvested in personal as well as familial economic development, thereby decreasing financial inequalities. Even if a market might lead to some initial losses in equal access to expensive health care, this may be compensated for at the social level by gains in individual liberty and personal and family wealth, and lessening of total human suffering.

Community solidarity and altruism are also likely supported by the creation of a market. While prohibition closes off options for increasing the supply of organs, the existence of a market creates social space for persons to interact in the pursuit of private family and social goals. These may include directed dona- tion to members of one's family or even to members of a particular minority, the sale of organs to raise funds to feed and house the poor, or the pooling of money to purchase organs for the impecunious. If it is altruistic for a parent to give a kid- ney to a child to save his life, it can similarly be altruistic for a parent to sell a kidney to pay for a lifesaving operation. A market in organs creates and respects further opportunities for the expression of social solidarity and private altruism.

With regard to health care outcomes, it is plausible that a market would fare better than current systems of donation. Commercial incentives have the promise of leading to greater organ availability, with organs of better quality, and more efficient organ procurement for transplantation. Legal safeguards from tort liability, which are unavailable under donation, gear in with market-based organ procurement, transplantation, and scientific research. Torts predicated on warranty or strict liability are only possible if the transplanted organ is understood as a good that is being sold to the recipient. Organs removed from living persons are also more likely to be of significant use to recipients. They have greater vitality and can be screened in advance for defects, disease, or other negative transplant indicators. If organs are primarily procured from the recently deceased, such as accident victims, one loses both vitality and, in the press of time, some screening opportunities. Organ quality may be problematic precisely because of insufficient commercialization. In addition, as has been explored, indirect health benefits and life expectancy associated with increases in income, or resources to support educational training, are advantages in favor of permitting such a market. Insofar as there exists a social commitment to provide all with access to adequate health care, including organ transplantation, this commitment will very likely be more effectively achieved with a market rather than through prohibition.

Finally, the purported moral repugnance of organ selling is neither a feeling nor an intuition all share. Feelings about the inappropriate nature of commerce in human organs can be countered by equally strong but contrary feelings. For example, those who object that organ vending is morally repugnant because the procurement operation is not performed for therapeutic purposes should recognize that such criticisms apply equally to procurement in the case of altruistic donation. The Hippocratic injunction "primum non nocere" is equally satisfied or violated in either situation.

The exploration of Locke's arguments concluded that given adequate medical and social safeguards, selling organs is not plausibly analogous to slavery or suicide. Therefore, comparisons with such practices are solely inflammatory, possessing at best rhetorical force. As with other ethical controversies, such as homosexuality, physician-assisted suicide, genetic engineering, and abortion, one must determine whether generalized feelings of moral repugnance or intuitions regarding the wrongness of an action are justified prior to presupposing that such ought to carry any weight in meeting the burden of proof, or lowering the standard of proof, to proscribe organ sales.

The arguments of the preceding chapters suggest in sum that there are good grounds for holding that the allegedly global "consensus" does not have the strength usually assumed. Indeed, there are strong reasons for reassessing the foundational arguments it claims for support. First, it fails adequately to appreciate the phenomenological and physiological distinctions among different body parts, the relative strength of ownership rights, and the general significance of forbearance, privacy, and property rights. Second, the "consensus" fails as well to take adequate account of the ways in which a market would likely maximize health care benefits; promote equality, liberty, altruism, and social solidarity; protect persons from exploitation; and preserve regard for human dignity more successfully than prohibition. Finally, with regard to Aquinas, Locke, and Kant, in each case their positions on closer examination do not globally preclude the selling of redundant internal organs. If certain premises are reexamined and recast in plausible ways, then their general positions can support the permissibility of organ sales.

CRAFTING HEALTH CARE POLICY AMID MORAL PLURALISM
The Failure to Secure a Particular Ethic

To establish a choice as preferable requires determining preferable according to whom and with respect to what set of criteria. An adequately articulated answer requires an actual determination of facts and a specification of the moral criteria employed. Insofar as one recognizes that there are a number of equally defensible but quite different moral perspectives, one loses hope of a unique authoritative secular viewpoint from which to justify certain decisions. Moral content is gained at the price of universality. Securing a particular ethic requires specification of premises and content that will not be acknowledged among moral strangers.

There have been many attempts to heal this rift in medical practice and moral reflection. Some have sought moral guidance, for example, in the lived phenomenological experience of illness or within the practical caring of nurses. Here the attempt is to secure a practical ethic in which abstract moral principles gain content through everyday understandings of what it means to the patient himself to be ill, to recover, or to move toward eventual death with a chronic illness, such as organ failure. It is argued that moral perspective is gained at the level of everyday consciousness, including all the thoughts, feelings, and actions that go into caring for oneself and others. Thoughts and feelings are fused with practical presence and human interaction, as Rosemarie Tong urges, "care (benevolence, human-heartedness) is the virtue without which true human community and, therefore, bona-fide moral relations are impossible."[15] "At the heart of the care orientation," contends Alisa Carse, "is a focus on the facts of human vulnerability and interdependency, particularly as they are expressed in asymmetries of need and dependency."[16] Deep empathetic connections with patients prompt the move from a dispassionate ethic of the primacy of individual freedom and the commodification of health care, to an ethic of a caring community; a "transformation of health care systems into caring communities"—systems in which the good for patients can be instantiated.[17]

The challenge remains, though, that particular understandings of the good for patients often conflict with notions of the good for providers, families, and society.[18] Patients and providers do not operate in a vacuum in which the good of the patient is the only interest that ought to be considered. Each treatment choice allocates resources to some patients at the expense of decreasing resource availability for others. As has been argued, this is very much the case in organ transplantation. Allocating extensive scarce medical resources to the identifiable patient out of compassion, while allowing "statistical persons" to go without, often leads to the death and suffering of many others. Statistical persons have names and faces, but are outside of the public eye; without efficient and effective use of scarce resources they die just the same. Policy regarding organ procurement and allocation necessarily changes the opportunities of potential recipients, privileging some over others. Medical choices themselves allocate resources away from nonmedical needs.

As Paul Menzel has noted, the fundamental drive behind rationing in the medical context is that there are other things in life besides health care on which we can use our finite resources. One might expect, for example, that the fewer resources to which individuals have access, the more likely they are to ration high-cost, low-impact care. "Thus poor people, if they can control the use of their resources (their own private resources plus any societal assisted ones to which they have access), would naturally ration care before wealthier people would."[19] Given limited available resources, those with lower income would very likely choose differently than wealthier ones.

In addition, such choices require taking into account the "best interests" of vendors, recipients, and their families. The difficulty is specifying the content of "best interests." Who ought to judge? Consider two conflicting resource allocation policies, each of which purports to secure the best interests of patients. The first policy offers high-morbidity/low-mortality health care. Resources are allocated to expensive life-prolonging treatments and end-of-life care, including organ transplantation, kidney dialysis, and intensive care for severely deformed and anencephalic neonates. Resource availability for nonemergency medical activities is limited. Treatments that increase mobility, such as knee and hip replacements, are either unavailable or must be paid for out of pocket. The second policy offers low-morbidity/high-mortality health care to enhance life options, limit pain, increase mobility, and enhance freedom from illness. Treatments include knee and hip replacements, vision and hearing care, inoculation from disease, and other forms of preventive medicine. Such a policy limits access to high-cost/low-yield end-of-life treatments, and allocates no resources to kidney dialysis or organ transplantation. As Allan Gibbard makes the point: "It may be a better prospect—rationally to be preferred, that is, on prudential grounds—to enjoy what the premium will buy if one is healthy and risk needing the treatment and not being able to get it, than to live less well if healthy and get the treatment if one needs it."[20] Advocates of each policy argue that it implements health care that is in patients' "best interests." Which type of policy should guide biomedical decision making?

Given the many possible responses, determining the patient's best interests requires defining "best interests," specifying "for whom" and "by what criteria." Physicians, nurses, families, policy makers, and patients each provide different perspectives on a multifaceted and differentiated set of consequences, rights, liberties, and ethical solutions. Being attentive to the physical and emotional needs of a patient may assist in the clarification of some sources of the "good" of the patient. But this will not wholly settle the question at issue because it will not justify a unique, much less necessarily true, understanding of the "good."

Emotive caring has the benefit of reaching toward the humanity of the patient with tenderness and compassion. It struggles, however, under the burden of needing to differentiate between the patient's and the provider's perhaps quite different notions of well-being and benevolence. Also, caring may involve disengagement from medical, societal, and familial reality. How is one to understand appropriately the humanity of the patient? In addition, such emotive accounts collide with moral theories, such as that of Kant, who argued for an objective rational morality, articulated without direct reference to human feelings and inclinations. A perfectly rational, autonomous, Kantian moral agent would necessarily act on the objective necessity of the moral imperatives. Acting on emotions or other inclinations assimilates content-full maxims that are subjectively contingent, would not be objectively universalizable for all rational agents, and would involve heteronomy, rather than free, autonomous, moral action. For Kant, acting on emotion (even deeply felt repugnance) or other personal inclination has no moral worth.[21]

Those who urge emotive bioethical accounts often regard this Kantian position as removing human feeling from the realm of morality as "a disreputable, arbitrary irrelevant partner weakening the authority of reason."[22] However, if one is to hold, contra Kant, that our natural feelings should be embraced as important, formative elements of morality—consider Kass's "The Wisdom of Repugnance"[23]—then one must presuppose a content-full account of the rules for identifying and ranking the emotions that are to qualify. Do all emotive reactions by all parties point to important moral features of a situation? Which emotions should we take as authoritative and how should we quantify them intra- and interpersonally? And if the emotive reactions of different persons and communities to particular types of health care—such as selling human organs for transplantation—are different, how should those that are canonical be identified?

Others have sought an internal morality of medicine from the insights and goals of physicians. As Keyserlingk argues: "It does appear to me slightly absurd that many of us seem quite prepared to accept a degree of moral guidance from many who have seen and shared far less of life, death, suffering, human frailty, commitment and courage than have many physicians."[24] The internal morality of medicine is believed to come from reflection of the goods and ends of the practice of medicine itself: medical practice, it is argued, is seen by those working in this field, as having "goods" or "ends" internal to it—that is, that certain ends are inherent to and constitutive of the behavior of physicians.[25] Clarifying the appropriate ends of medicine—such as the healing and health of patients—is believed to clarify the moral standards to guide medical practice.[26]

Yet why would medical authority and expertise necessarily entail moral authority and expertise? Does working closely with patients help one to develop appropriate ethical theory or moral judgment? Or does it harden one to the casual acceptance of immoral behavior? Does one begin to cloud the truth with emotive valences that make facing medical (and perhaps moral) reality more difficult? The latter is at times clearly the case with families whose emotional responses of love or guilt render them unable to accept the medical reality and finality of the dying patient. And as Baruch Brody points out, this emotional situation is also experienced by health care professionals.[27] The challenge is then to identify "good judgment." As has been noted, there are a variety of opinions, even within the medical community, regarding the moral appropriateness of commercializing organ appropriation and allocation. Even if we attempt to ground morality in the judgment of physicians, the problem of identifying good judgment remains.

We confront the problem not only of defining the "good" but also of determining how the "good" ought to be realized. Many appeal, as Veatch points out, to an emerging moral consensus that the patient is the best authority of his own best interests:

> Increasingly, a consensus is emerging over the underlying moral and legal principles for resolving these cases. Where there is agreement that the patient is competent to make his or her own medical decisions and the treatment is proposed for the patient's own good, the autonomous choice of the individual patient to refuse medical treatment has in every single case been found to take precedence over the desire to prolong the patient's life.[28]

According to Veatch, there is a consensus that insofar as the patient is competent, he is the best judge of his own best interests, and his decision (at least to refuse treatment) should in the end trump, as long as no significant interests of others are at stake.

Insofar as such a consensus exists, though, it should plausibly extend to allowing potential organ vendors to make judgments regarding their own best interests. It would thus support the existence of an organ market—rather than paternalistic prohibition.

However, here—as with all claims to the existence of a "consensus"—one must determine who is party to the consensus, as well as how and why it should bind those who do not concur with it. How in particular should one respond to conscientious objectors to the consensus? Does one use coercive force so that autonomous nonconsenters comply with the general consensus, or should they be allowed peaceably to ignore the community's moralistic viewpoint, acting on their own judgments of their own best interests? Why, for example, should those who wish to sell their redundant internal organs be forbidden on the grounds of a consensus to which they are not party?

Moreover, such an account of patient autonomy collides with an obligation of forbearance in the sense that the patient is in authority over his own person and ought not to be interfered with or touched without permission. Forbearance rights understood as part of the essential grammar of morality,[29] or as necessary side constraints,[30] do not have any particular content and do not depend on a moral consensus. Rather, forbearance rights are advanced as constitutive parts of the very practice of morality. As has been explored, they are meant to strictly limit the moral authority of physicians, health care workers, and society to interfere with patients except in those instances in which patients themselves consent to the treatment. By an appeal to such rights patients are able to refuse medical treatment that they find burdensome or inappropriate. Often captured under the terminology of autonomy, forbearance rights limit the moral authority of others to force nonconsenters to act in conformity with general agreement. Insofar as objectors to the consensus, which Veatch advances regarding patient autonomy, or which much of the world purportedly advances regarding the sale of human organs for transplantation, act peaceably with consenting collaborators, the moral authority for others, including the state, to interfere is limited.

The Unjustified Coercion of Legislative Moral Monism

Biomedical ethics has become an often willing agent of political power.[31] Indeed, the power vested in the medical and bioethical community has become increasingly significant. Bioethical commissions inform public policy at state, national, and international levels. Its authoritative judgment is sought on nearly all aspects of life: from copulation and birth, appropriate diet, sexual behaviors, and methods of child rearing, to abortion, infanticide, suffering, and death. Bioethical expertise serves as the basis of expert testimony in courts of law and is widely sought in the framing of public and institutional policy.[32] Since medicine is such a pervasive aspect of modern culture, this agency has significant potential to be particularly insidious.

Judged solely in terms of expenditures, health care commands nearly one out of every seven dollars in the United States. In 2002 this amounted to some 14.6 percent of the gross domestic product (GDP), roughly $5,627 per capita. In comparison, health care as a percentage of GDP in 2002 was 9.6 percent in Canada (US$2,931 per capita), 10.9 percent (US$2,817) in Germany, 9 percent (US$2,515) in Belgium, 7.7 percent (US$2,220) in Austria, and 7.7 percent (US$2,160) in the United Kingdom.[33] In the United States in 2003, health care spending rose to approximately $5,440 per capita, or about 15.3 percent of the GDP.[34] Such increasingly significant investment of personal and social resources is driven by a perceived technological and moral imperative to ameliorate the consequences of age, injury, and disease, and thereby extend life and alleviate suffering. Combined with the belief that rational argument delivers the particulars of medical morality, claims to global "moral consensus," and the denial of the existence of substantial moral difference, as well as assumptions regarding the importance of equality of condition and legitimate political authority to enforce such moral views, this technological imperative provides the secular equivalent of orthodox belief; bioethical disagreement is to be at least shunned, if not actively persecuted.[35]

As this study has shown, moral foundations and particular moral content forged through a consensus will likely form a stable structure for social policy only if it is coercively enforced upon dissenters, thus failing to respect the fundamental differences among persons and content-full moral communities. Endeavoring to bridge the gap among moral strangers and diverse moral communities, governments have attempted to establish a universal "moral culture" by decree. There is a concern to legislate and regulate a single moral culture that speaks with authority to all.[36] The establishment of moral values and goals is evermore being thrust into the political arena.

This attempt has been especially significant in Europe. Consider, for example, the basic human rights that the European Bioethics Convention, The Barcelona Declaration, enumerates: autonomy, dignity, integrity, and vulnerability. Respecting personal autonomy is spelled out in terms of protecting and enhancing individual capacities for (1) the "creation of ideas and goals of life," (2) "moral insight, 'self-legislation,' and privacy," (3) "reflexion (sic) and action without coercion," (4) "personal responsibility and political involvement," and (5) informed consent.[37] Similarly, dignity, integrity, and vulnerability are explicated in terms of preserving the material, psychological, and social conditions for individuals to achieve their own abilities and goals. Where consideration for personal dignity requires ensuring that individuals are able to express "autonomous action," individual integrity compasses the "basic condition of the dignified life, both physical and mental . . . respect for privacy and in particular for the patient's understanding of his or her own life and illness."[38] Respecting persons, it is held, consists in appreciating the finitude and fragility of human life, which in turn is seen as grounding a general obligation to care for those who are perceived as vulnerable.[39]

Thus, it is concluded, all must be guaranteed the material conditions as well as psychological and social support necessary to ameliorate physical, social, and health disadvantages. State regulations and institutional guidelines ought to be crafted to protect those whose autonomy, dignity, or integrity is perceived as threatened. Family, social, and community barriers (such as religious, racial, gender, or sexual bias) should be removed so that all are freed from situations in which they do not choose for themselves, are educated in the capacities of free choice, and enjoy the resources necessary to equally impact outcomes. All individuals are seen as possessing basic human rights to state assistance sufficient to enable them to release their potential,[40] including organ transplantation without income or social barriers.

Legislative action attempts to create a content-full biopolitics that binds all, with particular understandings of germ-line genetic engineering, artificial reproduction, transplantation, and so forth. As a consequence there have been significant attempts (often successful)[41] to prohibit genetic enhancement to increase personal performance, along with prohibition against any modification not directly related to disease, and, as documented throughout this study, to prohibit the sale of human organs for transplantation.

As I have argued, though, empirical evidence belies any claim to the existence of a universal morality. Rather, a significant diversity of moral viewpoints in contemporary society compete without an apparent principled basis for definitively establishing one as uniquely true. Medical practice is shaped by particular understandings of the reasonable amount of pain to be borne, the kinds of functions and abilities men and women should have at different points in their lives, what should count as deformities and disfigurements, what should be regarded as the normal ranges of life, how much of one's own or community resources ought to be spent to postpone death, and under what circumstances death should be accepted as natural or inevitable. Adequately to address such issues, health care policy must be fashioned out of the characteristics of the cultural and moral understandings of the underlying community. Attempts to frame uniform society-wide health care policy are thus significantly encumbered if moral pluralism is marked by real and substantive divisions.

The essential question, then, regards coping with such pluralism. On the one hand, there is the dominant political strategy of denying the significance of moral disagreement, to discount or marginalize those who disagree as nonmainstream or radical, or even to dismiss alternate views as hopelessly irrational. Yet, prima facie, such heavy-handedness simply imposes one moral viewpoint over others. Alternatively, one could honestly face the foundational challenges of biotechnology, health care financing, allocation of resources, and development of the biomedical sciences while preserving social space for diverse understandings of right conduct and human flourishing. As explored in previous chapters, here the market fares more successfully than governmental regulation and legalistic prohibition.

The general predicament lies in establishing the moral authority coercively to impose a particular moral culture through state legislation. If the state is to draw a morally authoritative line between appropriate and inappropriate uses of the body and its parts, then it must possess moral authority to impose such decisions. The commercialization of human organ procurement and allocation, even if limited to organs from brain-dead or cadaver sources, offers significant untapped potential for addressing this current health care crisis. If extended to include internal redundant organs, its potential for saving human life and reducing suffering appears markedly to increase. Without a valid demonstration that such legislation has moral authority, restrictions on the market are only legally, not morally, authoritative. In the absence of a successful sound rational argument or an appeal to a moral authority acceptable to all to demonstrate that this particular moral culture ought to be so privileged, such legislation will be without general moral authority.

However, as this study has explored, in many regards Western European and American bioethics appears committed to preserving significant elements of a moral vision that could only find deep justification in a religious account. This phenomenon appears to reflect a desperate attempt to recapture moral content and guidance that has been lost as the underlying Western cultures complete a profound transition toward becoming post-Christian. The bioethics project reflects an attempt to secure, by reason and legislation, elements of the Christian tradition outside of an exclusively Christian community and without acknowledgment of the Christian Deity. Aquinas could draw on the richness of a background religious morality in ways that are simply unavailable to Western secular bioethics. Contemporary bioethics finds itself in a position with great similarity to Kantian rationalism: the kingdom of grace becomes equivalent to the kingdom of reason,[42] with moral reason given a very particular content.

Europe, much less Northern America, can no longer claim that it is Christendom: a Christian community with a single, content-full, coherent, and all-encompassing morality. Instead it contains a plurality of moral cultures. Recasting moral controversies, such as human organ sales for transplantation, within the legal arena offers a sociopragmatic resolution to a complicated moral dilemma. The result, however, is a cardinal difficulty in providing a morally authoritative foundation for the content that is legally enforced.[43]

Moral controversies achieve closure through loss of interest, agreement, force, or sound rational argument.[44] While one might hope to resolve the controversy regarding organ sales through sound rational argument, this study provides significant grounds for concluding that the global "consensus" to proscribe organ sales fails to take adequate account of many of the issues central to the debate. Indeed, this study provides significant medical, moral, and social policy reasons for holding that legal prohibition of organ sales causes more harm than benefit. Despite the apparent potential of a market in human organs to increase the efficiency and effectiveness of organ procurement, as well as the number of organs available for transplantation, the global "consensus" continues to hold that such a market is morally impermissible and actively promotes global prohibition. Yet the urgent public health challenge due to the considerable disparity between the number of patients who could benefit from organ transplantation and the number of human organs that are available for transplant will not be resolved through a rhetoric of moral repugnancy, exploitation, and human dignity. All of these considerations leave us with a well-founded basis critically to approach current national and international proscription of payments for human organs for transplantation. If this public health crisis is to be adequately addressed and remedied, any future policy maker's assessment must honestly recognize the possibility that the market is the most efficient and effective—and morally justified—means of procuring and allocating organs for transplantation.

APPENDIX

Sample of International Legislation Restricting the Sale of Human Organs for Transplantation

Algeria: *On Health Protection and Promotion*, Law No. 85-05 (February 16, 1985) *Journal Official de la République Algérienne Démocratique et Populaire* 8 (February 17, 1985): 122–140; amended and supplemented (August 19, 1998), *Journal Officiel de la République Algérienne Démocratique et Populaire* 61 (August 23, 1998): 3–5.

Argentina: *On the Transplantation of Human Organs and Anatomical Materials. The Recording in National Identity Documents of the Holder's Wishes with Regard to the Authorization of Removal*, Resolution No. 1000 (R.N.P.) (December 14, 1993), *Anales de Legislación Argentina* LIV-A (1994): 560–561.

Australia (New South Wales): *An Act Relating to the Donation of Tissues by Living Persons, the Removal of Tissue from Deceased Persons, the Conduct of Post-mortem Examinations of Deceased Persons, and Certain Other Matters*, Law No. 164 (December 31, 1983), *Prohibition of Trading in Tissue*, chapter 6, section 32.

Australia (Northern Territory): *An Act to Make Provision for and In Relation to the Removal and Use of Human Tissues, for Post-mortem Examinations, for the Definition of Death and for Related Purposes*, Law No. 121 (1979), *Prohibition of Trading in Tissue*, part 5, paragraphs 24(1)–24(5).

Australia (Queensland): *The Transplantation and Anatomy Act* (1979–1984), *Prohibition of Trading in Tissue*, part 7, sections 40–44.

Australia (South Australia): *The Transplantation and Anatomy Act* (1983), *Prohibition of Trading in Tissue*, part 7, section 35(1)–35(6).

Australia (Tasmania): *The Human Tissue Act* (1985), *Prohibition of Trading in Tissue*, part 4, section 27(1)–27(5).

Australia (Western Australia): *The Human Tissue Act* (1982), *Prohibition of Trading in Tissue*, part 5, sections 29–30.

Austria: *Amending the Hospitals Law*, Federal Law of June 1, 1982 (Serial No. 273), *Bundesgesetzblatt für die Republik Österreich* 113 (June 18, 1982): pp. 1161–1162; chapter F: "Removal of Organs or Parts of Organs from the Bodies of Deceased Persons for Transplantation Purposes," section 62a(4).

Belgium: *On the Removal and Transplantation of Organs* (June 13, 1986), *Moniteur belge* 32 (February 14, 1987): 2129–2132, chapter 1, section 4(1)–4(2).

Belgium: *On the Removal and Allocation of Organs of Human Origin*, Crown Order of November 24, 1997, *Moniteur belge* (December 23, 1997, No. 243): 34527– 34531.

Bolivia: *On the Donation and Transplantation of Organs, Cells, and Tissues*, Law No. 1716 (November 5, 1996).

Brazil: Constitution of the Federative Republic of Brazil, *Diário Oficial* (October 5, 1988): section 199, item 4.

Brazil: *Organ Donation*, Law No. 9434 (February 1997) and Law No. 10211 (March 2001).

Bulgaria: Resolution No. 189 of (July 16, 2001) of the Council of Ministers amending the *Regulations* [as amended] *for the Implementation of the Law on Public Health* adopted by Resolution No. 23 (1974) of the Council of Ministers, *D'rzhaven Vestnik* (2001, No. 66), *Sluzheben Buletin* (2001, No. 13): 48–50.

Canada (New Brunswick): *An Act (Chapter 44) to Amend the Human Tissue Act* (date of assent: June 18, 1986), *Acts of New Brunswick*, 1986, section 8(3).

Canada (Ontario): *The Human Tissue Gift Act*, 1982, part 3, section 10.

Canada: *Trillium Gift of Life Network Act*, R.S.O. 1990, chapter H.20, Amended by 1998, c. 18, sched. G, s. 58; 1999, c. 6, s. 29; 2000, c. 39; 2002, c. 18, sched. I, s. 20.

Canada: *The Uniform Human Tissue Donation Act* (1990), section 15(1)–15(3).

Chile: Law No. 19451 [establishing rules governing the transplantation and donation of organs], March 29, 1996, *Diario Official de la República de Chile* (April 10, 1996, No. 35438): Article 145.

Colombia: Decree No. 1172, *For the Partial Implementation of Title IX of Law No. 9 of 1979, as Regards the Procurement, Preservation, Storage, Transplantation, Destination and Final Utilization of Anatomical Organs or Parts, and the Procedures for Their Transplantation in Human Beings, as well as of Law No. 73 of 1988*, June 6, 1989, *Legislation Económica*, Bogotá 74(881) (June 30, 1989): 760–776, chapter 2, section 17.

Costa Rica: Law No. 5560, *On Human Transplants*, August 20, 1974, *La Gaceta— Diário Oficial* 165 (3 September 1974): 4362, section 14; Law No. 7409 [authorizing the transplantation of human organs and anatomical materials], May 12, 1994, *Colección de Leyes, Decretos y Reglamentos* (1994, vol. 1): L255–L260.

Council of Europe: Resolution (78) 29, *On Harmonisation of Legislations of Member States to Removal, Grafting and Transplantation of Human Substances*, May 11, 1978, Article 9; Recommendation No. R (97) 16 of the Committee of Ministers to Member States, *Liver Transplantation from Living Related Donors*, adopted by the Committee of Ministers on September 30, 1997, at the 602nd meeting of the Ministers' Deputies; *Additional Protocol to the Convention on Human Rights and Biomedicine, on Transplantation of Organs and Tissues of Human Origin*, Strasbourg, January 24, 2002 (http://conventions.coe.int/treaty/EN/Treaties/Html/186.htm).

Cyprus: Law No. 97, Section 4, *On the Removal and Transplantation of Biological Materials of Human Origin*, 1987, *Episêmi Ephimerida tês Kypriakês Dêmokratias* 2230, supplement no. 1 (May 22, 1987): 921–926, section 4.

Czech Republic: Act 285/2002, *On Donation, Removal, and Transplantation of Organs and Tissues, and Amending Certain Acts (The Transplantation Act)*, coll. of May 30, 2002.

Denmark: Law No. 402, *On the Examination of Cadavers, Autopsies, and Transplantation, etc.*, June 13, 1976, *Lovtidende for Kongeriget Danmark* 63, part A (June 13, 1990): 1331–1334, chapter 6, section 20, subsection 3.

Dominican Republic: Law No. 60–88, *On the Donation of Corneas*, August 30, 1988, *Gaceta Oficial* 9742 (August 31, 1988): 5–8, sections 11–12.

Ecuador: Law No. 64, *Reforming the Health Code*, May 26, 1987, *Registro Oficial* 707 (15 June 1987): section 1: "Declaration of death and the transplantation of parts, tissues, and organs of the human body"; Law No. 58, *On Organ and Tissue Transplantation*, July 5, 1994, *Registro Oficial* (July 27, 1994, No. 492): 1–4.

Estonia: *The Transplantation of Organs and Tissues Act*, January 30, 2002, *Riigi Teataja* 1 (2002, 21): 118.

Finland: Law No. 355, *On the Removal of Human Organs and Tissues for Medical Purposes*, April 26, 1985, *Finlands Forfattningssamling* 355–358 (May 6, 1985): 741–743, section 11; Law No. 101, *On the Use of Human Organs and Tissues for Medical Purposes*, February 2, 2001, *Finlands Författningssamling* (February 8, 2001, Nos. 101–105): 249–256.

France: Law No. 76–1181, dated December 22, 1976, *On the Removal of Organs*, *Journal Officiel de la Republique française, Editiondes Lois et Decrets* 299 (December 23, 1976): 7365, section 39.

France: Decree No. 2000–409 of May 11, 2000, on the reimbursement of expenses incurred during the removal of elements or the collection of products of the human body for therapeutic purposes, and supplementing the Public Health Code (Second Part: Decrees made after consulting the Conseil d'Etat), *Journal oficiel de la République française, Lois et Décrets* (May 18, 2000, No. 115): 7433–7434.

Germany: Act of November 5, 1997, on the donation, removal, and transplantation of organs (*The Transplantation Act*), *Bundesgesetzblatt, Part I* (November 11, 1997, No. 74): 2631–2639.

Georgia: Law of Georgia of December 10, 1997, on health care, *Sakartvelos k'anoni* (December 31, 1997, Nos. 47–48): 126–145, Text No. 1139–Is, especially sections 121–122.

Greece: Law No. 1383, dated August 2, 1983, *On the Removal and Transplantation of Human Tissues and Organs, Ephêmeris tês Kybernêseôs tês Hellênikês Dêmokratias* 106 (August 5, 1983): part 1, 1917–1920, chapter 1, section 2.

Greece: *Removal and Transplantation of Biological Substances from Humans*, Act 2737 of 1999.

Hong Kong: *Human Organ Transplant Bill of 1992*, dated March 27, 1992.

Hong Kong: Cap 465 Human Organ Transplant Ordinance, Law of Hong Kong.

Hungary: Ordinance No. 18, dated November 4, 1972, *Of the Minister of Health for the Implementation of the Provisions of Law No. II of 1972 on Health Relating to the Removal and Transplantation of Organs and Tissues, Magyar Közlöny* 87 (November 4, 1972): 862–866, part 2, section 1.

Hungary: Law No. 154 of December 15, 1997, on public health, *Magyar Közlöny* (23 December 1997, No. 119): 9503–9558.

Italy: Law No. 64, dated December 2, 1975, *Regulating the Removal of Parts of Cadavers for Purposes of Therapeutic Transplantation and Prescribing Rules Governing the Removal of Pituitary Glands from Cadavers with a View to Producing Extracts for Therapeutic Purposes, Gazetta Officiale della Repubblica Italiana* 334 (December 19, 1975): Part I, 8869–8871, sections 19–20.

Italy: Law No. 91 of April 1, 1999, on the removal and transplantation of organs and tissues, *Gazzetta Ufficiale della Repubblica Italiana* (April 15, 1999, No. 87).

Japan: Law No. 104 of July 16, 1997, on organ transplantation, *Kanpo* (July 16, 1997, No. 2181): 3–5.

Kuwait: Decree-Law No. 55, dated December 20, 1987, *On Organ Transplantation, Al-Kuwait Al-Yom* 1751 (December 27, 1987): 3–4, section 7.

Lebanon: Decree No. 109, dated September 16, 1983, *On the Removal of Human Tissues and Organs for Therapeutic and Scientific Purposes, Al-Jaridah Al-Rasmiyah* 45 (November 10, 1983): 645–645, section 1.

Lithuania: Law (Text No. VIII-1484) of the Republic of Lithuania of December 21, 1999, on human tissue and organ donation and transplantation, as amended to 10 October 2000, Text No. VIII-1985 (http://www3.lrs.lt/c-bin / . . . /preps2? Condition1 =112278 &Condition2=health_insurance).

Malawi: *The Anatomy Act of 1990*, dated May 18, 1990, *An Act (No. 14 of 1990) to Make Provision for the Donation, Examination and Use of Bodies, or Parts of Bodies, of the Deceased Persons for Education, Scientific, Research, Therapeutic or Diagnostic Purposes: To Re-enact the Law Dealing with Human Tissue and to*

Provide for Matters Incidental Thereto or Connected Therewith, The Malawi Gazette Supplement 4C (June 4, 1990): part IV, section 16.

Mexico: Federal Regulations of August 16, 1976, *On the Use of Human Organs, Tissues and Cadavers, Salud Pública de México* 19 (1977): 59–68, sections 10 and 24.

Morocco: Dahir No. 1–99–208 of August 25, 1999, promulgating Law No. 16–98 on the donation, removal, and transplantation of human organs and tissues, *Bulletin officiel* (September 16, 1999, No. 4726).

The Netherlands: Law of February 6, 2003 (Stb. 90), promulgating rules concerning the safety and quality of human tissues that may be used in medical treatment (Law on the safety and quality of human tissues), *Staatsblad van het Koninkrijk der Nederlanden* (2003).

Norway: Law No. 31 of June 8, 2001, amending Law No. 6 of February 9, 1973, on transplantation, hospital autopsies, and the donation of cadavers, etc., *Norsk Lovtidend* (Part I, July 4, 2001, No. 7): 818–819.

Panama: Law No. 10, dated July 11, 1983, *Regulating the Transplantation of Organs and Anatomical Parts, and Laying Down Other Provisions, Gaceta Oficial* (July 15, 1983): 1–8, part 4.

Panama: Law No. 52 of December 12, 1998, *Regulating the Removal, Preservation, Storage, Transportation, Intended Use, and Final Disposal of Organs or Anatomical Parts, and Also the Procedures for Their Transplantation into Human Beings, Gaceta Oficial* (December 13, 1995, No. 22929): 143–190.

Peru: General Law No. 26842 of July 9, 1997, *On Health, El Peruano* (July 20, 1997, No. 6232): 151245–151252.

Poland: Law of October 26, 1995, *On the Removal and Transplantation of Cells, Tissues, and Organs, Dziennik Ustaw of: Rzeczypospolitej Polskiej* (December 6, 1995, No. 138): 2008–3012, Text No. 682.

Portugal: Order No. 31/2002 of January 8, 2002, prescribing that the activity of the collection of tissues and organs of human origin for the purposes of transplantation and the activity of transplantation are to be subject to prior authorization by the Minister of Health after consulting the Portuguese Transplant Organization (OPT), and repealing Order No. 1245/93 of 6 December 1993, *Diário da República*, Part I-B (January 8, 2002, No. 6): 150–152.

Republic of Singapore: Law No. 15, dated June 10, 1987, *Human Organ Transplant Act of 1987, Republic of Singapore Government Gazette, Acts Supplement* 16 (10 July1987): 411–421, part IV, sections 14–15. Chapter 131A of the 1998 Revised Edition (http://agcvldb4.agc.gov.sg/non_version/html/homepage .html).

Romania: Law of July 1978, *On Safeguarding of the Health of the Population,* sections 129–137.

Romania: Law of January 8, 1998, *On the Removal and Transplantation of Human Tissues or Organs, Monitorul al României* (13 January 1998, No. 8, http://www.cdep.ro/pls/legis/legis_pck.htp_act?ida=15976).

Russian Federation: Law of December 22, 1992, *Of the Russian Federation on the Transplantation of Human Organs and/or Tissues*, RF 93.12.

Slovenia: Regulations of October 8, 2001, on the procedure for the notification of the death of persons considered as donors of human body parts for transplantation, *Uradni list Republike Slovenije* (2001, No. 85).

Spain: Law No. 30, dated October 27, 1979, *On the Removal and Transplantation of Organs, Boletín Oficial de Estado, Gaceta de Madrid* 63, serial no. 5627 (March 13, 1980): 5705–5707, chapter 1, section 5.

Spain: Law No. 27–10–1979.núm.30/1979, sobre extracción y trasplante de órganos.

Sri Lanka: *The Transplantation of Human Tissues Act,* No. 48 of 1987, dated December 11, 1987, section 17(1)-17(3).

Switzerland: 01.057 Loi sur la transplantation, Transplantationsgesetz, Nationalrat Wintersession 2003, Elfte Sitzung 17.12.03 15h00.

Switzerland: Federal Order of December 18, 1998, on the revision of the Federal Constitution, *Recueil officiel des lois fédérales* (October 26, 1999, No. 42): 2556–2611.

Switzerland (Ticino): Law of April 18, 1989, *On Health Promotion and Coordination in the Health Sector (The Health Law)*, section 15.

Syrian Arab Republic: Law No. 31, dated August 23, 1972, *On the Removal and Transplantation of Organs from the Human Body, Recueil des Lois et de la Législation Financière de la République Arabe Syrienne* (September 1972): 2–4, part 2, section 6.

Turkey: Law No. 2238, dated May 29, 1979, *On the Removal, Storage, Transfer, and Grafting of Organs and Tissues, T.C. Resmî Gazete* 16655 (3 June 1979): 1–4, chapter 1, sections 3–4.

Turkey: Regulations [of 2000] on organ and tissue transplantation services, *Türkiye Cumhuriyeti, Remî Gazete* (1 June 2000, No. 24066): 2–10.

Union of Myanmar: *The State Peace and Development Council: The Body Organ Donation Law* (The State Peace and Development Council Law No. 1/2004), The 14th Waning Day of Tabodwe 1365 ME (19th February, 2004), Chapter VIII, Section 21.

United Kingdom: *The Human Organ Transplants Act of 1989*, dated July 27, 1989, Part I, section 1a-1d.

United States of America: USA: Public Law 98-507, *The National Organ Transplant Act*.

Zimbabwe: *Anatomical Donations and Post-mortem Examinations Act* (No. 34 of 1976, section 17).

List of Cases

Compassion in Dying v. State of Washington 79 F.3d 790 (9th cir. 1996)

Cruzan v. Director, Missouri Department of Health, 497 U.S. 261 (1990)

Gildiner v. Thomas Jefferson Univ. Hosp., 451 F. Supp. 692 (E.D.Pa. 1978)

In re President & Directors of Georgetown College Inc., 331, F.2d 1000, 1017 [D.C. Cir.] *cert. denied*, 337 U.S. 978 (1964), W. Burger dissenting

In re Winship, 397 U.S. 358 (1970)

Mohr v. Williams, 95 Minn. 261, 104 N.W. 12 (1905)

Moore v. Regents of the University of California et al., Supreme Court of California, 51 Cal. 3d 120 (July 9, 1990)

Olmstead v. United States, 277 U.S. 438 (1928); 48 S. Ct. 564; 72 L. Ed. 944; 1928 U.S. 89uujLEXIS 694; 66 A.L.R. 376 at 478. J. Brandeis dissenting

Phillips v. United States, 508 F. Supp. 544 (D.S.C. 1981)

Planned Parenthood v. Casey, 505 U.S. 833 (1992)

Robak v. United States, 658 F.2d 471 (7th Cir. 1981)

Roe v. Wade, 410 U.S. 113 (1973)

Rolater v. Strain, 39 Okla. 572, 137 (1913)

Santosky v. Kramer, 102 S. Ct. 1388 (1982)

Schloendorff v. Society of New York Hospital, 211 N.Y. 125, 105 N.E. 93, 133 N.Y.S. 1143 (1914)

Schmerber v. California, 382 U.S. 757 (1966)

Slater v. Baker and Stapleton, 95 Eng. Rep. 860, 2 Wils. K.B. 359 (1767)

Surrogate Parenting Associates Inc. v. Commonwealth of Kentucky, Supreme Court of Kentucky, Ky., 704, South West Reporter, 2nd series (1986)

Tina Smedley Reed, et al. v. Mary Campagnolo, et al. (810 f. Supp. 167; 1993 U.S. Dist. LEXIS 245)

Union Pacific R. Co. v. Botsford, 141 U.S. 250 (1891)

Winston v. Lee, 470 U.S. 753 (1985)

Notes

INTRODUCTION

1. UNOS, "2002 Annual Report of the U.S. Organ Procurement and Transplantation Network and the Scientific Registry of Transplant Recipients: Transplant Data 1992–2001" (Rockville, MD: HHS/HRSA/OSP/DOT, 2003).

2. UNOS, "2003 Annual Report of the U.S. Organ Procurement and Transplantation Network and the Scientific Registry of Transplant Recipients: Transplant Data 1992–2002" (Rockville, MD: HHS/HRSA/OSP/DOT; 2003), table 1.7, http://www.optn.org/data/annualreport.asp (last accessed August 9, 2004).

3. "Any financial incentive to organ procurement, even if government regulated, must be avoided as it dangerously undermines human dignity by obscuring the difference between being human and marketing. We recently expressed our concern about the American Medical Association's suggestion of exploring monetary incentives for organ donation, and we are frightened by the enthusiastic support for it." I. R. Mario, C. Cirillo, and A. Cattoi, "Market in Organs Is Unethical Under Any Circumstances," *British Medical Journal* 325 (2002): 835. See also A. Caplan, C. T. Van Buren, and N. L. Tilney, "Financial Compensation for Cadaver Organ Donation: Good Idea or Anathema?" *Transplantation Proceedings* 25, no. 4 (1993): 2270–72; reprinted in A. Caplan and D. Coelho, eds., *The Ethics of Organ Transplants: The Current Debate* (pp. 219–23) (Amherst: Prometheus Books, 1998); P. Adams et al., "The Nondirected Live-Kidney Donor: Ethical Considerations and Practice Guidelines: A National Conference Report," *Transplantation* 74, no. 4 (2002): 582–90.

4. Transplantation Society, "Statement of the Committee on Morals and Ethics of the Transplantation Society," *Annals of Internal Medicine* 75, no. 4 (1970): 631–33; reprinted in World Health Organization, *Legislative Responses to Organ Transplantation* (pp. 465–66) (Dordrecht: Martinus Nijhoff, Dordrecht, 1994); Transplantation Society, "Commercialization in Transplantation: The Problem and Some Guidelines for Practice," *Lancet* 2 (1985): 715–16; reprinted in World Health Organization, *Legislative Responses to Organ Transplantation* (pp. 459–64) (Dordrecht: Martinus Nijhoff, 1994); Transplantation Society, "Commercialization in Transplantation: The Problem and Some Guidelines for Practice," *Transplantation* 41 (1986): 1; Transplantation Society, "Position of the Transplantation Society on Paid Organ Donation," http://www.transplantation-soc.org (last accessed August 9, 2004); R. Sheil, "Position of the Transplantation Society on Paid Organ Donation," *The Transplantation Society Bulletin* 2 (1994): 22; R. Sheil, 1995, "Position of the Transplantation Society on Paid Organ Donation," *The Transplantation Society Bulletin* 3 (1995): 3.

5. World Health Organization, "Human Organ Transplantation: A Report on the Developments Under the Auspices of the WHO," *International Digest of Health Legislation*

42 (1991): 389–96; reprinted in World Health Organization, *Legislative Responses to Organ Transplantation* (pp. 468–74) (Dordrecht: Martinus Nijhoff, 1994).

6. Nuffield Council on Bioethics, *Human Tissue: Ethical and Legal Issues* (London: Nuffield Council on Bioethics, 1995).

7. United States Task Force on Organ Transplantation, *Organ Transplantation: Issues and Recommendations* (Washington, DC: U.S. Department of Health and Human Services, U.S. Government Printing Office, 1986).

8. R. Fox and J. Swazey, *Spare Parts: Organ Replacement in American Society* (New York: Oxford University Press, 1992), p. 65.

9. J. Childress, "Ethical Criteria for Procuring and Distributing Organs for Transplantation," *Journal of Health Policy and Law* 14 (1989): 87–113, p. 88.

10. P. Ramsey, *The Patient as Person* (New Haven, CT: Yale University Press, 1970), p. 209.

11. As representative examples, see H. Schlitt, "Paid Non-Related Living Organ Donation: Horn of Plenty or Pandora's Box?" *Lancet* 359 (2002): 906–7; M. M. Friedlaender, "The Right to Sell or Buy a Kidney: Are We Failing Our Patients?" *Lancet* 359 (2002): 971–73; M. B. Gill and R. M. Sade, "Paying for Kidneys: The Case Against Prohibition," *The Kennedy Institute of Ethics Journal* 12, no. 1 (2002): 17–45; J. Siegel-Itzkovich, "Israel Considers Paying People for Donating a Kidney," *British Medical Journal* 326, no. 7381 (2003): 126; J. Rapoport, A. Kagan, and M. M. Friedlaender, "Legalizing the Sale of Kidneys for Transplantation: Suggested Guidelines," *The Israel Medical Association Journal* 4, no. 12 (2002): 1132–34; R. Amerling, "Paying for Organs: Another Look," *Nephrology News and Issues* 17, no. 3 (2003): 23–24; L. D. Castro, "Commodification and Exploitation: Arguments in Favour of Compensated Organ Donation," *Journal of Medical Ethics* 29, no. 3 (2003): 142–46; M. M. Friedlaender, "A Protocol for Paid Kidney Donation in Israel," *The Israel Medical Association Journal* 5, no. 9 (2003): 611–14; Council on Ethical and Judicial Affairs, American Medical Association, "Financial Incentives for Organ Procurement: Ethical Aspects of Future Contracts for Cadaveric Donors," *Archives of Internal Medicine* 155 (1995): 581–89; F. L. Delmonico, R. Arnold, N. Scheper-Hughes, L. A. Siminoff, J. Kahn, and S. J. Youngner, "Ethical Incentives—Not Payment—for Organ Donation," *New England Journal of Medicine* 346, no. 25 (2002): 2002–5; R. V. Grazi and J. B. Wolowelsky, "Nonaltruistic Kidney Donations in Contemporary Jewish Law and Ethics," *Transplantation* 75, no. 2 (2003): 250–52.

12. C. Harris and S. Alcorn, "To Solve a Deadly Shortage: Economic Incentives for Human Organ Donation," *Issues in Law and Medicine* 16, no. 3 (2001): 213; J. Harris and C. Erin, "An Ethically Defensible Market in Organs: A Single Buyer Like the NHS Is an Answer," *British Medical Journal* 325 (2002): 114–15; R. Tavar and T. F. Murphy, "The Case for Compensation of Tissue Donors," *Archives of Internal Medicine* 161, no. 15 (2001): 1924–25.

13. The American Medical Association's Council on Ethical and Judicial Affairs concludes: "By entering into a future contract, an adult would agree while still competent to donate his or her organs after death. In return, the donor's family or estate would receive some financial remuneration after the organs have been retrieved and judged medically suitable for transplantation. Several other conditions would apply: (1) Only the potential donor, and not the donor's family or other third party, may be given the option of accepting financial incentives for cadaveric organ donation. In addition, the potential donor must be a competent adult when the decision to donate is made, and the donor must not

have committed suicide. (2) Any incentive should be of moderate value and should be the lowest amount that can reasonably be expected to encourage organ donation. By designating a state agency to administer the incentive, full control over the level of incentive can be maintained. (3) Payment should occur only after the organs have been retrieved and judged medically suitable for transplantation. Suitability should continue to be determined in accordance with the procedures of the Organ Procurement and Transplantation Network. (4) Incentives should play no part in the allocation of donated organs among potential transplant recipients." American Medical Association Council on Ethical and Judicial Affairs, *Code of Medical Ethics* (Chicago: American Medical Association, 2003), policy E-2.15, http://www.ama-assn.org/ama/pub/category/2704.html#ethics (last accessed August 9, 2004); issued June 1984; updated June 1994, based on the report "Financial Incentives for Organ Procurement: Ethical Aspects of Future Contracts," *Archives of Internal Medicine* 155 (1995): 581–89.

14. D. Josefson, "AMA Considers Whether to Pay for Donation of Organs," *British Medical Journal* 324 (2002): 1541.

15. R. Scott, *The Body as Property* (New York: Viking Press, 1981); R. Scott, "The Human Body: Belonging and Control," *Transplantation Proceedings* 22, no. 3 (1990): 1002–4.

CHAPTER 1

1. For the most recent United States Organ Procurement and Transplantation Network data, see www.unos.org.

2. The term "market" picks out a cluster of related practices, ranging from highly state-regulated systems of production and exchange to libertarian free markets. The *Oxford English Dictionary* presents markets as including the meeting or congregating together of people for the purchase and sale of provisions, the time during which such goods are exposed for sale, the action or business of buying and selling, to make an occasion of bargaining or profit, sale as controlled by supply and demand, to bring an enterprise to the notice of the public by interesting dealers in it, or the particular trade or traffic in the commodity specified in the context. J. A. Simpson and E. S. C. Weiner (preparers), *The Oxford English Dictionary*, 2nd ed. (Oxford: Clarendon Press, 1989), vol. 9, pp. 384–86.

The related terms "sale" and "payment" similarly encapsulate a range of meanings. "Sale" may refer to the action or act of making over to another for a price, the exchange of a commodity for money or other valuable consideration, or the disposal of goods for money or other valuable consideration (ibid., vol. 14, pp. 388–89). "Payment" includes remuneration of a person with money or its equivalent, the giving of money or other valuable consideration in discharge of a debt, including the act or rendering to a person anything due, deserved or befitting, or in discharge of an obligation, or the giving of reward or satisfaction (ibid., vol. 11, pp. 379–80).

For the purposes of this study, I will adopt a broad understanding of such terms to include both present and future markets, regulated and free markets, as well as sales and payments in the form of barter, financial income, reward, or other valuable consideration.

3. For general discussion of presumed consent proposals, see A. J. Matas and F. J. Veith, "Presumed Consent for Organ Retrieval," *Theoretical Medicine* 5 (1984): 155–66; R. A. Sells, "Let's Not Opt Out: Kidney Donation and Transplantation," *Journal of Medical Ethics* 5 (1979): 165–69; L. Roels, Y. Vanrenterghem, M. Waer, J. Gruwez, and P. Michielsen,

"Effect of a Presumed Consent Law on Organ Retrieval in Belgium," *Transplantation Proceedings* 22, no. 4 (1990): 2078–79; A. P. Monaco, "Transplantation: The State of the Art," *Transplantation Proceedings* 22, no. 3 (1990): 896–901.

4. UNOS, *2002 Annual Report of the U.S. Organ Procurement and Transplantation Network and the Scientific Registry of Transplant Recipients: Transplant Data 1992–2001* (Rockville, MD: HHS/HRSA/OSP/DOT; 2003). Additional data for the 2003 transplants and 2004 registrants was obtained from the United States Organ Procurement and Transplantation Network: www.unos.org (last accessed August 12, 2004).

5. T. M. Chan, "Donor Shortage in Organ Transplantation: Perspective from Hong Kong," *Transplantation Proceedings* 34, no. 7 (2002): 2558–59.

6. D. Divakar, C. M. Thiagarajan, and K. C. Reddy, "Ethical Aspects of Renal Transplantation in India," *Transplantation Proceedings* 30, no. 7 (1998): 3626. In one study of 463 end-stage renal disease patients undergoing dialysis in India, the mortality rate was 9.5 percent. M. Rao, R. Juneja, R. Shirly, and C. Jacob, "Haemodialysis for End-Stage Renal Disease in Southern India—A Perspective from a Tertiary Referral Care Centre," *Nephrology, Dialysis, Transplantation* 13, no. 10 (1998): 2494–500. Similar challenges to increased transplantable organs access is experienced worldwide. See, for example, C. L. Milanés, E. Bellorín-Font, and B. Rodríguez-Iturbe, "Renal Transplantation in Venezuela, 2001," *Transplantation Proceedings* 34, no. 7 (2002): 2529–30; N. K. Chou, W. J. Ko, and C. J. Lee, "How to Promote Organ Donation: A Successful Experience at the National Taiwan University Hospital," *Transplantation Proceedings* 34, no. 7 (2002): 2556–57; L. Bäckman, A.-C. Croon, U. Feuk, and N. H. Persson, "Organ Donation in Sweden," *Transplantation Proceedings* 34, no. 7 (2002): 2560; T. P. Thulo, M. C. M. Modiba, A. Kobryn, S. Ndlovu, and P. Becker, "Five-Year Results of Living Related Renal Donation Are Similar to Cadaveric Transplantation in Black South Africans," *Transplantation Proceedings* 34, no. 7 (2002): 2565–66; S. Frew, A. Tavakoli, S. Al-Maket, S. Woodcock, S. Duncalf, D. Lee, A. Asderakis, N. R. Parrott, and H. N. Riad, "Review of Cadaveric Kidney Donation Programme at Manchester Royal Infirmary," *Transplantation Proceedings* 34, no. 1 (2002): 17; F. M. de Cabo, C. Cabrer, D. Paredes, A. Navarro, E. Trias, and M. Manyalich, "Timing Comparison of Donation Process After the New Real Decreto of Transplantation in Spain," *Transplantation Proceedings* 34, no. 1 (2002): 18; I. Osio, M. Escobedo, U. Chavarría, E. Pérez, A. Martinez, A. Rodriguez, M. Guedea, J. P. Maldonado, and C. Rodriguez-Montalvo, "Experience with Transplant Coordination in Northern Mexico Following the Spanish Model," *Transplantation Proceedings* 34, no. 1 2002: 19; G. R. Schütt, "25 Years of Organ Donation: European Initiatives to Increase Organ Donation," *Transplantation Proceedings* 34, no. 6 (2002): 2005–6; O. Erdoğan, L. Yücetin, M. Tuncer, N. Keçecioğlu, A. Gürkan, M. Akaydin, and G. Yakupoğlu, "Attitudes and Knowledge of Turkish Physicians about Organ Donation and Transplantation," *Transplantation Proceedings* 34, no. 6 (2002): 2007–8; K. C. Reddy, C. M. Thiagarajan, D. Shunmugasundaram, R. Jayachandran, P. Nayar, S. Thomas, and V. Ramachandran, "Unconventional Renal Transplantation in India," *Transplantation Proceedings* 22, no. 3 (1990): 910–11; C. M. Thiagarajan, K. C. Reddy, D. Shunmugasundaram, R. Jayachandran, P. Nayar, S. Thomas, and V. Ramachandran, "The Practice of Unconventional Renal Transplantation (UCRT) at a Single Centre in India," *Transplantation Proceedings* 22, no. 3 (1990): 912–14; J. B. Dossetor, "Discussion," *Transplantation Proceedings* 22, no. 3 (1990): 933–38; K. V. Johny, J. Nesim, N. Namboori, and R. K. Gupta, "Values Gained and Lost in Live Unrelated Renal Transplantation," *Transplantation Proceedings* 22, no. 3 (1990): 915–17.

7. As obtained from the UNOS 1998 and 2003 annual reports, together with additional data compiled by UNOS and published on their Web site in August 2004: UNOS, *1998 Annual Report of the U.S. Scientific Registry of Transplant Recipients and the Organ Procurement and Transplantation Network*; and *2003 Annual Report of the U.S. Scientific Registry of Transplant Recipients and the Organ Procurement and Transplantation Network: Transplant Data 1992–2002* (Rockville, MD, and Richmond, VA: HHS/HRSA/OSP/DOT and UNOS); http://www.unos.org.

8. A. Capron, "Reexamining Organ Transplantation," *Journal of the American Medical Association* 285, no. 3 (2001): 334.

9. Donors recovered in the United States by donor type and donors recovered: January 1, 1988–September 30, 2003; based on OPTN data as of December 12, 2003; www.unos.org.

10. As Johnson et al. document, nationally donor mortality has been estimated at 0.03 percent. Overall complication rate was 8.2 percent with only 2 (0.2 percent) major complications. In one study, major complications for living kidney donation included femoral nerve compression with resulting weakness and a retained sponge, which required further surgery for removal. Minor complications included suspected wound infections (2.4 percent of donors), pneumothoraces (1.5 percent), unexplained fever (1.3 percent), operative blood loss greater than or equal to 750 ml (0.9 percent), pneumonias (0.9 percent), wound hematomas (0.6 percent), phlebitic intravenous sites (0.5 percent), urinary tract infections (0.3 percent), readmission for pain and mild confusion (0.3 percent), atelectasis (0.3 percent), corneal abrasions (0.2 percent), urethral trauma from catheter placement (0.1 percent) with other minor complications occurring with a frequency of 0.1 percent or less. E. M. Johnson, M. J. Remucal, K. J. Gillingham, R. A. Dahms, J. S. Najarian, and A. J. Matas, "Complications and Risks of Living Donor Nephrectomy," *Transplantation* 64, no. 8 (1997), 1124–28; E. M. Johnson, J. S. Najarian, and A. J. Matas, "Living Kidney Donation: Donors Risks and Quality of Life," *Clinical Transplantation* (1997): 231–40. See also M. J. Waples, F. O. Belzer, and D. T. Uehling, "Living Donor Nephrectomy: A 20 Year Experience," *Urology* 45, no. 2 (1995): 207–10; J. S. Najarian, B. M. Chavers, L. E. McHugh, and A. J. Matas, "20 Years or More of Follow-up of Living Kidney Donors," *Lancet* 340 (1992): 807–10; I. Blohme, H. Gabel, and H. Brynger, "The Living Donor in Renal Transplantation," *Scandinavian Journal of Urology and Nephrology* 64 (Supplement) (1981): 143–51; C. Troppmann, A. C. Grussner, D. E. Sutherland, and R. W. Grussner, "Organ Donation by Living Donors in Isolated Pancreas and Simultaneous Pancreas-Kidney Transplantation," *Zentralblatt fur Chirurgie* 124, no. 8 (1999): 734–38; M. Siebels, J. Theodorakis, N. Schmeller, S. Corvin, N. Mistry-Burchardi, G. Hillebrand, D. Frimberger, O. Reich, W. Land, and A. Hofstetter, "Risks and Complications in 160 Living Kidney Donors Who Underwent Nephroureterectomy," *Nephrolology, Dialysis, Transplant* 18, no. 12 (2003): 2648–54.

11. P. A. Singer, M. Siegler, P. F. Whitington, J. D. Lantos, J. C. Emond, J. R. Thistlethwaite, and C. E. Broelsch, "Ethics of Liver Transplantation with Living Donors," *New England Journal of Medicine* 321 (1989): 620–22; P. A. Singer, M. Siegler, J. D. Lantos, J. C. Emond, P. F. Whitington, J. R. Thistlethwaite, and C. E. Broelsch, "The Ethical Assessment of Innovative Therapies: Liver Transplantation Using Living Donors," *Theoretical Medicine* 11, no. 4 (1990): 343–46; M. Siegler, "Liver Transplantation Using Living Donors," *Transplantation Proceedings* 24, no. 5 (1992): 2223–24.

12. W. V. McDermott and L. W. Ottinger, "Elective Hepatic Resection," *American Journal of Surgery* 112 (1966): 376–81; T. E. Starzl, L. J. Koep, R. Weil III, J. R. Lilly, C. W.

Putnam, and J. A. Aldrete, "Right Trisegmentectomy for Hepatic Neoplasms," *Surgery for Gynecology and Obstetrics* 150 (1980): 208–14; M. A. Adson, "Diagnosis and Surgical Treatment of Primary and Secondary Solid Hepatic Tumors in the Adult," *The Surgical Clinics of North America* 61, no. 1 (1981): 181–96.

13. For example, in one study of thirty-five patients there were no operative deaths or serious postoperative complications for patients who underwent hepatic resection for tumors. P. A. Singer, M. Siegler, P. F. Whitington, J. D. Lantos, J. C. Emond, J. R. Thistlethwaite, and C. E. Broelsch, "Ethics of Liver Transplantation with Living Donors," *New England Journal of Medicine* 321 (1989): 620–22. In a study of 120 cases of adult living donors utilizing the right lobe, Egawa and Tanaka reported, "One patient had jaundice 6 months after the donor operation due to stricture of the bile duct, which was treated by radiologic intervention. Other complications were sub-ileus (1), pancreatitis (1), long-term elevation of biliary enzyme (2), and portal thrombus (1), which was treated by thrombectomy on day 5. No donor died to date." H. Egawa and K. Tanaka, "Adult Living Donor Liver Transplantation Using Right Lobe," *Transplantation Proceedings* 34, no. 1 (2002): 235–36. See also J. C. Garcia-Valdecasas, J. Fuster, L. Grande, C. Fondevila, A. Rimola, M. Navasa, E. Bombuy, J. Ferrer, and J. Visa, "Adult Living Donor Liver Transplantation: Initial Results of a Starting Program," *Transplantation Proceedings* 34, no. 1 (2002): 237–38; R. Robles, P. Ramirez, F. S. Bueno, J. A. Fernandez , J. M. Rodriguez, J. A. Lujan, V. Munitiz, C. Marin, and P. Parrilla, "Importance of Training in Liver Resection Surgery to Implement Programs of Living Donor Liver Transplantation," *Transplantation Proceedings* 34, no. 1 (2002): 240; M. J. Waples, F. O. Belzer, and D. T. Uehling, "Living Donor Nephrectomy: A 20 Year Experience," *Urology* 45, no. 2 (1995): 207–10; S. Iwatsuki, B. W. Shaw Jr., and T. E. Starzl, "Experience with 150 Liver Resections," *American Surgery* 197, no. 3 (1983): 247–53; T. Nagao, S. Inoue, T. Mizuta, H. Saito, N. Kawano, and Y. Morioka, "One Hundred Hepatic Resections: Indications and Operative Results," *American Surgery* 202, no. 1 (1985): 42–49.

In a study of 871 kidney donors, there were no operative deaths and only two major complications. E. M. Johnson, M. J. Remucal, K. J. Gillingham, R. A. Dahms, J. S. Najarian, and A. J. Matas, "Complications and Risks of Living Donor Nephrectomy," *Transplantation* 64, no. 8 (1997), 1124–28; E. M. Johnson, J. S. Najarian, and A. J. Matas, "Living Kidney Donation: Donors Risks and Quality of Life," *Clinical Transplantation* (1997): 231–40.

14. R. Scott, *The Body as Property* (New York: Viking Press, 1981); R. Scott, "The Human Body: Belonging and Control," *Transplantation Proceedings* 22, no. 3 (1990): 1002–4.

15. Transplantation Society, "Statement of the Committee on Morals and Ethics of the Transplantation Society," *Annals of Internal Medicine* 75, no. 4 (1970): 631–33; reprinted in World Health Organization, *Legislative Responses to Organ Transplantation* (pp. 465–66) (Dordrecht: Martinus Nijhoff, 1994).

16. World Health Organization, *Human Organ Transplantation: A Report on Developments Under the Auspices of WHO (1987–1991)* (Geneva: World Health Organization, 1991), pp. 5, 7. Guiding Principle 5: "The human body and its parts cannot be the subject of commercial transactions. Accordingly, giving or receiving payment (including any other compensation or reward) for organs should be prohibited" (p. 8).

17. World Health Organization, "Human Organ Transplantation: A Report on the Developments Under the Auspices of the WHO," *International Digest of Health Legislation*

42 (1991): 389–96; reprinted in World Health Organization, *Legislative Responses to Organ Transplantation* (pp. 468–74) (Dordrecht: Martinus Nijhoff, 1994).

18. The Committee on Organ Procurement and Transplantation Policy of the United States National Institutes of Medicine opined: "The committee views organ transplantation as a valuable, often life saving process that should be managed equitably across the nation. It also believes the federal government has a legitimate and appropriate oversight role to ensure that reasonable standards of equity and quality are met." Committee on Organ Procurement and Transplantation Policy, *Organ Procurement and Transplantation Policy: Appraising Current Policies and the Potential Impact of the DHHS Final Rule* (Washington, DC: National Academy Press, 1999), p. 5.

For a historical perspective on the ownership of human bodies, see D. Gracia, "Ownership of the Human Body: Some Historical Remarks," in *Ownership of the Human Body* (pp. 67–80), ed. H. ten Have and J. Welie (Dordrecht: Kluwer Academic Publishers, 1998); and Z. Szawarski, "The Stick, the Eye, and Ownership of the Body," in *Ownership of the Human Body* (pp. 81–98), ed. H. ten Have and J. Welie (Dordrecht: Kluwer Academic Publishers, 1998).

Others offer legal accounts of body ownership from the perspectives of France and The Netherlands. See A. Fagot-Largeault, "Ownership of the Human Body: Judicial and Legislative Responses in France," in *Ownership of the Human Body* (pp. 115–42), ed. H. ten Have and J. Welie (Dordrecht: Kluwer Academic Publishers, 1998); as well as J. Welie and H. ten Have, "Ownership of the Human Body: The Dutch Context," in *Ownership of the Human Body* (pp. 99–114), ed. H. ten Have and J. Welie (Dordrecht: Kluwer Academic Publishers, 1998).

19. Transplantation Society, "Commercialization in Transplantation: The Problem and Some Guidelines for Practice," *Lancet* 2, no. 8457 (1985): 715–16; reprinted in World Health Organization, *Legislative Responses to Organ Transplantation* (pp. 459–64) (Dordrecht: Martinus Nijhoff, 1994), p. 462.

20. United States Task Force on Organ Transplantation, *Organ Transplantation: Issues and Recommendations* (Washington, DC: U.S. Department of Health and Human Services, U.S. Government Printing Office, 1986), p. 9.

21. Ibid., p. 86.

22. Prior to 1988, the Danish policy was one of taking "the body away for autopsy and of taking organs from the body before it was 'delivered' back to the family since this was considered justified since it advanced medical research." U. Jensen, "Property, Rights, and the Body: The Danish Context—A Democratic Ethics or Recourse to Abstract right?" in *Ownership of the Human Body* (pp. 173–86), ed. H. ten Have and J. Welie (Dordrecht: Kluwer Academic Publishers, 1998), p. 173.

Similarly, "some countries, Austria for instance, attempting to avoid the problem of organ scarcity, favor regulating organ donation by countermand. According to this regulation the consent of the newly deceased will be presumed in the absence of a certificate expressly stating the subject's disapproval." F. Illhardt, "Ownership of the Human Body: Deontological Approaches," in *Ownership of the Human Body* (pp. 187–206), ed. H. ten Have and J. Welie (Dordrecht: Kluwer Academic Publishers, 1998), 188–89. See also P. Schotsmans, "Ownership of the Body: A Personalist Perspective," *Ownership of the Human Body* (pp. 159–72), ed. H. ten Have and J. Welie (Dordrecht: Kluwer Academic Publishers, 1998).

In contrast, Kevin Wm. Wildes argues that the general assumption that available organs are a public rather than a private resource is misguided and unjustified. K. Wildes,

"Libertarianism and Ownership of the Human Body," in *Ownership of the Human Body* (pp. 143–58), ed. H. ten Have and J. Welie (Dordrecht: Kluwer Academic Publishers, 1998). See also S. Gorovitz, "Ethical Implications of Reimbursement Policies," in *Human Organ Transplantation: Societal, Medical-Legal, Regulatory, and Reimbursement Issues* (pp. 173–78), ed. D. Cowan et al. (Ann Arbor: Health Administration Press, 1987).

23. Transplantation Society, "Statement of the Committee on Morals and Ethics of the Transplantation Society," *Annals of Internal Medicine* 75, no. 4 (1970): 631–33; reprinted in World Health Organization, *Legislative Responses to Organ Transplantation* (pp. 465–66) (Dordrecht: Martinus Nijhoff, 1994); Transplantation Society, "Commercialization in Transplantation: The Problem and Some Guidelines for Practice," *Lancet* 2, no. 8457 (1985): 715–16; reprinted in World Health Organization, *Legislative Responses to Organ Transplantation* (pp. 459–64) (Dordrecht: Martinus Nijhoff, 1994); Transplantation Society, "Commercialization in Transplantation: The Problem and Some Guidelines for Practice," *Transplantation* 41 (1986): 1–3; Transplantation Society, 2002: "Position of the Transplantation Society on Paid Organ Donation," http://www.transplantation-soc.org (last accessed August 9, 2004).

24. World Medical Association, "Statement on Live Organ Trade," adopted by the 37th World Medical Assembly, Brussels, Belgium, October 1985; reprinted in World Health Organization, *Legislative Responses to Organ Transplantation* (Dordrecht: Martinus Nijhoff, 1994), p. 475; World Medical Association, "Declaration on Human Organ Transplantation," adopted by the 39th World Medical Assembly, Madrid Spain, October 1987; reprinted in World Health Organization, *Legislative Responses to Organ Transplantation* (pp. 475–76) (Dordrecht: Martinus Nijhoff, 1994).World Medical Association, "Statement on Human Organ and Tissue Donation and Transplantation," adopted by the 52nd World Medical Assembly, Edinburgh Scotland, October 2000, http://www.wma.net/e /policy (last accessed August 9, 2004).

25. World Health Organization, "Human Organ Transplantation: A Report on the Developments Under the Auspices of the WHO," *International Digest of Health Legislation* 42 (1991): 389–96; reprinted in World Health Organization, *Legislative Responses to Organ Transplantation* (pp. 468–74) (Dordrecht: Martinus Nijhoff, 1994).

26. Nuffield Council on Bioethics, *Human Tissue: Ethical and Legal Issues* (London: Nuffield Council on Bioethics, 1995).

27. United States Task Force on Organ Transplantation, *Organ Transplantation: Issues and Recommendations* (Washington, DC: U.S. Department of Health and Human Services, U.S. Government Printing Office, 1986).

28. World Health Organization, "Human Organ Transplantation: A Report on the Developments Under the Auspices of the WHO," *International Digest of Health Legislation* 42 (1991): 389–96; reprinted in World Health Organization, *Legislative Responses to Organ Transplantation* (pp. 468–74) (Dordrecht: Martinus Nijhoff, 1994), p. 472.

29. Office of Technology Assessment, *New Developments in Biotechnology: Ownership of Human Tissues and Cells* (Washington, DC: U.S. Government Printing Office, 1987), p. 96.

30. Transplantation Society, "Commercialization in Transplantation: The Problem and Some Guidelines for Practice," *Lancet* 2, no. 8457 (1985): 715–16; reprinted in World Health Organization, *Legislative Responses to Organ Transplantation* (pp. 459–64) (Dordrecht: Martinus Nijhoff, 1994), pp. 461–62.

31. The Ethics Committee of the American Society of Transplant Surgeons urged: "The purchase of organs for the purpose of human transplantation could encounter formidable

opposition from governmental, medical, and religious segments of our society because of the following undesirable consequences that such a policy might foster:

- It could exploit the poor as an economic underclass of organ donors to serve the wealthy
- It could risk the withholding of medical information that results in the transmission of donor disease (malignancy or infection) to the recipient . . .
- It could influence the family of a patient to prematurely withdraw care (if the death of a person is linked to the sale of their organs, and the payment is made to the next of kin . . .)
- It could result in the perception of the human organ as a commodity."

R. Arnold, S. Bartlett, J. Bernat, J. Colonna, D. Dafoe, N. Dubler, S. Gruber, J. Kahn, R. Luskin, H. Nathan, S. Orloff, J. Prottas, R. Shapiro, C. Ricordi, S. Youngner, and F. L. Delmonico, "Financial Incentives for Cadaver Organ Donation: An Ethical Reappraisal," *Transplantation* 73, no. 8 (2002): 1361–7, p. 1362.

See also R. A. Sells, "Organ Commerce: Ethics and Expediency," *Transplantation Proceedings* 22, no. 3 (1990): 931–32; R. A. Sells, "The Case Against Buying Organs and a Future's Market in Transplantation," *Transplantation Proceedings* 24, no. 5 (1992): 2198–2202; R. A. Sells, "Transplants," *Principles of Health Care Ethics* (pp. 1003–25), ed. R. Gillon (Chichester, NY: John Wiley & Sons, 1994); A. S. Daar, A. K. Salahudeen, A. Pingle, and H. F. Woods, "Ethics and Commerce in Live Donor Renal Transplantation: Classification of the Issues," *Transplantation Proceedings* 22, no. 3 (1990): 922–24; G. M. Abouna, M. S. Kumar, M. Samhan, S. K. Dadah, P. John, and N. M. Sabawi, "Commercialization in Human Organs: A Middle Eastern Perspective," *Transplantation Proceedings* 22, no. 3 (1990): 918–21.

32. United States Task Force on Organ Transplantation, *Organ Transplantation: Issues and Recommendations* (Washington, DC: U.S. Department of Health and Human Services, U.S. Government Printing Office, 1986), p. 10.

33. Guiding Principle 6: "Advertising the need for or availability of organs, with a view to offering or seeking payment should be prohibited." World Health Organization, *Human Organ Transplantation: A Report on Developments Under the Auspices of WHO (1987–1991)* (Geneva: World Health Organization, 1991), p. 9.

34. Transplantation Society, "Commercialization in Transplantation: The Problem and Some Guidelines for Practice," *Lancet* 2, no. 8457 (1985): 715–16; reprinted in World Health Organization, *Legislative Responses to Organ Transplantation* (pp. 459–64) (Dordrecht: Martinus Nijhoff, 1994), p. 463.

35. The American Medical Association admits the moral possibility of purchasing organs from cadaver sources. "By entering into a future contract, an adult would agree while still competent to donate his or her organs after death. In return, the donor's family or estate would receive some financial remuneration after the organs have been retrieved and judged medically suitable for transplantation." They require that adequate safeguards be in place to ensure that the health of donors and recipients is not jeopardized and that the quality of the organs procured is not degraded. "The voluntary donation of organs in appropriate circumstances is to be encouraged. However, it is not ethical to participate in a procedure to enable a living donor to receive payment, other than for the reimbursement of expenses necessarily incurred in connection with removal, for any of the donor's non-renewable organs." American Medical Association Council on Ethical and Judicial Affairs, *Code of Medical Ethics* (Chicago: American Medical Association, 2003), policy E-2.15, http://www.ama-assn.org/ama/pub/category/2704.html#ethics (last accessed August 9, 2004).

36. Transplantation Society, "Statement of the Committee on Morals and Ethics of the Transplantation Society," *Annals of Internal Medicine* 75, no. 4 (1970): 631–33; reprinted in World Health Organization, *Legislative Responses to Organ Transplantation* (pp. 465–66) (Dordrecht: Martinus Nijhoff, 1994), p. 466.

37. Transplantation Society, "Commercialization in Transplantation: The Problem and Some Guidelines for Practice," *Lancet* 2, no. 8457 (1985): 715–16; reprinted in World Health Organization, *Legislative Responses to Organ Transplantation* (pp. 459–64) (Dordrecht: Martinus Nijhoff, 1994), p. 463.

38. R. Fox and J. Swazey, *Spare Parts: Organ Replacement in American Society* (New York: Oxford University Press, 1992), p. 207.

39. Ibid.

40. Ibid.

41. S. Gorovitz, "Against Selling Body Parts," *Report from the Center for Philosophy and Public Policy* 4 (1984): 9–12, p. 12.

42. Daar argues: "The altruistic stranger might have internalized the concept of altruism being linked to 'brotherly love,' as it is in some definitions of altruism, and might, in a cosmic sense, consider all human beings to be an extended family. After all, the Human Genome Project demonstrated that our DNA is 99.9% identical. This leads us to conclude that the very distinction . . . between intimates and strangers, based on existence of duty/obligation, may not exist in the mind and calculations of the altruistic stranger, and surely that is what should matter." A. S. Daar, "Strangers, Intimates, and Altruism in Organ Donation," *Transplantation* 74, no. 3 (2002): 424–25, p. 425.

Similarly, Leder holds: "If the body itself is seen as a gift, never simply a possession, then the act of organ donation becomes itself a way of graciously fulfilling such obligations. The gift is, as it were, reciprocated in a way that benefits others. With the living donor, interdependence is confirmed and manifested in the most vital way through the sharing of what one has received. In the case of cadaver donation, new life springs from death through a passing on of the gift. One participates in a larger circulation that both enfolds and out runs the individual self." D. Leder, "Whose Body? What Body? The Metaphysics of Organ Transplantation," in *Persons and Their Bodies: Rights, Responsibilities, Relationships* (pp. 233–64), ed. M. J. Cherry (Dordrecht: Kluwer Academic Publishers, 1999), p. 262.

43. R. A. Sells, "Transplants," *Principles of Health Care Ethics* (1003–25), ed. R. Gillon (Chichester, NY: John Wiley & Sons, 1994), p. 1017.

44. J. B. Dossetor et al., "Discussion," *Transplantation Proceedings* 22, no. 3 (1990): 933–38, p. 933.

45. T. Peters, "Life or Death: The Issue of Payment in Cadaveric Organ Donation," *Journal of the American Medical Association* 265 (1991): 1302–5, p. 1305.

46. E. D. Pellegrino, "Families' Self Interest and the Cadaver's Organs: What Price Consent?" *Journal of the American Medical Association* 265 (1991): 1305–6, p. 1305.

47. See also A. Caplan, "Obtaining and Allocating Organs for Transplantation," in *Human Organ Transplantation: Societal, Medical-Legal, Regulatory, and Reimbursement Issues* (pp. 5–17), ed. D. Cowan et al. (Ann Arbor: Health Administration Press, 1987); T. Cooper, "Survey of Development, Current Status, and Future Prospects for Organ Transplantation," in *Human Organ Transplantation: Societal, Medical-Legal, Regulatory, and Reimbursement Issues* (pp. 18–26), ed. D. Cowan et al. (Ann Arbor: Health Administration Press, 1987); R. Evans and J. Yagi, "Social and Medical Considerations Affecting

Selection of Transplant Recipients: The Case of Heart Transplants," in *Human Organ Transplantation: Societal, Medical-Legal, Regulatory, and Reimbursement Issues* (pp. 27–41), ed. D. Cowan et al. (Ann Arbor: Health Administration Press, 1987); C. Callender, "Legal and Ethical Issues Surrounding Transplantation: The Transplant Team Perspective," in *Human Organ Transplantation: Societal, Medical-Legal, Regulatory, and Reimbursement Issues* (pp. 42–54), ed. D. Cowan et al. (Ann Arbor: Health Administration Press, 1987); B. Brecher, "Buying Human Kidneys: Autonomy, Commodity and Power," *Journal of Medical Ethics* 19 (1991): 99; B. Brecher, "Organs for Transplant: Donation or Payment?" in *Principles of Health Care Ethics* (pp. 993–1002), ed. R. Gillon (Chichester, NY: John Wiley & Sons, 1994).

48. R. A. Sells, "Transplants," *Principles of Health Care Ethics* (pp. 1003–25), ed. R. Gillon (Chichester, NY: John Wiley & Sons, 1994), p. 1016. See also A. M. Sadler and B. Sadler, "Organ Donation: Is Volunteerism Still Valid?" *Hastings Center Report* 14 (1984): 6–9.

49. "Nevertheless, research on attitudes indicates a broad consensus that the gift of a kidney to a stranger is reasonable and proper—a clear challenge to the medical profession's reluctance to use living unrelated donors . . . the donation of a kidney to a stranger does not involve so much risk to the donor that questions should automatically be raised about his or her competence to decide . . . [P]roponents . . . argue that giving a kidney enhances the donor's self-esteem and, in this light, is neither irrational nor unreasonable." T. Beauchamp and J. Childress, *Principle of Biomedical Ethics*, 4th ed. (New York: Oxford University Press, 1994), p. 371. See also R. Simmons, "Psychological Reactions to Giving a Kidney," in *Psychonephrology* (pp. 227–45), ed. N. Levy (New York: Plenum, 1981).

For contrasting conclusions, see C. H. Fellner, "Organ Donation: For Whose Sake?" *Annals of Internal Medicine* 79 (1973): 590; T. E. Starzl, "Will Live Organ Donation No Longer Be Justified?" *Hastings Center Report* 15 (April 1985): 5; C. H. Fellner and S. H. Schwartz, "Altruism in Disrepute," *New England Journal of Medicine* 284 (1971): 582–85.

50. R. Arnold, S. Bartlett, J. Bernat, J. Colonna, D. Dafoe, N. Dubler, S. Gruber, J. Kahn, R. Luskin, H. Nathan, S. Orloff, J. Prottas, R. Shapiro, C. Ricordi, S. Youngner, and F. L. Delmonico, "Financial Incentives for Cadaver Organ Donation: An Ethical Reappraisal," *Transplantation* 73, no. 8 (2002): 1361–67.

51. R. Scott, "The Human Body: Belonging and Control," *Transplantation Proceedings* 22, no. 3 (1990): 1002–4, p. 1003. Even the *National Geographic* has published the direct comparison of organ vending and human slavery. See A. Cockburn, "21st-Century Slaves," *National Geographic* 204, no. 3, (September 2003): 2–26.

52. J. Childress, "Ethical Criteria for Procuring and Distributing Organs for Transplantation," *Journal of Health Policy and Law* 14 (1989): 87–113, p. 88. See also Office of Technology Assessment, *New Developments in Biotechnology: Ownership of Human Tissues and Cells* (Washington, DC: U.S. Government Printing Office, 1987), pp. 130–32.

53. P. Ramsey, *The Patient as Person* (New Haven, CT: Yale University Press, 1970), p. 209. See also S. Scorsone, "Christianity and the Significance of the Human Body," *Transplantation Proceedings* 22, no. 3 (1990): 943–44. For a thoughtful analysis of the importance of religion to health care policy and bioethics, see G. McKenny, *To Relieve the Human Condition* (Albany: State University of New York Press, 1997).

54. In the context of human cloning, for example, Kass urges that there is a "narcissism of those who would clone themselves and the arrogance of others who think they know who deserves to be cloned or which genotype any child-to-be should be thrilled to receive; the Frankensteinian hubris to create human life and increasingly to control its

destiny; man playing God. Almost no one finds any of the suggested reasons for human cloning compelling; almost everyone anticipates its possible abuses. Moreover, many people feel oppressed by the sense that there is probably nothing we can do to prevent it from happening. This makes the prospect all the more revolting. . . . Shallow are the souls that have forgotten how to shudder." L. Kass, "The Wisdom of Repugnance," *The New Republic*, June 2, 1997, 17–25, p. 20. See also L. Kass, *Toward a More Natural Science* (New York: Free Press, 1985).

55. World Health Assembly, "Development of Guiding Principles for Human Organ Transplantation" (WHA 40.13), in World Health Organization, *Human Organ Transplantation: A Report on Developments Under the Auspices of WHO (1987–1991)* (Geneva: World Health Organization, 1991), p. 5.

The Universal Declaration of Human Rights adopted by the General Assembly of the United Nations in Paris on December 10, 1948, combined forbearance rights (e.g., "Everyone has the right to life, liberty and security of person" [article 3]) and procedural rights (e.g., "No one shall be subjected to arbitrary arrest, detention, or exile" [article 9]) with claim rights (e.g., "Everyone . . . has the right to social security and is entitled to realization . . . of the economic, social and cultural rights indispensable for his dignity and the free development of his personality" [article 22]). The clearest statement of human dignity appears in the "Preamble": "Whereas recognition of the inherent dignity and of the equal and inalienable rights of all members of the human family is the foundation of freedom, justice and peace in the world." It is unclear which particular articles of this declaration the WHO believes are contravened by selling organs. Without further argument the WHO's various declarations at best point toward moral considerations. They are not, however, conclusive; nor should they be understood as morally authoritative or prescriptively binding. http://www.un.org/Overview/rights.html (last accessed August 9, 2004).

56. World Health Assembly, "Preventing the Purchase and Sale of Human Organs" (WHA 42.5) (Geneva: World Health Organization, 1989), p. 1; reprinted in World Health Organization, *Legislative Responses to Organ Transplantation* (pp. 467–68) (Dordrecht: Martinus Nijhoff, 1994), p. 467.

57. United States Task Force on Organ Transplantation, *Organ Transplantation: Issues and Recommendations* (Washington, DC: U.S. Department of Health and Human Services, U.S. Government Printing Office, 1986), p. 98.

58. G. M. Abouna, M. S. Kumar, M. Samhan, S. K. Dadah, P. John, and N. M. Sabawi, "Commercialization in Human Organs: A Middle Eastern Perspective," *Transplantation Proceedings* 22, no. 3 (1990): 918–21, p. 919; J. B. Dossetor and C. R. Stiller, "Ethics, Justice, and Commerce in Transplantation," *Transplantation Proceedings* 22, no. 3 (1990): 892–95.

59. Nuffield Council on Bioethics, *Human Tissue: Ethical and Legal Issues* (London: Nuffield Council, 1995), para 6.7.

60. Ibid., para 6.4.

61. A. Caplan, C. T. Van Buren, and N. L. Tilney, "Financial Compensation for Cadaver Organ Donation: Good Idea or Anathema?" *Transplantation Proceedings* 25, no. 4 (1993): 2270–42. Reprinted in A. Caplan and D. Coelho, eds., *The Ethics of Organ Transplants: The Current Debate* (pp. 219–23) (Amherst: Prometheus Books), p. 220.

62. See, for example, M. J. Meyer, "Dignity, Death, and Modern Virtue," *American Philosophical Quarterly* 32 (1995): 45–55; A. Grubb, "The Nuffield Council Report on Human Tissue," *Medical Law Review* 3 (1995): 235–36, p. 235; P. Walsh, "Principles and Pragmatism," *Medical Law Review* 3 (1995): 237–50.

63. My emphasis. E. Keyserlingk, "Human Dignity and Donor Altruism—Are They Compatible with Efficiency in Cadaveric Human Organ Procurement?" *Transplantation Proceedings* 22, no. 3 (1990): 1005–6, p. 1005.

64. See, for example, W. Dekkers and H. ten Have, "Biomedical Research with Human Body 'Parts,'" in *Ownership of the Human Body* (pp. 49–66), ed. H. ten Have and J. Welie (Dordrecht: Kluwer Academic Publishers, 1998); B. Blasszauer, "Autopsy," in *Ownership of the Human Body* (pp. 19–26), ed. H. ten Have and J. Welie (Dordrecht: Kluwer Academic Publishers, 1998).

65. M. Finkel, "Complications," *New York Times Magazine*, May 27, 2001, p. 32.

66. B. Brecher, "Organs for Transplant: Donation or Payment?" in *Principles of Health Care Ethics* (pp. 993–1002), ed. R. Gillon (Chichester, NY: John Wiley & Sons, 1994), pp. 1001–2. See also B. Brecher, "The Kidney Trade; Or, The Customer Is Always Wrong," *Journal of Medical Ethics* 16 (1990): 123.

67. J. Childress, "Ethical Criteria for Procuring and Distributing Organs for Transplantation," *Journal of Health Policy and Law* 14 (1989): 87–113, p. 88. See also J. Childress, "The Implication of Major Western Religious Traditions for Policies Regarding Human Biological Materials," contract paper prepared for the Office of Technology Assessment, Washington, DC, 1986, p. 4; J. Childress, "Who Shall Live When All Cannot Live?" *Soundings* 53 (1970): 339–55. For religious accounts of organ donation, see W. F. May, "Religious Justifications for Donating Body Parts," *Hastings Center Report* 15 (1985): 38–42; R. McCormick and P. Ramsey, *Doing Evil to Achieve Good* (Chicago: Loyola University Press, 1978); N. L. Rabinovitch, "What Is the Halakhah for Organ Transplants?" in *Challenge: Torah Views on Science and Its Problems* (pp. 482–90), ed. A. Carmell and C. Domb (Jerusalem: Feildham Publishers, 1978); F. Rosner and J. Bleich, *Jewish Bioethics* (New York: Hebrew Publishing Company, 1979); F. Rosner and M. Tendler, *Practical Medical Halacha*, 2nd ed. (New York: Feldheim, 1980).

68. Transplantation Society, "Commercialization in Transplantation: The Problem and Some Guidelines for Practice," *Lancet* 2, no. 8457 (1985): 715–16; reprinted in World Health Organization, *Legislative Responses to Organ Transplantation* (pp. 459–64) (Dordrecht: Martinus Nijhoff, 1994), p. 460.

69. B. M. Dickens, "Human Rights and Commerce in Health Care," *Transplantation Proceedings* 22, no. 3 (1990): 904–5; A. Jonsen, "Organ Transplants and the Principle of Fairness," in *Human Organ Transplantation: Societal, Medical-Legal, Regulatory, and Reimbursement Issues* (pp. 266–71), ed. D. Cowan et al. (Ann Arbor: Health Administration Press, 1987); J. F. Blumstein, "Government's Role in Organ Transplantation Policy," in *Organ Transplantation Policy Issues and Prospects*, ed. J. F. Blumstein and F. Sloan (Durham: Duke University Press, 1990), p. 5; J. F. Blumstein, "The Case of Commerce in Organ Transplantation," *Transplantation Proceedings* 24 (1992): 2190–97.

70. President's Commission for Study of Ethical Problems in Medicine and Biomedical and Behavioral Research, *Securing Access to Health Care* (Washington, DC: U.S. Government Printing Office, 1983), p. 4.

71. Norman Daniels opines: "The most promising strategy for extending Rawls's theory without tampering with useful assumptions about the index of primary goods simply includes health-care institutions among the background institutions involved in providing for fair equality of opportunity. Once we note the special connection of normal species functioning to the opportunity range open to an individual, this strategy seems the natural way to extend Rawls's view that the subject of theories of social justice are the basic

institutions which provide a framework of liberties and opportunities within which individuals can use fair income shares to pursue their own conceptions of the good. Insofar as meeting health care needs has an important effect on the distribution of health, and more to the point, on the distribution of opportunity, the health-care institutions are plausibly included on the list of basic institutions a fair equality of opportunity principle should regulate." N. Daniels, *Justice and Justification* (Cambridge: Cambridge University Press, 1996), p. 192.

See also N. Daniels, *Just Health Care* (New York: Cambridge University Press, 1985); M. Ignatieff, *The Needs of Strangers* (London: Chatto and Windus, 1984); D. L. Jackson, "The Role of State Health Departments in Assuring Equitable Selection and Regulation of Resources," in *Human Organ Transplantation: Societal, Medical-Legal, Regulatory, and Reimbursement Issues* (pp. 159–65), ed. D. Cowan et al. (Ann Arbor: Health Administration Press, 1987); G. Vlastos, "Justice and Equality," in *Social Justice* (pp. 31–72), ed. R. Brandt (Englewood Cliffs, NJ: Prentice-Hall, 1962); A. Schneider and M. P. Flaherty, *The Challenge of a Miracle: Selling the Gift* (Pittsburgh: Pittsburgh Press, 1985); C. Davis, "Paying for Organ Transplants Under Medicare," in *Human Organ Transplantation: Societal, Medical-Legal, Regulatory, and Reimbursement Issues* (pp. 179–86), ed. D. Cowan et al. (Ann Arbor: Health Administration Press, 1987); B. Mayers, "Blue Cross and Blue Shield Coverage for Major Organ Transplants," in *Human Organ Transplantation: Societal, Medical-Legal, Regulatory, and Reimbursement Issues* (pp. 187–92), ed. D. Cowan et al. (Ann Arbor: Health Administration Press, 1987).

72. United States Task Force on Organ Transplantation, *Organ Transplantation: Issues and Recommendations* (Washington, DC: U.S. Department of Health and Human Services, U.S. Government Printing Office, 1986), pp. xxi; 9–11.

73. Ibid., p. xxi.

74. Ibid., p. 105.

75. Massachusetts Task Force on Organ Transplantation: 1984, "Report of the Task Force, G. Annas, Chairman," reprinted in *Human Organ Transplantation: Societal, Medical-Legal, Regulatory, and Reimbursement Issues*, ed. D. Cowan et al. (Ann Arbor: Health Administration Press, 1984), p. 233.

76. P. Townsend and N. Davidson, eds., *Inequalities in Health: The Black Report* (Harmondsworth: Penguin Press, 1982).

77. H. T. Engelhardt Jr., "Shattuck Lecture: Allocating Scarce Medical Resources and the Availability of Organ Transplantation," in *Human Organ Transplantation: Societal, Medical-Legal, Regulatory, and Reimbursement Issues* (pp. 339–53), ed. D. Cowan et al. (Ann Arbor: Health Administration Press, 1987); H. T. Engelhardt, "Allocating Scarce Medical Resources and the Availability of Organ Transplantation: Some Moral Presuppositions," *New England Journal of Medicine* 311 (1984): 66–71.

78. F. Cantarovich, "Values Sacrificed and Values Gained by the Commerce of Organs: The Argentine Experience," *Transplantation Proceedings* 22, no. 3 (1990): 925–27, especially 927; M. Pauly, "Equity and Costs," in *Human Organ Transplantation: Societal, Medical-Legal, Regulatory, and Reimbursement Issues* (pp. 251–56), ed. D. Cowan et al. (Ann Arbor: Health Administration Press, 1987).

79. R. Evans, "Health Care Technology and the Inevitability of Resource Allocation and Rationing Decisions, part I," in *Human Organ Transplantation: Societal, Medical-Legal, Regulatory, and Reimbursement Issues* (pp. 277–97), ed. D. Cowan et al. (Ann Arbor: Health Administration Press, 1987); R. Evans, "Health Care Technology and the

Inevitability of Resource Allocation and Rationing Decisions, part II," in *Human Organ Transplantation: Societal, Medical-Legal, Regulatory, and Reimbursement Issues* (pp. 298–330), ed. D. Cowan et al. (Ann Arbor: Health Administration Press, 1987).

80. G. Annas, "The Prostitute, the Playboy and the Poet: Rationing Schemes for Organ Transplantation," in *Human Organ Transplantation: Societal, Medical-Legal, Regulatory, and Reimbursement Issues* (pp. 331–38), ed. D. Cowan et al. (Ann Arbor: Health Administration Press, 1987), p. 332. See also Massachusetts Task Force on Organ Transplantation, *Report of the Massachusetts Task Force on Organ Transplantation*, G. Annas, Chairman (Boston: Boston University School of Public Health, 1983); M. Basson, "Choosing Among Candidates for a Scarce Medical Resource," *Journal of Medicine and Philosophy* 4 (1979): 313–34.

81. A. Caplan, "Organ Transplants: The Cost of Success," *Hastings Center Report* 13 (1983): 23–32, p. 23. See also A. Caplan, "Ethical and Policy Issues in the Procurement of Cadaver Organs for Transplantation," *New England Journal of Medicine* 311 (1984): 981–84; A. Caplan, *If I Were a Rich Man, Could I Buy a Pancreas?* (Bloomington: Indiana University Press, 1992).

82. United States Task Force on Organ Transplantation, *Organ Transplantation: Issues and Recommendations* (Washington, DC: U.S. Department of Health and Human Services, U.S. Government Printing Office, 1986), p. 104.

83. For a detailed discussion of justice-related issues and organ distribution policies, see F. Kamm, *Morality, Mortality*, vol. 1, part 3 (New York: Oxford University Press, 1993); N. Daniels, "Justice and the Dissemination of 'Big-Ticket' Technologies," in *Organ Substitution Technology: Ethical, Legal, and Public Policy Issues* (pp. 211–20), ed. D. Mathieu (Boulder: Westview Press, 1988); P. Menzel, *Medical Costs, Moral Choices: A Philosophy of Health Care Economics in America* (New Haven, CT: Yale University Press, 1983).

84. For an analysis of the difficulties of redistributive justice addressing historical wrongs see G. Sher, "Reverse Discrimination, The Future and the Past," *Ethics* 90 (1979): 81–87; G. Sher, "Ancient Wrongs and Modern Rights," *Philosophy and Public Affairs* 10 (1981): 3–17. For historical analysis of social justice in health care see L. McCullough, "Justice and Health Care: Historical Perspectives and Precedents," *Justice and Health Care* (pp. 51–71), ed. E. Shelp (Boston: Reidel Publishers, 1981); G. Outka, "Social Justice and Equal Access to Health Care," *Journal of Religious Ethics* 2 (1974): 11–32.

85. United States Task Force on Organ Transplantation, *Organ Transplantation: Issues and Recommendations* (Washington, DC: U.S. Department of Health and Human Services, U.S. Government Printing Office, 1986), p. xxi.

86. Transplantation Society, "Commercialization in Transplantation: The Problem and Some Guidelines for Practice," *Lancet* 2, no. 8457 (1985): 715–16; reprinted in World Health Organization, *Legislative Responses to Organ Transplantation* (pp. 459–64) (Dordrecht: Martinus Nijhoff, 1994), p. 462.

87. A. Caplan, "Organ Transplants: The Cost of Success," *Hastings Center Report* 13 (1983): 23–32, p. 23.

88. D. Frier and G. Mavrodes, "The Morality of Selling Human Organs," in *Ethics, Humanism, and Medicine*, ed. M. Basson (New York: Alan R. Liss, 1980). See also A. Jonsen, "Ethical Issues in Organ Transplantation," in *Medical Ethics*, 2nd ed. (pp. 229–52), ed. R. Veatch (Sudbury, MA: Jones and Barlett, 1997); I. Kennedy, "The Donation and Transplantation of Kidneys: Should the Law Be Changed?" *Journal of Medical Ethics* 5 (1979): 13–21.

89. G. M. Abouna, M. S. Kumar, M. Samhan, S. K. Dadah, P. John, and N. M. Sabawi, "Commercialization in Human Organs: A Middle Eastern Perspective," *Transplantation Proceedings* 22, no. 3 (1990): 918–21, p. 918.

90. R. A. Sells, "Organ Commerce: Ethics and Expediency," *Transplantation Proceedings* 22, no. 3 (1990): 931–32, p. 931. See also R. Fox and J. Swazey, *Spare Parts: Organ Replacement in American Society* (New York: Oxford University Press, 1992), p. 208.

91. G. M. Abouna, M. S. Kumar, M. Samhan, S. K. Dadah, P. John, and N. M. Sabawi, "Commercialization in Human Organs: A Middle Eastern Perspective," *Transplantation Proceedings* 22, no. 3 (1990): 918–21, p. 919.

92. A. S. Daar, A. K. Salahudeen, A. Pingle, and H. F. Woods, "Ethics and Commerce in Live Donor Renal Transplantation: Classification of the Issues," *Transplantation Proceedings* 22, no. 3 (1990): 922–24.

93. C. M. Thiagarajan, K. C. Reddy, D. Shunmugasundaram, R. Jayachandran, P. Nayar, S. Thomas, and V. Ramachandran, "The Practice of Unconventional Renal Transplantation (UCRT) at a Single Centre in India," *Transplantation Proceedings* 22, no. 3 (1990): 912–14, p. 913; K. C. Reddy, C. M. Thiagarajan, D. Shunmugasundaram, R. Jayachandran, P. Nayar, S. Thomas, and V. Ramachandran, "Unconventional Renal Transplantation in India," *Transplantation Proceedings* 22, no. 3 (1990): 910–11.

94. Organ Procurement and Transplantation Network, "All Kaplan-Meier Graft Survival Rates for Transplants Performed: 1996–2001," based on OPTN data as of July 30, 2004, http://www.optn.org/latestData/rptStrat.asp (last accessed August 12, 2004).

95. "The physician must be able to tell the antecedents, know the present, and foretell the future—must mediate these things, and have two special objects in view with regard to disease, namely to do good or to do no harm." Hippocrates, "On the Epidemics," in *The Genuine Works of Hippocrates*, trans. F. Adams (Baltimore: Williams & Wood Co. 1946), book 1, chapter 5. For discussion of this injunction, see L. Edelstein, "The Genuine Works of Hippocrates," *Ancient Medicine* (pp. 133–44), ed. O. Temkin and C. L. Temkin (Baltimore: Johns Hopkins University Press, 1967); A. Jonsen, "Do No Harm: Axiom of Medical Ethics," in *Philosophical Medical Ethics: Its Nature and Significance* (pp. 27–42), ed. S. Spicker and H. T. Engelhardt Jr. (Dordrecht: Kluwer Academic Publishers, 1977).

96. R. A. Sells, "Organ Commerce: Ethics and Expediency," *Transplantation Proceedings* 22, no. 3 (1990): 931–32, p. 931. See also F. Cantarovich, "Values Sacrificed and Values Gained by the Commerce of Organs: The Argentine Experience," *Transplantation Proceedings* 22, no. 3 (1990): 925–27.

97. G. M. Abouna, M. S. Kumar, M. Samhan, S. K. Dadah, P. John, and N. M. Sabawi, "Commercialization in Human Organs: A Middle Eastern Perspective," *Transplantation Proceedings* 22, no. 3 (1990): 918–21.

98. A. Jonsen, "Ethical Issues in Organ Transplantation," in *Medical Ethics*, 2nd ed. (pp. 229–52), ed. R. Veatch (Sudbury, MA: Jones and Barlett Publishers, 1997), p. 242; J. F. Blumstein and F. A. Sloan, eds., *Organ Transplantation Policy: Issues and Prospects* (Durham: Duke University Press, 1989).

99. The President's Commission reminded policy makers that a reasoned judgment must be concerned "not only about impact of the condition on the welfare and opportunity of the individual but also about the efficacy and the costs of the care itself in relation to other conditions and the efficacy and cost of the care that is available for them . . . and the cost of each proposed option in terms of foregone opportunities to apply the same resources to social goals other than that of ensuring access [to health care]." President's

Commission for Study of Ethical Problems in Medicine and Biomedical and Behavioral Research, *Securing Access to Health Care* (Washington, DC: U.S. Government Printing Office, 1983), pp. 36–37. The effects of particular policy decisions can both directly and indirectly impact health care outcomes.

100. S. Youngner, "Organ Retrieval: Can We Ignore the Dark Side," *Transplantation Proceedings* 22, no. 3 (1990): 1014–15, p. 1015.

101. Veatch presents a similar possibility with regard to directed donation: "Occasionally, a sophisticated utilitarian may oppose directed donation claiming that the overall transplant enterprise could be jeopardized if a dramatic directed donation case such as that of the Ku Klux Klan member or donation limited to a gay recipient turned the public against the organ transplant system." R. Veatch, "Egalitarian and Maximin Theories of Justice: Directed Donation of Organs for Transplant," *Journal of Medicine and Philosophy* 23, no. 5 (1998): 456–76, p. 461.

102. G. M. Abouna, M. S. Kumar, M. Samhan, S. K. Dadah, P. John, and N. M. Sabawi, "Commercialization in Human Organs: A Middle Eastern Perspective," *Transplantation Proceedings* 22, no. 3 (1990): 918–21, p. 919. See also J. B. Dossetor et al., "Discussion," *Transplantation Proceedings* 22, no. 3 (1990): 933–38, pp. 933–34.

103. L. Skelly, "Practical Issues in Obtaining Organs for Transplantation," in *Human Organ Transplantation: Societal, Medical-Legal, Regulatory, and Reimbursement Issues* (pp. 261–65), ed. D. Cowan et al. (Ann Arbor: Health Administration Press, 1987).

104. Office of Technology Assessment, *New Developments in Biotechnology: Ownership of Human Tissues and Cells* (Washington, DC: U.S. Government Printing Office, 1987), p. 116.

105. M. A. Baily, "Economic Issues in Organ Substitution Technology," in *Organ Substitution Technology: Ethical, Legal and Public Policy Issues* (pp. 198–210), ed. D. Mathieu (Boulder: Westview Press, 1988).

106. J. B. Dossetor et al., "Discussion," *Transplantation Proceedings* 22, no. 3 (1990): 933–38, pp. 934–35.

107. C. M. Thiagarajan, K. C. Reddy, D. Shunmugasundaram, R. Jayachandran, P. Nayar, S. Thomas, and V. Ramachandran, "The Practice of Unconventional Renal Transplantation (UCRT) at a Single Centre in India," *Transplantation Proceedings* 22, no. 3 (1990): 912–14, p. 914.

108. K. C. Reddy, C. M. Thiagarajan, D. Shunmugasundaram, R. Jayachandran, P. Nayar, S. Thomas, and V. Ramachandran, "Unconventional Renal Transplantation in India," *Transplantation Proceedings* 22, no. 3 (1990): 910–11, p. 911.

109. Ibid.

110. J. B. Dossetor et al., "Discussion," *Transplantation Proceedings* 22, no. 3 (1990): 933–38, p. 935.

111. Transplantation Society, "Commercialization in Transplantation: The Problem and Some Guidelines for Practice," *Lancet* 2, no. 8457 (1985): 715–16; reprinted in World Health Organization, *Legislative Responses to Organ Transplantation* (pp. 459–64) (Dordrecht: Martinus Nijhoff, 1994). See also Transplantation Society, "Commercialization in Transplantation: The Problem and Some Guidelines for Practice," *Transplantation* 41 (1986): 1–3; R. Sheil, "Position of the Transplantation Society on Paid Organ Donation," *The Transplantation Society Bulletin* 2 (1994): 22; R. Sheil, "Position of the Transplantation Society on Paid Organ Donation," *The Transplantation Society Bulletin* 3 (1995): 3.

112. Available at http://www.transplantation-soc.org (last accessed August 9, 2004).

113. United Network for Organ Sharing, "UNOS Board Condemns Organ Brokering," *UNOS News Bureau*, June 29 (2001). See also United Network for Organ Sharing, "Financial Incentives for Organ Donation; A Report of the UNOS Ethics Committee Payment Subcommittee" (UNOS: 1993); United Network for Organ Sharing, "News Release: National Minority Donor Awareness Day" (UNOS: 2002); United Network for Organ Sharing, "UNOS Responds to *48 Hours* Assertions of Illegal Organ Trade in the U.S." *UNOS News Bureau*, Feb 12, 2002.

114. Rabbi Tendler contends: "The leading medical journals (*New England Journal of Medicine* in the United States and *Lancet* in England) have published thoughtful articles suggesting that remuneration will not lead to the commodification (treating as a commodity) of body parts or exploitation of the indigent if the organs are donated to the national organ bank and not directed to a specified individual. The Jewish tradition reluctantly concurs with this analysis because of the over-arching considerations of 'saving a life'" M. Tendler, "The Judeo-Biblical Perspective on Organ Donation: You Shall Choose Life," *UNOS Update*, September–October 2002, 19. See also J. Harris and C. Erin, "An Ethically Defensible Market in Organs: A Single Buyer Like the NHS Is an Answer," *British Medical Journal* 325 (2002): 114–15.

115. K. V. Johny, J. Nesim, N. Namboori, and R. K. Gupta, "Values Gained and Lost in Live Unrelated Renal Transplantation," *Transplantation Proceedings* 22, no. 3 (1990): 915–17, p. 917.

CHAPTER 2

1. L. Pennekamp, "Recent Case: Before a State May Sever Permanently the Rights of Parents in Their Natural Child, Due Process Requires That the State Support Its Allegations by at Least Clear and Convincing Evidence," *University of Cincinnati Law Review* 51 (1982): 933–44, p. 943.

2. *Santosky v. Kramer*, 102 S. Ct. 1388 (1982).

3. *In re Winship*, 397 U.S. 358 (1970).

4. The significance of the rights and liberties at stake is not the only difference between tort law and criminal law. Criminal conviction usually includes a mens rea requirement, or demonstration of intention to harm, whereas intention to harm is generally speaking immaterial in tort law. Richard Epstein summarizes: "Briefly put, the position must be that the intention to harm is immaterial (to the *prima facie* case) in the tort law, whereas the actual harm itself is immaterial to the criminal law. Common acts, such as street muggings, may well be actionable as torts and punishable as crimes. Yet that fact should not obscure the essential point that the grounds for liability are never the same. The act itself may be a unitary phenomenon, but the descriptions under which it is judged in the two systems do and should diverge." R. A. Epstein, "Crime and Tort: Old Wine in Old Bottles," in *Assessing the Criminal: Restitution, Retribution, and the Legal Process* (pp. 231–57), ed. R. E. Barnet and J. Hagel (Cambridge: Ballinger , 1977), p. 248.

Nor is this to suggest that one ought to be more careful with criminal prosecution simply because the penalties are always perceived as more severe. Perhaps some would prefer criminal conviction resulting in only several weeks in prison to a multimillion-dollar civil judgment. When considered in toto as systems of law, however, civil and criminal cases have quite different net costs, especially considering the risks of false positive determinations of guilt. Raising the standard of proof lowers the risk of innocent conviction, while raising the likelihood of guilty acquittal. Whether increasing the standard of proof is justified depends on an all things considered judgment of the net costs of the two types of mistakes. Whereas loss of a civil suit typically results in a cash payment from defendant to plaintiff, criminal conviction may impose not merely fines but also lengthy imprisonment or execution, depending on jurisdiction and the relative severity of the offense. While errors in civil cases unjustly transfer financial resources from one party to another, errors in criminal cases result in loss of years, perhaps decades, of personal freedom, if not loss of life itself. Such costs, especially if in error, are not rectifiable. Hence, ordinarily in criminal cases erroneous conviction is deemed much worse than erroneous acquittal. R. S. Bell, "Criminal Law: Decision Theory and Due Process: A Critique of the Supreme Court's Lawmaking for Burdens of Proof," *Journal of Criminal Law & Criminology* 78 (1987): 557–85.

Thus, William Blackstone's famous assertion: "It is better that ten guilty persons escape than that one innocent suffer." W. Blackstone, *Commentaries on the Laws of England* (Oxford: Clarendon Press, 1765–69), chapter 27, p. 353; http://www.yale.edu /lawweb/avalon/blackstone/blacksto.htm (last accessed August 10, 2004). Indeed, where one can often purchase insurance against personal and civil liability, to protect oneself against judgment errors (e.g., medical malpractice insurance, personal or corporate umbrella policies, and other forms of liability insurance), one cannot purchase insurance protection against criminal prosecution.

5. J. Locke, "An Essay Concerning Human Understanding," in *Classics of Western Philosophy* (pp. 479–574), 2nd ed., ed. S. Cahn (Indianapolis: Hackett, 1977 [1690]), p. 518, book 2, chapter 27.

6. I. Kant, *The Metaphysics of Morals*, trans. M. Gregor (Cambridge: Cambridge University Press, 1991 [1797]), p. 50, AK 223.

7. The common law of the twelfth and thirteenth centuries was in large measure the law of property rights. The protection of possessions was at the center of Henry II's legislation between 1164 and 1179. A. Hogue, *Origins of the Common Law* (Indianapolis: Liberty Press, 1966), pp. 161–63.

In the nineteenth century, Blackstone, reflecting on the common law of England, argued: "There is nothing which so generally strikes the imagination and engages the affections of mankind, as the right of property; or that sole and despotic dominion which one man claims and exercises over the external things of the world, in total exclusion of the right of any other individual in the universe." W. Blackstone, *Commentaries on the Laws of England* (Oxford: Clarendon Press, 1765–69), book 2, chapter 1, p. 3; http://www.yale.edu/lawweb/avalon/blackstone/blacksto.htm (last accessed August 10, 2004). See also S. Buckle, *Natural Law and the Theory of Property: Grotius to Hume* (Oxford: Clarendon Press, 1991).

8. W. Prosser, *Law of Torts* (St. Paul: West, 1971), p. 34.

9. P. Matthews, "The Man of Property," *Medical Law Review* 3 (1995): 251–74, p. 251.

10. *Slater v. Baker and Stapleton*, 95 Eng. Rep. 860, 2 Wils. K.B. 359 (1767).

11. *Union Pacific R. Co. v. Botsford*, 141 U.S. 250 (1891); at 251.

12. *Mohr v. Williams*, 95 Minn. 261, 104 N.W. 12 (1905) at 14.

13. *Rolater v. Strain*, 39 Okla. 572, 137 (1913) at 96.

14. *Schloendorff v. Society of New York Hospital*, 211 N.Y. 125, 105 N.E. 93, 133 N.Y.S. 1143 (1914) at 129–30.

15. *Olmstead v. United States*, 277 U.S. 438 (1928); 48 S. Ct. 564; 72 L. Ed. 944; 1928 U.S. LEXIS 694; 66 A.L.R. 376 at 478. J. Brandeis dissenting.

16. *In re President & Directors of Georgetown College Inc.*, 331, F.2d 1000, 1017 [DC Cir.] *cert. denied*, 337 U.S. 978 (1964), W. Burger dissenting.

17. *Planned Parenthood v. Casey*, 505 U.S. 833 (1992).

18. *Cruzan v. Director, Missouri Department of Health*, 497 U.S. 261 (1990) at 287.

19. *Schmerber v. California*, 382 U.S. 757 (1966) at 772.

20. *Winston v. Lee*, 470 U.S. 753 (1985) at 759.

21. *Planned Parenthood v. Casey*, 505 U.S. 833 (1992) at 857–59.

22. R. Puccetti, "Brain Transplantation and Personal Identity," *Analysis* 29 (1969): 65.

23. D. Leder, *The Absent Body* (Chicago: University of Chicago Press, 1990), pp. 107, 111, 115.

24. In 1984 a surgeon transplanted the heart of a baboon into an infant whose heart lacked a left ventricle. The girl died several days later. Perhaps the most famous case occurred in 1985 at Loma Linda University, when Leonard Bailey transplanted a baboon heart into Baby Fae—a neonate who thereby survived for four weeks following the transplant. In the early 1990s at the University of Pittsburgh, Thomas Starzl implanted baboon livers into two patients, who were each dying of advanced hepatitis B. Both died from complications due to extensive immunosuppression. One survived twenty days, the other twenty-six days, posttransplant. A third patient with advanced AIDS was implanted with baboon bone marrow, but it did not engraft. Committee on Xenotransplantation, *Xenotransplantation: Science, Ethics, and Public Policy* (Washington, DC: National Academy Press, 1996). See also L. K. Altman, "Learning from Baby Fae," *The New York Times*, Nov. 18, 1985, 1, 30; A. Jonsen, "Ethical Issues in Organ Transplantation," in *Medical Ethics*, 2nd ed. (pp. 229–52), ed. R. Veatch (Sudbury, MA: Jones and Barlett Publishers, 1997), 253; R. A. Sells, "Transplants," *Principles of Health Care Ethics* (pp. 1003–25), ed. R. Gillon (Chichester, NY: John Wiley & Sons, 1994); D. Mollevi, Y. Ribas, M. Ginesta, and T. Serrano et al., "Heart and Liver Xenotransplantation Under Low-Dose Tacrolimus: Graft Survival After Withdrawal of Immunosuppression," *Transplantation* 71, no. 2 (2001): 217–24; W. Parker, S. Lin, and J. Platt, "Antigen Expression in Xenotransplantation: How Low Must It Go?" *Transplantation* 71, no. 2 (2001): 313–19.

25. Numerous researchers have urged caution to prevent interspecies disease transmission. Those viruses of greatest concern are the porcine endogenous retroviruses (PERV), which belong to the same family of retroviruses that causes AIDS. Utilizing test tube experiments, investigators have shown that pig PERVs can infect human cells. "The genetic coding of pig viruses lie in the DNA of all pig cells, including the cells of the transplanted organ. While we do not know how many pig viral sequences exist that could be of concern to us, we do know from laboratory experiments that some pig viruses can infect human cells. Of course this laboratory demonstration of infection is a long way from the natural world, and a simple, isolated, real life infection is in turn a long way from an epidemic. Nonetheless, the risk, however remote, that a pandemic could result as a consequence of pig-to-human organ transplantation exists." F. Bach, A. Ivinson, and H. Weeramantry, "Ethical and Legal Issues in Technology: Xenotransplantation," *American Journal of Law and Medicine* 2–3 (Summer–Fall 2001): 283–300, pp. 285–86. See also A. Caplan, "Is Xenografting Morally Wrong?" *Transplantation Proceedings* 24, no. 2 (1992): 722–27; S. J. Tacke, R. Kurth, and J. Denner, "Porcine Endogenous Retroviruses Inhibit Human Immune Cell Function: Risk for Xenotransplantation?" *Virology* 268, no. 1 (2000): 87–93.

As the Committee on Xenotransplantation of the U.S. Institute of Medicine concluded: "although the degree of risk cannot be quantified, it is unequivocally greater than zero. Hence, the committee recommends that guidelines for human trails of xenotransplantation address four major areas: (1) procedures to screen source animals for the presence of infectious organisms and consideration of the development of specific pathogen-free animals for use in xenotransplants; (2) continued surveillance throughout their lifetimes of patients and periodic surveillance of their contacts (families, health care workers and others) for evidence of infectious diseases; (3) establishment of tissue banks containing tissue and blood samples from source animals and patients; and (4) establishment of national and local registries of patients receiving xenotransplants." Committee on Xenotransplantation, *Xenotransplantation: Science, Ethics, and Public Policy* (Washington, DC: National Academy Press, 1996), p. 2.

For more concerns regarding animal rights and xenotransplantation, see G. Fracione, "Xenografts and Animal Rights," *Transplantation Proceedings* 22 (1990): 1044–45; K. Reemtsma, "Ethical Aspects of Xenotransplantation," *Transplantation Proceedings* 22 (1990): 1042–43.

For discussion of animal rights more generally, see F. Loew, "Animals in Research," in *Birth to Death: Science and Bioethics* (pp. 301–12), ed. D. Thomasma and T. Kushner (Cambridge: Cambridge University Press, 1996); D. Moros, "Taking Duties Seriously: Medical Experimentation, Animal Rights, and Moral Incoherence," in *Birth to Death: Science and Bioethics* (pp. 313–23), ed. D. Thomasma and T. Kushner (Cambridge: Cambridge University Press, 1996); T. Benton, "Animal Rights and Social Practices," in *Birth to Death: Science and Bioethics* (pp. 324–37), ed. D. Thomasma and T. Kushner (Cambridge: Cambridge University Press, 1996); T. Regan, "The Case for Animal Rights," in *In Defense of Animals* (pp. 13–26), ed. P. Singer (Oxford: Basil Blackwell, Inc., 1985); P. Singer, ed., *In Defense of Animals* (Oxford: Basil Blackwell, 1985).

26. The now classic fourth edition of *Black's Law Dictionary* (4th ed., rev. [St. Paul, MN: West, 1968]) defined death as "the cessation of life; the ceasing to exist; defined by physicians as a total stoppage of the circulation of the blood and a cessation of the animal and vital functions consequent thereon, such as respiration, pulsation, etc." This description of whole body death emphasizes the presence of circulatory and respiratory functions. The advent of intensive care units and respirators capable of sustaining brain-dead but biologically alive bodies, and the costs such treatments engendered, placed whole body definitions under intense conceptual scrutiny. Developments in kidney transplantation in the 1950s and heart transplantation in 1967 further underscored the medical need for a brain oriented definition of death, because brain-dead, but otherwise biologically alive, human bodies are excellent sources of transplantable organs. In 1981, the President's Commission for the Study of Ethical Problems in Medicine and Biomedical and Behavioral Research explicitly endorsed a change that would incorporate an addition to the circulatory and respiratory definition of the importance of brain stem function for the life of persons. "An individual who has sustained either (1) irreversible cessation of circulatory and respiratory functions, or (2) irreversible cessation of all functions of the entire brain, including the brain stem is dead. A determination of death must be made in accordance with accepted medical standards." *Defining Death* (Washington, DC: U.S. Government Printing Office, 1981), p. 3. Brain death places the death of the person over against the death of the biological human body. With brain death, whatever is distinctly personal in the organism is dead. See also S. Youngner, R. Arnold, and R. Shapiro, *The Definition of Death* (Baltimore: Johns Hopkins University Press, 1999).

27. Samuel Pufendorf, for example, characterizes ownership as "a right, by which what one may call the substance of a thing belongs to someone in such a way that it does not belong in its entirety to anyone else in the same manner." It follows, he adds, that "we may dispose as we will of things which belong to us as property and bar all others from using them, except insofar as they may acquire a particular right from us by agreement." S. Pufendorf, *On the Duty of Man and Citizen According to Natural Law*, ed. J. Tully and trans. M. Silverthorne (Cambridge: Cambridge University Press, 1991 [1672]), p. 85. See also L. Becker, "The Moral Basis of Property," in *Property* (pp. 187–220), ed. J. R. Pennock and J. Chapman (New York: New York University Press, 1980); A. M. Honoré, "Ownership," in *Oxford Essays in Jurisprudence* (pp. 370–433), ed. A. Guest (Oxford: Oxford University Press, 1961).

28. M. Friedman, "Freedom under Capitalism," in *The Libertarian Reader* (pp.76–85), ed. T. R. Machan (Totowa, NJ: Rowman and Littlefield, 1982 [1962]), p. 77.

29. Regarding coercive offers, see M. Bayles, "Coercive Offers and Public Benefits," *The Personalist* 55 (1974); T. Benditt, "Threats and Offers," *The Personalist* 58 (1978); M. Gorr, "Toward a Theory of Coercion," *Canadian Journal of Philosophy* 16, no. 3 (1986): 383–406.

30. As Sidgwick notes regarding the ownership of land: it should only be confirmed insofar as it maximizes utility. "The theoretical question is simply whether the whole among of utility obtainable when the land is allotted to the exclusive use of individuals, is clearly greater or less than the whole among of utility that maybe expected to result from leaving it in common." H. Sidgwick, *The Elements of Politics* (London: Macmillan, 1919; reprint, New York: Kraus, 1969), chapter 5, §3. See also P. Singer, "The Right to Be Rich or Poor," in *Reading Nozick: Essays on Anarchy, State and Utopia* (pp. 37–53), ed. J. Paul (Totowa, NJ: Rowman & Littlefield, 1981); H. Sidgwick, 1969 [1901], *The Principles of Political Economy* (London: Macmillan, 1901; reprint, New York: Kraus, 1969), especially book 3, chapter 3, §6.

31. "Among the basic rights is the right to hold and to have the exclusive use of personal property. One ground of this is to allow a sufficient material basis for personal independence and a sense of self-respect, both of which are essential for the adequate development and exercise of the moral powers. Having this right and being able effectively to exercise it is one of the social bases of self-respect. Thus this right is a general right: a right all citizens have in virtue of their fundamental interests." J. Rawls, *Justice as Fairness: A Restatement* (Cambridge, MA: Harvard University Press: 2001), p. 114.

Wider understandings of private property, such as ownership of natural resources and the means of production, are excluded as nonbasic because they are not understood as necessary for the adequate development and exercise of the moral powers. They are not, therefore, an essential basis of self-respect. See also J. Rawls, *Political Liberalism* (New York: Columbia University Press, 1993); J. Rawls, *A Theory of Justice*, rev. ed. (Cambridge, MA: Harvard University Press, 1999).

32. "[W]hen they have observ'd that the principal disturbance in society arises from those goods, which we call external, and from their looseness and easy transition from one person to another; they must seek a remedy . . . this can be done after no other manner, than by a convention enter'd into by all the members of the society to bestow stability of the possession of those external goods, and leave everyone in the peaceful enjoyment of what he may acquire by his fortune or industry." Cited in S. Buckle, *Natural Law and the Theory of Property: Grotius to Hume* (Oxford: Clarendon Press, 1991), p. 489.

33. R. Posner, *The Economic Analysis of Law*, 3rd ed. (Boston: Little, Brown and Co., 1986), p. 27.

34. Here one ought to consider the costs and benefits of varying policies of organ allocation. One of the most contentious issues regarding the fairness of the UNOS system of organ allocation concerns disparities in the amount of time that potential recipients wait for a transplant, which varies significantly according to geographic location. In response to such perceived inequalities the U.S. Department of Health and Human Services published a new regulation in April 1988 (42 CFR Part 121) to assure that allocation of scarce organs will be based on common medical criteria, not accidents of geography. The ruling required that organ allocation be based only on patient medical need rather than on variance in individual practice or any emphasis on keeping donated organs in the area in which they were procured. The ruling called for standardized medical criteria for determining the status of a patient's illness and their place on the waiting list. The question, though, was whether this would lead to fewer organs, less viable organs, and thus more deaths.

As a report from the Committee on Organ Procurement and Transplantation Policy argued, issuance of this Final Rule generated considerable controversy. Whereas its stated aims were to improve fairness and equal access, it was seen as likely leading to increased transplantation costs, forced closure of the smaller transplant centers, adverse affects on access to transplantation, less organ donation, and fewer lives saved. They urged that median waiting time is a poor and artificial measure of differences in access to transplantation. "Status—specific rates of pre-transplantation mortality and transplantation—are more meaningful indicators of equitable access" and permit a focus on lives saved rather than on the artificial standard of waiting time. Committee on Organ Procurement and Transplantation Policy, *Organ Procurement and Transplantation Policy: Appraising Current Policies and the Potential Impact of the DHHS Final Rule* (Washington, DC: National Academy Press, 1999), p. 10.

35. David Friedman provocatively illustrates this point: "the market is, generally speaking, the best set of institutions we know of for producing and distributing things. The more important a good is, the stronger the argument for having it produced by the market. Both barbers and physicians are licensed, both professions have for decades used licensing to keep their numbers down and their salaries up. Governmental regulation of barbers makes haircuts more expensive; one result presumably is that we have fewer haircuts and longer hair. Governmental regulation of physicians makes medical care more expensive; one result presumably is that we have less medical care and shorter lives. Given the choice of deregulating one profession or the other, I would choose the physicians." D. Friedman, "Should Medical Care Be a Commodity?" in *Rights to Health Care* (pp. 259–306), ed. T. Bole and W. Bondeson (Dordrecht: Kluwer Academic Publishers, 1991), p. 302.

36. See, for example, N. Daniels, "Equal Liberty and Unequal Worth of Liberty," in *Reading Rawls* (pp. 253–81), ed. N. Daniels (New York: Basic Books, 1975); N. Daniels, *Just Health Care* (New York: Cambridge University Press, 1985); N. Daniels, *Justice and Justification* (Cambridge: Cambridge University Press, 1996).

37. R. Nozick, *Anarchy, State and Utopia* (New York: Basic Books, 1974), pp. 161–62.

38. Cohen presents arguments concerning the ways in which enforcing such patterning of economic distribution might preserve liberty. G. A. Cohen, "Robert Nozick and Wilt Chamberlain: How Patterns Preserve Liberty," *Erkenntnis* 11 (1977): 5–23.

39. J. Rawls, *A Theory of Justice*, rev. ed. (Cambridge, MA: Harvard University Press, 1999), p. 64.

40. Ibid., p. 89.

41. J. Rawls, *Political Liberalism* (New York: Columbia University Press, 1993), p. 184. Here one might consider Norman Daniels's argument that society ought to secure the normal opportunity range for its citizens: "I want to emphasize a relationship between normal functioning and opportunity, one of the primary social goods. Impairments of normal species functioning reduce the range of opportunity open to the individual in which he may construct his 'plan of life' or conception of the good. Life plans for which we are otherwise suited are rendered unreasonable by impairments of normal functioning. Consequently, if persons have a fundamental interest in preserving the opportunity to revise their conceptions of the good through time, then they will have a pressing interest in maintaining normal species functioning by establishing institutions, such as health-care systems, which do just that." N. Daniels, *Justice and Justification* (Cambridge: Cambridge University Press, 1996), p. 214.

42. Hastings Center, *Ethical, Legal, and Policy Issues Pertaining to Solid Organ Procurement: A Report to the Project on Organ Transplantation* (New York: The Hastings Center, 1985), pp. 3–4.

43. P. Ramsey, *The Patient as Person* (New Haven, CT: Yale University Press, 1970), p. 168.

44. Two encyclical letters of the pope of Rome signal recognition of these significant changes. In *Veritatis Splendor* the Roman pontiff characterizes the antitraditional character of much of contemporary moral reflection as marked by "an overall and systematic calling into question of traditional moral doctrine, on the basis of certain anthropological and ethical presuppositions." John Paul II, *Veritatis Splendor* (Vatican City: Libreria Editrice Vaticana, 1993), p. 8. In *Evangelium Vitae*, John Paul II places this difficulty within a major cultural crisis and a shift in the presuppositions of moral theory. "In the background there is the profound crisis of culture, which generates skepticism in relation to the very foundations of knowledge and ethics, and which makes it increasingly difficult to grasp clearly the meaning of what man is, the meaning of his rights and his duties." John Paul II, *Evangelium Vitae* (Vatican City: Libreria Editrice Vaticanna, 1995), p. 21. The result is, as the pontiff recognizes, a transformation and fragmentation of culture, a fragmentation that sets the stage for the emergence of fundamental moral differences that divide morality into not merely different but mutually antagonistic accounts of proper moral conduct.

45. Prenatal diagnosis of Down syndrome and hemophilia in many countries is almost invariably followed by abortion. Moreover, failure to inform the pregnant woman of the possibility of nontherapeutic abortion has, at times, opened genetic counselors to civil liability under the law of torts. Such suits have typically alleged malpractice on grounds of either "wrongful life" or "wrongful birth." Civil claims for "wrongful life" involve parental suit on behalf of the child alleging that his nonexistence would have been preferable to his current existence with defects, such that his existence is a wrong done to him as a result of the negligence of the genetic counselor. Under a wrongful birth civil suit, the parents allege emotional and financial harms associated with caring for a defective newborn that they would have chosen to abort if they had been informed of the appropriateness of the option. Such legally supported torts require Christian counselors to encourage patients to seek abortions based on very secular quality of life judgments and in violation of deeply held religious convictions. See A. Milunsky and G. Atkins, "Prenatal Diagnosis of Genetic Disorders: An Analysis of Experience with 600 Cases," *Journal of the American Medical Association* 230, no. 2 (1974): 232–35; G. Atkinson and A. Moraczewski, eds.,

Genetic Counseling, the Church and the Law; A Task Force Report of the Pope John Center (St. Louis: Pope John XXIII Medical-Moral Research and Education Center, 1980), pp. 27–29.

46. In response to a possible counterexample in which being born male in a particular society was sufficient to ensure that a child will lead a miserable life, a life judged not worth living, Peter Singer stated: "But if this were the case—and there were nothing one could do about it—then I would indeed accept that the parents of newborn males should be allowed to kill them painlessly, so as to be able to raise a girl." P. Singer and H. Kuhse, "More on Euthanasia: A Response to Pauer-Studer," *Monist* 76, no. 2 (1993): 158–75, p. 162.

   Similarly, Singer has argued elsewhere that life is a journey and that, when the current prospects for that journey are seriously unfavorable, it may be better for the parents to choose not to let that journey continue—to wait instead for another time when the outlook is more favorable. "Parents will grieve when a newborn child dies, just as when a pregnancy miscarries at a late stage, but in most cases they will be able to have another child, and if that child's prospects are better, both they and 'their child' will be better off in the long run." P. Singer and P. Ratiu, "The Ethics and Economics of Heroic Surgery," *Hastings Center Report* 31, no. 2 (2001): 47–48, p. 48.

47. J. T. McHugh, "Building a Culture of Life: A Catholic Perspective," *Christian Bioethics* 7, no. 3 (2001): 441–52, p. 442.

48. S. T. Poppema, *Why I Am an Abortion Doctor* (Amherst: Prometheus Books, 1996), p. 11.

49. Many contemporary nontraditional Christian moralists have adopted a similar stance. As Beverly Harrison describes the challenges of abortion: "We are only at the beginning of the public political dispute over procreative choice in human history. If we do not obliterate ourselves with other life-destructive technologies in the meanwhile, the abortion debate probably will continue in one form or another for decades, perhaps for generations. This is because all of the intricate social systems that characterize human life—our institutions, mores, and customs and all the varied religious sacralization of these systems through all recorded history—have been shaped inherently to control women's procreative power. This control will not be relinquished without a struggle." B. Harrison, *Our Right to Choose: Toward a New Ethic of Abortion* (Boston: Beacon Press, 1983), p. 3.

50. "I understand oppression to mean any social situation that systematically requires heroism on the part of a class of people based on gender, race or other such identification. Given the gendered structure of society at present and the resultant lack of communal support for women, the absolute prohibition on taking the life of the fetus, however protective of the right to life of that fetus, remains oppressive of women." T. Whitmore, "Notes for a 'New, Fresh Compelling' Statement," *America* 171, no. 10 (1994): 14.

51. Maguire and Burtchaell argue, in addition, that the anti-abortion statements of the ancient traditional Christian Church must be placed fully within a particular cultural context: "(1) All occurred before the beginning of any formal theology on abortion. (2) They rose from a period of ignorance of the processes of generation, the ovum having been discovered only in the nineteenth century. (3) They came at a time of under population. (4) They came in a time of notable sexism and negativity to sexuality. (5) Abortion was often condemned as a violation of the procreative nature of sex and not as murder." D. Maguire and J. Burtchaell, "The Catholic Legacy and Abortion: A Debate," in *On Moral Medicine*, 2nd ed. (pp. 586–98), ed. S. Lammers and A. Verhey (Grand Rapids: Eerdsmans, 1998), p. 589. This moral tradition, they urge, can only be adequately understood as part of a regrettable history of the oppression of women.

52. National Academy of Sciences, *Confronting AIDS: Directions for Public Health, Health Care, and Research* (Washington, DC: National Academy Press, 1986).

53. Office of the Surgeon General, "Surgeon General's Report on Acquired Immune Deficiency Syndrome" (Washington, DC: Public Health Service, Office of the Surgeon General, 1986).

54. See generally Task Force on Pediatric AIDS, "Adolescents and the Human Immuno-deficiency Virus Infection: The Role of the Pediatrician in Prevention and Intervention," *Pediatrics* 92 (1993): 626–30; and Committee on Adolescence, "Homosexuality and Adolescence," *Pediatrics* 92 (1993): 631–34.

55. N. Bell, "Ethical Issues in AIDS Education," in *AIDS & Ethics* (pp. 128–54), ed. F. Reamer (New York: Columbia University Press, 1991), p. 150.

56. As Gunderson and Mayo note, as a discipline bioethics generally holds that competent individuals have the right to determine their own fates. "The autonomy-based argument for physician-assisted death is straightforward: as illness begins to seriously compromise the quality of a person's life, few issues could be more profound and personal for that person than determining the point at which his or her life is no longer worth living." M. Gunderson and D. Mayo, "Restricting Physician-Assisted Death to the Terminally Ill," *Hastings Center Report* 30, no. 6 (2000): 17–23, p. 18.

57. *Compassion in Dying v. State of Washington* 79 F.3d 790 (9th cir. 1996): 810–39 at 839.

58. In response to two cases, one involving a woman who committed suicide, the other a woman with seemingly suicidal intent who sought to end all medical care so that she would die—though with treatment she would likely live another fifteen to twenty years—a Presbyterian Minister stated: "But should we not also respond compassionately to a Diane or an Elizabeth, not condemning, but valuing a different kind of courage and faithfulness?" E. Bay, "The Christian Faith and Euthanasia," in *In Life and Death We Belong to God* (appendix 2, pp. 52–56), Christian Faith and Life Area, Congregational Ministries Division, PC (USA) (Louisville: Presbyterian Distributions Services, 1995), p. 55.

The Presbyterian Church (USA) has stepped back from absolute condemnation of euthanasia: "'Active Euthanasia' is extremely difficult to defend morally. There are, however, extreme circumstances in which we may have to at least raise the question of a fundamental conflict of obligations. There is an analogy between such cases of 'active euthanasia' and abortions, questions that are based on the circumstances of the fetus. There is an accompanying prejudice against the taking of life in both cases, since the conflict between doing no harm and protecting from harm has reference to one and the same individual. The ambiguity of this situation serves to reinforce what has already been said about cautious and consultative decision making." 121st General Assembly of the Presbyterian Church in the United States, "The Nature and Value of Human Life," in *In Life and Death We Belong to God* (Appendix 3, pp. 61–65), Christian Faith and Life Area, Congregational Ministries Division, PC (USA) (Louisville: Presbyterian Distributions Services, 1981), p. 62.

59. K. Wildes, "Sanctity of Life: A Study in Ambiguity and Confusion," in *Japanese and Western Bioethics: Studies in Moral Diversity* (pp. 89–101), ed. K. Hoshino (Dordrecht: Kluwer Academic Publishers, 1996), p. 89.

60. For example, while traditional Christianity has always condemned suicide and assisted suicide, as with abortion many contemporary Christians have begun following secular bioethics in adopting this nontraditional stance. In one survey of Protestant pas-

tors, 17 percent supported laws in favor of assisted suicide, with over 33 percent of those surveyed who were also associated with the National Council of Churches in favor. "Protestant Pastors Support Death Penalty," *Christian Century*, September 27–October 4, 2000, pp. 948–49. According to Frasen and Walters, if quality of life is sufficiently minimal, assisted suicide may be permissible since "the traditional concept of life after death would seem to question the value of eking out every moment of life when the whole of existence goes far beyond temporal death. The Bible portrays a God who values quality of life." S. Frasen and J. Walters, "Death—Whose Decision? Euthanasia and the Terminally Ill," *Journal of Medical Ethics* 26, no. 2 (2000): 121–25, p. 124. Or as Karen Lebacqz argues: "And yet I am also a Christian. I know that death is not the last word, not the greatest evil. Failure to live, to care, to enact justice, to be in proper relationship—those are greater evils. Death can serve evil or it can serve the values of life. As a way of bringing about death, active euthanasia can serve evil or it can serve the values of life. When it serves the values of life, it can be morally justified." K. Lebacqz, "Reflection," in *On Moral Medicine*, 2nd ed. (pp. 666–67), ed. S. Lammers and A. Verhey (Grand Rapids: Eerdmans,1998), p. 667.

Episcopal bishop John S. Spong also favorably regards assisted suicide: "My conclusions are based on the conviction that the sacredness of my life is not ultimately found in my biological extension. It is found rather in the touch, the smile, and the love of those to whom I can knowingly respond. When that ability to respond disappears permanently, so, I believe, does the meaning and the value of my biological life. Even my hope of life beyond biological death is vested in a living relationship with the God who, my faith tradition teaches me, calls me by name. I believe that the image of God is formed in me by my ability to respond to that calling Deity. If that is so, then the image of God has moved beyond my mortal body when my ability to respond consciously to that Divine Presence disappears. So nothing sacred is compromised by assisting my death in those circumstances." J. Spong, "In Defense of Assisted Suicide," *The Voice of the Diocese of Newark*, January–February 1996, pp. 3–4.

61. L. Torcello and S. Wear, "The Commercialization of Human Body Parts: A Reappraisal from a Protestant Perspective," *Christian Bioethics* 6 (2000): 153–69, p. 161.

62. Ibid., p. 163.

63. Ibid., p. 164.

64. K. Wildes, "Sanctity of Life: A Study in Ambiguity and Confusion," *Japanese and Western Bioethics: Studies in Moral Diversity* (pp. 89–101), ed. K. Hoshino (Dordrecht: Kluwer Academic Publishers, 1996), p. 91.

65. One suggestion for breaking through the fragmented character of moral theory has been to secure a practical ethic of care. For example, Joy Penticuff has argued that nursing ethics are straightforwardly practical. It is an ethics in which abstract moral principles gain content through everyday understandings of what it means to the patient himself to be ill, to recover, or to move toward eventual death with a chronic terminal illness. It is argued that a nurse's moral perspective is gained at the level of everyday consciousness. Nurses deal directly with patients with a closeness and intimacy. "Nursing perspectives therefore are practical and include all the thoughts, feelings, and actions that go into caring and being responsible for those who need nursing." J. H. Penticuff, "Nursing Perspectives in Bioethics," in *Japanese and Western Bioethics: Studies in Moral Diversity* (pp. 49–60), ed. K. Hoshino (Dordrecht: Kluwer Academic Publishers, 1996), p. 50. Thoughts and feeling are fused with practical presence and human interaction. Deep empathetic connections with patients prompt the move from a dispassionate ethic of the primacy of

individual freedom and the commodification of health care, to an ethic of a caring community, a "transformation of health care systems into caring communities—places and systems in which the good for patients can be instantiated and worked out." Ibid., p. 55.

Yet, caring is contextual. What it means to care for someone, or to practice an ethic of care, presupposes a context in which to understand how one individual ought to show compassion for another. For example, in "The Truth about Caring," by Judith Shelly, and "What Is Caring?" by Irene B. Alyn and Janet A. Conway, each argues that the nurse's commitment to caring and compassion arises out of a particular account of Christian revelation and Christian duties. J. Shelly, "The Truth about Caring," *Journal of Christian Nursing* (Summer 1995): 3, 46; I. B. Alyn and J. A. Conway, "What Is Caring?" *Journal of Christian Nursing* (Summer 1995): 7–12, 45.

Contrast a particularly Christian sense of caring to that for which Howard Curzer argues in "Is Care a Virtue for Health Care Professionals?" Curzer concludes that health care professionals do not have a duty to care for their patients. Rather, the notion of "care" should be deconstructed into notions of benevolence and "acting in a caring manner." H. J. Curzer, "Is Care a Virtue for Health Care Professionals?" *Journal of Medicine and Philosophy* 18 (1993): 51–69. These two categories again, however, require particular contextual notions of what it means to be benevolent and to "act in a caring manner" to be of use in determining appropriate codes of conduct. The particular Christian commitments of Alyn and Conway will not be authoritatively available outside of their particular religious contexts.

66. T. Murray, "Organ Vendors, Families, and the Gift of Life," in *Organ Transplantation: Meanings and Realities* (pp. 101–25), ed. S. Youngner, R. C. Fox, and L. O'Connell (Madison: University of Wisconsin Press, 1996), p. 111.

67. R. Arnold, S. Bartlett, J. Bernat, J. Colonna, D. Dafoe, N. Dubler, S. Gruber, J. Kahn, R. Luskin, H. Nathan, S. Orloff, J. Prottas, R. Shapiro, C. Ricordi, S. Youngner, F. L. Delmonico, "Financial Incentives for Cadaver Organ Donation: An Ethical Reappraisal," *Transplantation* 73, no. 8 (2002): 1361–67; B. Kahan, "Organ Donation and Transplantation—A Surgeon's View," in *Organ Transplantation: Meanings and Realities* (pp. 126–41), ed. S. Youngner, R. C. Fox, and L. O'Connell (Madison: University of Wisconsin Press, 1996); L. Barkan, "Cosmas and Damian: Of Medicine, Miracles, and the Economics of the Body," in *Organ Transplantation: Meanings and Realities* (pp. 221–51), ed. S. Youngner, R. C. Fox, and L. O'Connell (Madison: University of Wisconsin Press, 1996).

68. Office of Technology Assessment, *New Developments in Biotechnology: Ownership of Human Tissues and Cells* (Washington, DC: U.S. Government Printing Office, 1987), p. 124.

69. R. Nozick, *Anarchy, State and Utopia* (New York: Basic Books, 1974), especially chapter 3.

70. J. S. Mill, *On Representative Government*, in *Three Essays* (Oxford: Oxford University Press, 1975 [1861]), p. 145.

71. P. Singer, "The Right to Be Rich or Poor," in *Reading Nozick: Essays on Anarchy, State and Utopia* (pp. 37–53), ed. J. Paul (Totowa, NJ: Rowman & Littlefield, 1981).

72. Consider Edmund Pellegrino's denouncement of markets and managed care: "I refer here to how the books are 'balanced,' and profits reaped—by the denial of claims, cutting of payments to physicians and hospitals, erecting new barriers to care, disenrolling patients and physicians who cost too much, and refusing grievances and appeals by defin-

ing medical necessity and experimental therapy in terms favorable to managed care organizations. I refer, too, to the legitimation of self-interest and profit-making on the part of physicians, investors, and managed care organizations." E. D. Pellegrino, "The Good Samaritan in the Marketplace: Managed Care's Challenge to Christian Charity," in *The Changing face of Health Care* (pp. 103–18), ed. J. Kilner, R. Orr, and J. Shelly (Grand Rapids: Eerdmans, 1998), p. 106.

An ad hoc committee of the American Medical Association expressed similar sentiments: "Mounting shadows darken our calling and threaten to transform healing from a covenant into a business contract. Canons of commerce are displacing dictates of healing, trampling our profession's most sacred values. Market medicine treats patients as profit centers. The time we are allowed to spend with the sick shrinks under the pressure to increase throughput, as though we were dealing with industrial commodities rather than afflicted human beings in need of compassion and caring." American Medical Association, Ad Hoc Committee to Defend Health Care, "For Our Patients, Not for Profits: A Call to Action," *Journal of the American Medical Association* 278, no. 21 (1997): 1733–8, p. 1733.

Similarly, Patricia Brenner claims: "There is something radically wrong with treating health care as one more product in a free-market economy. It is unrealistic to expect patients to be consumers who will aggressively hunt for the best bargain and be wise in their 'product choice.' Viewing health care as a commodity to be bought and sold does not work in many situations. For example, if we are frail elderly persons, children, busy adults seeking to make a living for our family, in an automobile accident, under anesthesia, able to speak English only as a second language, or poor and uninsured, we are in no condition to be alert, smart consumers, protecting our investments and demanding our rights. We are at the mercy of our fellow citizens who we can only hope will be wise and compassionate strangers. Health care based on profit guidelines estranges patients from health care workers." P. Brenner, "When Health Care Becomes a Commodity: The Need for Compassionate Strangers," in *The Changing Face of Health Care* (pp. 119–35), ed. J. Kilner, R. Orr, and J. Shelly (Grand Rapids: Eerdmans, 1998), pp. 119–20.

73. J. Iglehart, "Canada's Health Care System Faces Its Problems," *New England Journal of Medicine* 322, no. 8 (1990): 562–68; R. Wilkins, O. Adams, and A. Brancker, "Changes in Mortality by Income in Urban Canada from 1971 to 1986: Findings of a Joint Study Undertaken by the Policy, Communications, and Information Branch, Health and Welfare Canada, and the Canadian Centre for Health Information," Statistics Canada, *Health Reports* 1, no. 2 (1989): 137–74; R. Wilkins, G. Sherman, and P. A. F. Best, "Birth Outcomes and Infant Mortality by Income in Urban Canada, 1986," Statistics Canada, *Health Reports* 3, no. 1 (1991): 7–31.

74. J. Rawls, *A Theory of Justice*, rev. ed. (Cambridge, MA: Harvard University Press, 1999), pp. 63–64.

75. Ibid., p. 87.

76. Ibid., p. 63.

77. Kai Nielsen encapsulates the view: "If we want a world of moral equals, we also need a world in which people stand to each other in a rough equality of condition. To have a world in which a condition of equal respect and concern obtain, we need . . . a rough equality of resources. If equality as a right is to be secure; that is, if that is a right that people actually can securely exercise, we must obtain the good of equality of condition." K. Nielsen, *Equality and Liberty: A Defense of Radical Egalitarianism* (Totowa, NJ: Rowman & Allenheld, 1985), p. 10.

78. N. Daniels, "Equal Liberty and Unequal Worth of Liberty," in *Reading Rawls* (pp. 253–81), ed. N. Daniels (New York: Basic Books, 1975); N. Daniels, *Justice and Justification* (Cambridge: Cambridge University Press, 1996).

79. D. Callahan, *Setting Limits: Medical Goals in an Aging Society* (New York: Simon and Schuster, 1987), 136–37. See also D. Sulmasy, "Do the Bishops Have It Right on Health Care Reform?" *Christian Bioethics* 2, no. 3 (1996): 309–25, p. 317.

80. Consider: "Health care needs are basic insofar as they promote fair equality of opportunity. Health care for children is especially important in relation to other social goods, because diseases and disabilities inhibit children's capacities to use and develop their talents, thereby curtailing their opportunities." L. Kopelman, "On Duties to Provide Basic Health and Dental Care to Children," *Journal of Medicine and Philosophy* 26 (2001): 193–209, p. 202.

81. The United States Catholic Bishops have urged: "Our nation's health care system serves too few and costs too much. . . . Every person has a right to adequate health care. This right flows from the sanctity of human life and the dignity that belongs to all human persons, who are made in the image of God. Health care is more than a commodity; it is a basic human right, an essential safeguard of human life and dignity." National Conference of Catholic Bishops, "Resolution on Health Care Reform," *Origins* 23 (1993): 97, 99–101, p. 97.

82. The five-year patient survival rate for kidneys transplanted from a deceased donor is 79.9 percent (with graft survival at 63.3 percent) and from a living donor is 89.7 percent (with graft survival at 76.5 percent). UNOS, *2002 Annual Report of the U.S. Scientific Registry of Transplant Recipients and the Organ Procurement and Transplantation Network: Transplant Data 1992–2001* (Rockville, MD, and Richmond, VA: HHS/HRSA/OSP/DOT and UNOS, 2002), table 1.14.

83. D. Brock and N. Daniels, "Ethical Foundations of the Clinton Administration's Proposed Health Care System," *Journal of the American Medical Association* 271 (1994): 1189–96, p. 1189.

84. J. Rawls, *Political Liberalism* (New York: Columbia University Press, 1993), pp. 58–62, 194ff.

85. Habermas's idea of discourse ethics and political decision making is illustrative:
"Discourse ethics rests on the intuition that the application of the principle of universalization, properly understood, calls for a joint process of 'ideal role taking.' . . . Under the pragmatic presuppositions of an inclusive and noncoercive rational discourse among free and equal participants, everyone is required to take the perspective of everyone else, and thus project herself into the understandings of self and world of all others; from this interlocking of perspectives there emerges an ideally extended we-perspective from which all can test in common whether they wish to make a controversial norm the basis of their shared practice." J. Habermas, "Reconciliation Through the Public Use of Reason: Remarks on John Rawls's *Political Liberalism*," *Journal of Philosophy* 92, no. 3 (1995): 109–31, p. 117.

86. J. Rawls, *A Theory of Justice*, rev. ed. (Cambridge, MA: Harvard University Press, 1999), p. 394.

87. See, for example, G. Khushf, "Intolerant Tolerance," *Journal of Medicine and Philosophy* 19 (1994): 161–81.

88. J. Rawls, *Political Liberalism* (New York: Columbia University Press, 1993), p. 243.

89. This ethos is similar to Habermas's concept of a *herrschaftsfreier Diskurs*, where all whose interests are touched by a course of action have a voice in stating their particular needs: "Citizens are politically autonomous only if they can view themselves jointly as authors of the laws to which they are subject as individual addressees." J. Habermas, "Reconciliation Through the Public Use of Reason: Remarks on John Rawls's *Political Liberalism*," *Journal of Philosophy* 92, no. 3 (1995): 109–31, p. 130. Habermas admits that his model of political discourse requires that all participants free themselves from too deep an involvement with any particular values and principles: "the truth claims of all reasonable worldviews have equal weight, where those worldviews count as reasonable which compete with one another in a reflexive attitude, that is, on the assumption that one's own truth claim could prevail in public discourse in the long run only though the force of better reasons." Ibid., p. 125. They must not be burdened with the absolutist constraints of traditional religions and cultures.

90. Ibid., p. 130.

91. H. T. Engelhardt Jr., *The Foundations of Christian Bioethics* (Lisse: Swets and Zeitlinger, 2000), p. 30.

92. R. N. Rankin, "Magnetic Resonance Imaging in Canada: Dissemination and Funding," *Canadian Association of Radiology Journal* 50, no. 2 (1999): 89–92.

93. These six countries are Australia, Iceland, Japan, Norway, Sweden, and Switzerland. N. Esmail and M. Walker, *How Good Is Canadian Health Care* (Vancouver: The Fraser Institute, 2002), pp. 5–6.

94. See J. V. Pappachan, B. Miller, E. D. Bennett, and G. B. Smith, "Comparison of APACHE III Outcome from Intensive Care Admission after Adjustment for Case Mix by the APACHE III Prognostic System," *Chest* 115, no. 3 (1999): 802–10; K. Wood, D. B. Coursin, and R. M. Grounds, "Critical Care Outcomes in the United Kingdom: Sobering Wake-Up Call or Stability of the Lamppost?" *Chest* 115, no. 3 (1999): 614–16.

ICUs were developed medically to support compromised patients requiring extensive and advanced support of their respiration, support of two or more organ systems, and those with chronic impairment of one or more organ systems who also require support for acute reversible failure of additional organ system(s). ICUs focus on two primary categories of patients: (1) those with a high risk of imminent death (e.g., critically ill patients with respiratory failure, heart failure, and so forth) and (2) those who are potentially at high risk of imminent death (e.g., those admitted for supervision of a high-risk procedure, such as management of cardiac arrhythmias). Consider critical care: because of the significant expense of such intense and technologically sophisticated care, it may not be economically feasible to provide universal, unlimited access to all those who might receive some marginal benefit. Choices regarding the use of ICU resources will have to be honestly faced. If the choice is to forgo access since it cannot be provided equally to everyone, this will lower the standard of care, permitting the death and suffering of many salvageable patients. Even different macro-allocations to health care, and within health care to critical care units, will result in significant variation in outcome. See P. Taboada, "What Is Appropriate Intensive Care: A Roman Catholic Perspective," in *Allocating Scarce Medical Resources: Roman Catholic Perspectives* (pp. 53–73), ed. H. T. Engelhardt Jr. and M. J. Cherry (Washington, DC: Georgetown University Press, 2002).

95. As critical care resources become more constrained, individual caregivers and institutions must become more diligent regarding the selection of patients who should not receive intensive care, whether too healthy to require such care or too sick for the ICU to

offer significant hope of recovery. Moreover, greater diligence must be given to tracking patients whose need for intensive care could have been prevented through provision of inexpensive therapeutic interventions. For example, Michael Rie argues that approximately 80 percent of the readmissions to the ICU for respiratory failure were potentially preventable. In most instances, the need for intensive care was precipitated by the absence or inadequacy of direct care to remove secretions from patients. As he somewhat rhetorically frames the concern: "This is low-quality, low-cost, fraudulent sale of health services, which may meet criminal negligence standards." M. Rie, "Respect for Human Life in the World of Intensive Care Units: Secular and Reform Jewish Reflections on the Roman Catholic View," in *Allocating Scarce Medical Resources: Roman Catholic Perspectives* (pp. 43–52), ed. H. T. Engelhardt Jr. and M. J. Cherry (Washington, DC: Georgetown University Press, 2002), p. 45. An initial criterion, he concludes, for the moral provision of critical care ought to be careful stewardship of the available resources, which would require providing inexpensive respiratory care beyond the ICU to prevent readmission costs and to reduce patient mortality.

96. As Alexis de Tocqueville frames this concern: "After having thus successively taken each member of the community in its powerful grasp and fashioned him at will, the supreme power then extends its arm over the whole community. It covers the surface of society with a network of small complicated rules, minute and uniform, through which the most original minds and the most energetic characters cannot penetrate, to rise above the crowd. The will of man is not shattered, but softened, bent, and guided. . . . Such a power does not destroy, but it prevents existence; it . . . compresses, enervates, extinguishes, and stupefies a people, till each nation is reduced to nothing better than a flock of timid and industrious animals, of which the government is the shepherd." A. de Tocqueville, *Democracy in America* (London: David Campbell Publishers, Ltd., 1994 [1835]), vol. 2, p. 319.

Here also John Stuart Mill illuminates the ways in which governmental and social paternalism inhibit the creation of genius: "Persons of genius, it is true, are, and are always likely to be, a small minority; but in order to have them, it is necessary to preserve the soil in which they grow. Genius can only breathe freely in an *atmosphere* of freedom. Persons of genius are, *ex vi termini, more* individual than any other people—less capable, consequently, of fitting themselves, without hurtful compression, into any of the small number of moulds which society provides in order to save its members the trouble of forming their own character." J. S. Mill, *On Liberty*, in *On Liberty and Other Essays* (pp. 5–130), ed. J. Gray (Oxford: Oxford University Press, 1998 [1859]), p. 72.

97. "Even if it were most efficiently distributed via market mechanisms, efficiency and individual liberty ought not to be given moral hegemony over the fundamental respect for human dignity that is required of a just system of health care." D. Sulmasy, "Do the Bishops Have It Right on Health Care Reform?" *Christian Bioethics* 2, no. 3 (1996): 309–25, p. 312; see also p. 317.

98. J. Rawls, *Political Liberalism* (New York: Columbia University Press, 1993), pp. 243ff.

99. The Roman Catholic Church considers abortion morally wrong both for the woman who obtains an abortion and for those who provide the service, especially doctors and health care institutions. Universal single-tier health care poses a particular difficulty because "if the position of pro-abortion advocates prevails in the formulation of a national health care plan, then all Catholic hospitals will be required to provide abortions, Catholic physicians and health care workers will be required to perform or assist in abortions, and Catholic citizens and others conscientiously opposed to abortion will be

required to subsidize abortion with their taxes or their contributions to a health care alliance." J. McHugh, "Health Care Reform and Abortion: A Catholic Moral Perspective," *Journal of Medicine and Philosophy* 19 (1994): 491–500, p. 496.

100. According to Health Canada, in British Columbia, Alberta, Ontario, Newfoundland, and most facilities in Quebec, hospital and clinic fees for abortion are paid by the province. In the other provinces and territories, only abortions performed in hospitals are funded. http://www.hc-sc.gc.ca (last accessed August 10, 2004).

101. K. Schmidt, "Stabilizing or Changing Identity? The Ethical Problem of Sex Reassignment Surgery as a Conflict Among the Individual, Community, and Society," in *Cross-Cultural Perspectives on the (Im)Possibility of Global Bioethics* (pp. 237–64), ed. J. Tao (Dordrecht: Kluwer Academic Publishers, 2002).

102. As Lord Acton noted, private property is central to the preservation of liberty. It protects one's liberty of conscience regarding the use of oneself, one's talents and abilities. Even when defense of conscience does not directly arise, property is always exposed to interference; it is the constant object of public policy. L. Acton, *Essays in Religion, Politics, and Morality*, ed. J. Rufus Fears (Indianapolis: Liberty Classics, 1988), p. 572.

John C. Calhoun noted that "the effect, then, of every increase is, to enrich and strengthen the one and impoverish and weaken the other. This, indeed, may be carried to such an extent, that one class or portion of the community may be elevated to wealth and power, and the other depressed to abject poverty and dependence, simply by the fiscal action of the government; and this too, through disbursements only—even under a system of equal taxes imposed for revenue only. If such may be the effect of taxes and disbursements, when confined to their legitimate objects—that of raising revenue for the public service—some conception may be formed, how one portion of the community may be crushed, and another elevated on its ruins, by systematically perverting the power of taxation and disbursement, for the purpose of aggrandizing and building up one portion of the community at the expense of the other." J. C. Calhoun, *Union and Liberty: The Political Philosophy of John C. Calhoun*, ed. R. Lence (Indianapolis: Liberty Classics, 1992), p. 19.

Taxing traditional Roman Catholics for support of abortion rights enhances the liberty of those who wish access to abortion at the expense of the former.

103. See, for example, the American Society for Bioethics and the Humanities publication *Core Competencies for Health Care Ethics Consultation* (Glenview, IL: American Society for Bioethics and Humanities, 1996).

104. Consider the following as representative examples: the United Nations published "HIV/AIDS and Human Rights," guidelines that specifically call for unfettered access to abortion: "Laws should also be enacted to ensure women's reproductive and sexual rights, including the right of . . . means of contraception, including safe and legal abortion and the freedom to choose among these, the right to determine number and spacing of children." Failing to provide safe and legal abortion as a matter of positive right is understood as a violation of basic human rights. Office of the United Nations High Commissioner for Human Rights and the Joint United National Programme on HIV/AIDS, "HIV/AIDS and Human Rights: International Guidelines" (Geneva: United Nations, September 23–25, 1996).

The Council of Europe's Convention for the Protection of Human Rights and Dignity of the Human Being with regard to the Application of Biology and Medicine: Convention on Human Rights and Biomedicine held signing parties to protect the dignity and identity of all human beings, guaranteeing everyone, without discrimination, "respect for their integrity and other rights and fundamental freedoms with regard to the applications of biology and medicine." Chapter 1, article 1 (Geneva: Council of Europe, 1997). Such rights and freedoms included individual-oriented free and informed consent, restrictions on the use of genetic testing, protections for human research subjects, and prohibitions on the sale of human organs for transplantation. http://conventions.coe.int/treaty/en/treaties/html/164.htm (last accessed August 10, 2004).

105. H. T. Engelhardt Jr., *The Foundations of Bioethics*, 2nd ed. (New York: Oxford University Press, 1996), especially chapters 3 and 4.

106. P. Applebaum, C. Lidz, and A. Meisel, *Informed Consent: Legal Theory and Clinical Practice* (New York: Oxford University Press, 1987); President's Commission for the Study of Ethical Problems in Medicine and Biomedical and Behavioral Research, *Making Health Care Decisions* (3 vols.) (Washington, DC: U.S. Government Printing Office, 1982).

107. R. Faden and T. Beauchamp, *A History and Theory of Informed Consent* (New York: Oxford University Press, 1986); S. Wear, *Informed Consent: Patient Autonomy and Physician Beneficence within Clinical Medicine* (Dordrecht: Kluwer Academic Publishers, 1993).

108. J. Tao Lai Po-wah, "Is Just Caring Possible? Challenge to Bioethics in the New Century," in *Cross-Cultural Perspectives on the (Im)Possibility of Global Bioethics* (pp. 41–58), ed. J. Tao Lai Po-wah (Dordrecht: Kluwer Academic Publishers, 2002), pp. 54–55.

109. As Qiu Ren-Zong elaborates, for Confucianism, "keeping familial integrity and orderly familial relations may be even more important than keeping bodily integrity." R.-Z. Qiu, "The Tension Between Biomedical Technology and Confucian Values," in *Cross-Cultural Perspectives on the (Im)Possibility of Global Bioethics* (pp. 71–88), ed. J. Tao Lai Po-wah (Dordrecht: Kluwer Academic Publishers, 2002), p. 77.

110. H. T. Engelhardt, Jr., *The Foundations of Bioethics*, 2nd ed. (New York: Oxford University Press, 1996).

111. R.-Z. Qiu, "The Tension Between Biomedical Technology and Confucian Values," in *Cross-Cultural Perspectives on the (Im)Possibility of Global Bioethics* (pp. 71–88), ed. J. Tao Lai Po-wah (Dordrecht: Kluwer Academic Publishers, 2002), p. 84.

112. H. T. Engelhardt Jr., "Morality, Universality, and Particularity: Rethinking the Role of Community in the Foundations of Bioethics," in *Cross-Cultural Perspectives on the (Im)Possibility of Global Bioethics* (pp. 19–38), ed. J. Tao Lai Po-wah (Dordrecht: Kluwer Academic Publishers, 2002), pp. 24–25.

113. See, for example, A. tan Alora and J. Lumitao, eds., *Beyond a Western Bioethics: Voices from the Developing World* (Washington, DC: Georgetown University Press, 2001).

114. While the dominant legal and moral structure is individual oriented, with the individual himself as the presumptive decision maker, there are exceptions in Western health care law that carve out default family-oriented positions for decision making. In Texas, for example, at the surface level there is an affirmation of the centrality of individuals, yet space is also made for families as the presumed locus for appropriate medical decision making. As a default approach to medical decision making, when patients lose decisional capacity and have failed to appoint a formal proxy or establish their wishes, the law establishes a defeasible presumption in favor of what the law characterizes as "qualified relatives" (Texas Statutes, §166.081 [9]) who can function as decision makers for those terminal family members who lose decisional capacity. Such "qualified relatives" are in the following priority: the patient's spouse, the patient's reasonably available adult children, the patient's parents or the patient's nearest living relative (Texas Statutes, §166.039 [b]).

115. J. Rawls, *Justice as Fairness: A Restatement* (Cambridge, MA: Harvard University Press: 2001), p. 166.

116. J. Rawls, *Political Liberalism* (New York: Columbia University Press, 1993), p. 199.

117. Ibid., p. 122.

118. Ibid., p. 199.

119. A. Gutmann, "Civic Education and Social Diversity," *Ethics* 105 (1995): 557–79, p. 559. As Will Kymlicka notes, this is precisely why traditional religious communities seek to find exemption from such requirements: The aim is "to integrate citizens into a modern societal culture, with its common academic, economic, and political institutions, and this is precisely what ethno-religious sects wish to avoid. Moreover, the sorts of laws from which these groups seek exemption are precisely the sorts of laws which lie at the heart of modern nation-building—for example, mass education." W. Kymlicka, "Western Political Theory and Ethnic Relations in Eastern Europe," in *Can Liberal Pluralism Be Exported? Western Political Theory and Ethnic Relations in Eastern Europe* (pp. 13–106), ed. W. Kymlicka and M. Opalski (New York: Oxford University Press, 2001), p. 37.

120. John Harris encapsulates the position: "we need to remind ourselves of the point of valuing liberty—freedom of choice. The point of autonomy, the point of choosing and having the freedom to choose between competing conceptions of how, and indeed why, to live, is simply that it is only thus that our lives become in any real sense our own. The value of our lives is the value we give to our lives. And we do this, so far as this is possible at all, by shaping our lives for ourselves." J. Harris, "Euthanasia and the Value of Life," in *Euthanasia Examined* (pp. 6–22), ed. J. Keown (Cambridge: Cambridge University Press, 1995), p. 11.

121. H. T. Engelhardt Jr., "Morality, Universality, and Particularity: Rethinking the Role of Community in the Foundations of Bioethics," in *Cross-Cultural Perspectives on the (Im)Possibility of Global Bioethics* (pp. 19–38), ed. J. Tao Lai Po-wah (Dordrecht: Kluwer Academic Publishers, 2002), p. 25.

122. J. Rawls, *A Theory of Justice*, rev. ed. (Cambridge, MA: Harvard University Press, 1999), p. 89.

123. Ibid., p. 64.

124. Ibid., p. 448.

125. The United Nations *HIV/AIDS and Human Rights: International Guidelines*, for example, specifically calls for unfettered access to abortion: "Laws should also be enacted to ensure women's reproductive and sexual rights, including the right of . . . means of contraception, including safe and legal abortion and the freedom to choose among these, the right to determine number and spacing of children." Office of the United Nations High Commissioner for Human Rights and the Joint United National Programme on HIV/AIDS. *HIV/AIDS and Human Rights: International Guidelines* (Geneva: United Nations, September 23–25, 1996). Failing to provide safe and legal abortion as a matter of positive right is understood as a violation of basic human rights.

126. G. Becker, "The Ethics of Prenatal Screening and the Search for Global Bioethics," in *Cross-Cultural Perspectives on the (Im)Possibility of Global Bioethics* (pp. 105–30), ed. J. Tao Lai Po-wah (Dordrecht: Kluwer Academic Publishers, 2002), pp. 118–24.

127. Ibid., pp. 119–20.

128. A. Milunsky and G. Atkins, "Prenatal Diagnosis of Genetic Disorders: An Analysis of Experience with 600 Cases," *Journal of the American Medical Association* 230, no. 2 (1974): 232–35.

129. In *Tina Smedley Reed, et al. v. Mary Campagnolo, et al.* (810 f. Supp. 167; 1993 U.S. Dist. LEXIS 245), the plaintiffs sought damages resulting from the birth of their child who suffers from genetic birth defects. The plaintiffs contended that the physicians failed to inform Mrs. Reed of the existence and need for prenatal testing, which would have revealed the child's defects in utero. Mrs. Reed's claim was that she would have then terminated her pregnancy. In *Phillips v. United States*, 508 F. Supp. 544 (D.S.C. 1981), the court held that based on "both the trend of authorities and the applicable policy considerations" (at 551), a claim predicated upon the alleged failure to provide adequate genetic counseling and prenatal testing did present a viable cause of action predicated upon negligence or medical malpractice. See also *Robak v. United States*, 658 F.2d 471 (7th Cir. 1981) (applying Alabama law), and *Gildiner v. Thomas Jefferson Univ. Hosp.*, 451 F. Supp. 692 (E.D.Pa. 1978), among others. For a detailed discussion of such cases, see G. Atkinson and A. Moraczewski, eds., *Genetic Counseling, the Church and the Law; A Task Force Report of the Pope John Center* (St. Louis: Pope John XXIII Medical-Moral Research and Education Center, 1980), pp. 27–29.

130. G. Becker, "The Ethics of Prenatal Screening and the Search for Global Bioethics," in *Cross-Cultural Perspectives on the (Im)Possibility of Global Bioethics* (pp. 105–30), ed. J. Tao Lai Po-wah (Dordrecht: Kluwer Academic Publishers, 2002), p. 115.

131. W. V. D'Antonio, "Trends in U.S. Roman Catholic Attitudes, Beliefs, Behavior," *National Catholic Reporter*, October 29 (1999).

132. "Protestant Pastors Support Death Penalty," *Christian Century*, September 27–October 4 (2000): 948–49.

133. Qiu Ren-Zong argues that as Western bioethics has become the basis of "global bioethics," it has thereby become the basis for imperialistic war: "A so-called global bioethics may borrow some canons of morality from existing bioethics or invent something new. The fact is that Western bioethics is dominant in the world. So, the newly articulated global bioethics may be tainted with a strong color of Western culture, or may be just . . . another version of Western bioethics within the clothes of global bioethics. When it is imposed on the non-Western communities or heretic communities within Western culture, this constitutes ethical imperialism. Now the warning has become reality. When some country or a number of countries makes a military action somewhere using the excuse of protecting the universal value of human rights, it is claimed that it is an ethical war, but it is a war of ethical imperialism." R.-Z. Qiu, "The Tension Between Biomedical Technology and Confucian Values," in *Cross-Cultural Perspectives on the (Im)Possibility of Global Bioethics* (pp. 71–88), ed. J. Tao Lai Po-wah (Dordrecht: Kluwer Academic Publishers, 2002), p. 85.

Here, one might also consider the established European norms on minority rights, as adopted by the Organisation for Security and Co-operation in Europe: *OSCE Handbook* (Geneva: Organisation for Security and Co-operation in Europe, 1990); or the *Framework Convention for the Protection of National Minorities* adopted by the Council of Europe (Geneva: Council of Europe, 1995). According to an OSCE report, minority rights "are matters of legitimate international concern and consequently do not constitute exclusively an internal affair of the respective State." Quoted in W. Kymlicka and M. Opalski, introduction to *Can Liberal Pluralism Be Exported? Western Political Theory and Ethnic Relations in Eastern Europe*, ed. W. Kymlicka and M. Opalski (New York: Oxford University Press, 2001), p. 4. Failure to accommodate to the Western liberal cosmopolitan understandings of liberty is seen as a violation of basic human rights and, thereby, potentially justification for international response.

134. T. Joseph, "Living and Dying in a Post-Traditional World," in *Cross-Cultural Perspectives on the (Im)Possibility of Global Bioethics* (pp. 59–67), ed. J. Tao Lai Po-wah (Dordrecht: Kluwer Academic Publishers, 2002), p. 61.

135. Ruiping Fan captures the idea of a content-full moral community: "A moral perspective is the image of a real moral life lived by a group of people. It is concrete, canonical and content-full; it cannot be entirely discursive. It is composed of abstract statements that are inevitably vague, ambiguous, and underdetermined without further interpretations." R. Fan, "Moral Theories vs. Moral Perspectives: The Need for a New Strategy for Bioethical Exploration," in *Cross-Cultural Perspectives on the (Im)Possibility of Global Bioethics* (pp. 369–90), ed. J. Tao Lai Po-wah (Dordrecht: Kluwer Academic Publishers, 2002), p. 370.

136. Similarly, traditional Filipino culture does not share Western obsessions for individuality, equality, and personal autonomy. Instead, the family is the basic social unit: it is the primary means of financial and emotional support, education, career, and health care. As Kuan and Lumitao note: "Family interests take precedence over those of the individual members." L. Kuan and J. Lumitao, "The Family and Health Care Practices," in *Beyond a Western Bioethics: Voices from the Developing World* (pp. 23–29), (Washington, DC: Georgetown University Press, 2001), p. 23. Families as a whole participate in successes, honors, and shames. As a result, Filipino health care does not support patient-based confidentiality or individual-oriented informed consent. Consent is fully family oriented: "When a family member falls ill, he or she is considered to be in need of protection from the harmful effects of knowing the diagnosis, as well as the stress of decision-making. Family members automatically take the role of patient advocate, even requesting that the patient not be told the diagnosis. The dominant authority figure (the mother or father) together with older extended relatives take it upon themselves to talk with the physician and decide among treatment options." Ibid., p. 24. Benevolent paternalism is thoroughly characteristic of the Filipino medical context.

137. The nature of property rights, their character, scope, and form, was drawn from the nature of persons. Under the traditional law of torts, the person includes any part of the body as well as anything attached to it and practically identified with it. Violation of a person included nonconsensual contact with the individual's "clothing, or with a cane, a paper, or any other object held in his hand." W. Prosser, *Law of Torts* (St. Paul: West, 1971), p. 34. Interest in the integrity of the person included his body and all the things intimately associated with it. As such, property is an extension of the person and is protected as part of the individual's forbearance rights against battery, unauthorized touching, or use.

138. See, for example, M. Cherry, "Polymorphic Medical Ontologies: Fashioning Concepts of Disease," *The Journal of Medicine and Philosophy* 25, no. 5 (2000): 519–38; K. Sadegh-Zadeh, "Fuzzy Health, Illness, and Disease," *Journal of Medicine and Philosophy* 25, no. 5 (2000): 605–38.

139. Note that such an account is consistent with understanding persons as free to choose to participate in insurance schemes that create welfare rights for the poor, ill, or disadvantaged—however "disadvantaged" is defined. One could imagine Atheistcare as including rights to third-party assisted reproduction, human cloning, abortion, organ vending for transplantation, and assisted suicide, to protect those "disadvantaged" in such areas of life, while members of Vaticare might accept lower standards of care in deference to providing more care or equal care for the poor. State authority would not exist to force insurance plans to offer compatible comprehensive levels of coverage. In general, it would be

an illicit use of force to compel either participation or taxpayer financing of any such scheme, even through majority democratic rule. The moral authority to interfere with such rights is limited to peaceable consent among persons and communities.

140. As Locke notes, governments that use the property of their citizens without permission are not conceptually different from thieves: "Wherever law ends, tyranny begins, if the law be transgressed to another's harm; and whosoever in authority exceeds the power given him by the law, and makes use of the force he has under his command to compass that upon the subject which the law allows not, ceases in that to be a magistrate, and acting without authority may be opposed, as any other man who by force invades the right of another." J. Locke, *Second Treatise of Government*, ed. C. B. Macpherson (Indianapolis: Hackett, 1980 [1690]), p. 103, §202.

141. See also T. Bole, "The Perversity of Thomistic Natural Law Theory," in *Natural Law and the Possibility of a Global Ethics* (pp. 141–47), ed. M. J. Cherry (Dordrecht: Kluwer Academic Publishers, 2004).

142. Hegel recognized that the body is the preeminent example of property precisely because it is the embodiment of one's will. "As a person, I am myself an *immediate individual* [*Einzelner*]; in its further determination, this means in the first place that I am *alive* in this organic body, which is my undivided external existence [*Dasein*]. . . . But, as a person, I at the same time possess *my life and body*, like other things [*Sachen*], only *in so far as I so will it*." G. W. F. Hegel, *Philosophy of Right*, ed. A. Wood, trans. H. B. Nisbet (Cambridge: Cambridge University Press, 1991 [1821]), p. 78, § 47 (emphasis in original). The body is the direct immediate embodiment of a person's freedom (ibid., p. 79, § 48). It is the means through which one appears to others as a self-conscious, self-conspicuously rational moral being.

143. See, for example, the model for moral decision making developed in B. A. Brody, *Life and Death Decision Making* (New York: Oxford University Press, 1988). Brody argues for a method of pluralistic casuistry as an approach for gaining insight into and resolving complex ethics cases. The theory holds that there are many different irreducible moral appeals, which are often in conflict and yet necessary to complement each other. Moreover, it takes as its point of departure particular cases, applying the moral appeals in different ways appropriate to the myriad factors and subtle complexities of the specific cases that challenge medical decision making. The theory is developed in detail in *Life and Death Decision Making*, with further development and application to research ethics in *Ethical Issues in Drug Testing, Approval, and Pricing* (New York: Oxford University Press, 1995), *The Ethics of Biomedical Research* (New York: Oxford University Press, 1998), and *Taking Issue* (Washington DC: Georgetown University Press, 2003).

CHAPTER 3

1. R. Titmuss, *The Gift Relationship* (New York: Vintage Books, 1971), p. 246. Whereas Titmuss's conclusion from such claims is that the professional donor must be eliminated entirely (ibid., p. 152), it is unclear that such problems would not be effectively resolved with appropriate screening measures. See also P. J. Hagen, *Blood; Gift or Merchandise* (New York: Alan R. Liss, 1982); and Office of Technology Assessment, *Blood Policy and Technology* (Washington, DC: U.S. Government Printing Office, 1985).

2. R. Titmuss, *The Gift Relationship* (New York: Vintage Books, 1971), pp. 245–46.

3. See, for example, J. Blumstein, who argues for legalizing payment for transplantable cadaveric organs on similar grounds. J. Blumstein, "Legalizing Payment for Transplantable Cadaveric Organs," in *Birth to Death: Science and Bioethics* (pp. 119–32), ed. D. Thomasma and T. Kushner (Cambridge: Cambridge University Press, 1996). See also J. Radcliffe-Richards, "From Him That Hath Not," in *Ethical Problems in Dialysis and Transplantation* (pp. 53–60), ed. C. M. Kjellstrand and J. Dossetor (Dordrecht: Kluwer Academic Publishers, 1992); and R. Gillon, "Transplantation and Ethics," in *Birth to Death: Science and Bioethics* (pp. 106–18), ed. D. Thomasma and T. Kushner (Cambridge: Cambridge University Press, 1996).

4. See R. A. Sells, "Clinical Transplantation," in *Birth to Death: Science and Bioethics* (pp. 99–105), ed. D. Thomasma and T. Kushner (Cambridge: Cambridge University Press, 1996); C. M. Kjellstrand and J. B. Dossetor, eds., *Ethical Problems in Dialysis and Transplantation* (Dordrecht: Kluwer Academic Publishers, 1992); P. J. Morris, ed., *Kidney Transplantation: Principle and Practice*, 3rd ed. (Philadelphia: W. B. Saunders and Company, 1988).

5. According to a recent, albeit limited, survey, this concern may be unwarranted. Adams et al. surveyed a broad sample of undergraduates at Auburn University, which, they acknowledge, restricts the scope of their conclusions, since the individuals in this sample are generally younger and more highly educated than the average member of the population of potential organ donors. Moreover, "because younger, more highly educated people tend to be more receptive to the idea of donating organs (and perhaps less opposed to the formation of organ markets), this sample is likely to produce an upward biased estimate of a national organ supply curve." A. F. Adams, A. H. Barnett and D. Kaserman, "Markets for Organs: The Question of Supply," *Contemporary Economic Policy* 17, no. 2 (1999): 147–55, p. 150. Nevertheless, the evidence was compelling enough to conclude "that the provision of financial incentives has the potential to eliminate completely the organ shortage at very modest levels of remuneration. Specifically, payments to organ donors would not cause a substantial shift in the quantity intercept, and positive (but relatively modest) prices would call forth a substantial increase in the number of organs supplied." Ibid., p. 155.

6. N. Wallace, "Wealthy Donors Could Increase Giving by $107–Billion, Nonprofit Group Says," *Chronicle of Philanthropy* 16, no. 6 (2004): 25–27.

7. M. Gumprich, G. Woeste, K. Kohlhaw, J. T. Epplen, and W. O. Bechstein, "Living Related Kidney Transplantation between Identical Twins," *Transplantation Proceedings* 34, no. 6 (2002): 2205–6; P. Painter, J. Taylor, S. Wolcott, J. Krasnoff, D. Adey, S. Tomlanovich, P. Stock, and K. Topp, "Exercise Capacity and Muscle Structure in Kidney Recipient and Twin Donor," *Clinical Transplantation* 17, no. 3 (2003): 225–30.

8. R. Emiroglu, M. C. Yagmurdur, H. Karakayali, G. Moray, and G. Arslan, "Results with Living-Donor Kidney Transplants from Spouses: Fourteen Years of Experience at Our Center," *Transplantation Proceedings* 34, no. 6 (2002): 2060–61; M. Haberal, R. Emiroglu, M. C. Yagmurdur, H. Karakayali, G. Moray, G. Arslan, and N. Bilgin, "Results with Living-Donor Kidney Transplants from Spouses: Fourteen Years of Experience at Our Center," *Transplantation Proceedings* 34, no. 6 (2002): 2410–11.

For additional reflection on the reasons individuals provide for donating, see M. Haberal, R. Emiroglu, G. Moray, H. Karakayali, and G. Arslan, "Living-Donor Transplantation: Single Center Experience," *Transplantation Proceedings* 34, no. 6 (2002): 2056–59; M. Haberal, R. Emiroglu, S. Boyactoglu, and B. Demirhan, "Donor Evaluation for Living-Donor Transplantation," *Transplantation Proceedings* 34, no. 6 (2002): 2145–47; H. H. Wolters, T. Vowinkel, J. Brockmann, D. Palmes, S. Heidenreich, and K. H. Dietl, "Living Donor Renal Transplantation: Experience with Fifty Patients in Five Years," *Transplantation Proceedings* 34, no. 6 (2002): 2216; M. Karliova, M. Malago, C. Valentin-Gamazo, J. Reimer, U. Treichel, G. H. Franke, S. Nadalin, A. Frilling, G. Gerken, and C. E. Broelsch, "Living-Related Liver Transplantation from the View of the Donor: A One-Year Follow-Up Survey," *Transplantation* 73, no. 11 (2002): 1799–1805; S. J. Wigmore and J. J. Forsythe, "Living-Related Liver Transplantation from the View of the Donor: A One-Year Follow-Up Survey," *Transplantation* 73 (2002): 1799.

9. As Monaco makes the point: "society and the government should consider institutions of further financial incentives to the living-related donor in the form of direct federal grants, tax rebates or credits, tuition subsidies for children, etc." A. P. Monaco, "Transplantation: The State of the Art," *Transplantation Proceedings* 22, no. 3 (1990): 896–901, p. 901. See also A. P. Monaco, "A Transplant Surgeon's Views on Social Factors in Organ Transplantation," *Transplantation Proceedings* 21 (1989): 3403–6; J. B. Dossetor et al., "Discussion," *Transplantation Proceedings* 22, no. 3 (1990): 933–38; and J. B. Dossetor and C. R. Stiller, "Ethics, Justice, and Commerce in Transplantation," *Transplantation Proceedings* 22, no. 3 (1990): 892–95.

10. For example, in 2000, General Motors announced that it would spend more than one million dollars within a six month period to launch organ, bone marrow, and stem-cell drives among its nearly 400,000 employees. "General Motors Launches Organ, Marrow Donor Campaign," *Transplant & Tissue Weekly*, May 28 2000.

11. R. A. Sells, "Paired-Kidney Exchange Program," *New England Journal of Medicine* 337 (1997): 1392–93.

12. K. Blum, "Johns Hopkins Surgeons Perform World's First 'Triple Swap' Kidney Transplant Operation," August 1, 2003, http://www.Hopkinsmedicine.org/press/2003/August/030801.htm (last accessed August 10, 2004).

13. C. Perry, "Human Organs and the Open Market," *Ethics* 91 (1980): 63–71; P. Manga, "A Commercial Market for Organs? Why Not?" *Bioethics* 1, no. 4 (1987): 321–38, p. 324.

14. Similarly, many conclude that there exists significant gender imbalances in living donor kidney transplantation. In the United States, for 2000 the percentages by gender were as follows: heart transplants: 73.3 percent male, 26.7 percent female; lung: 49.9 percent male, 50.1 percent female; heart-lung: 35.4 percent male, 64.6 percent female; liver: 60.9 percent male, 39.1 percent female; kidney: 59.4 percent male, 40.6 percent female; pancreas: 53.6 percent male, 46.4 percent female; kidney-pancreas: 57.2 percent male, 42.8 percent female. R. H. Hauboldt and N. J. Ortner, "2002 Organ and Tissue Transplant Costs and Discussion, A Milliman Research Report," Milliman USA Consultants and Actuaries. www.milliman.com/health/publications/research_reports.asp (last accessed August 10, 2004). See also L. K. Kayler, H. U. Meier-Kriesche, J. D. Punch, D. A. Campbell Jr., A. B. Leichtman, J. C. Magee, S. M. Rudich, J. D. Arenas, and R. M. Merion, "Gender Imbalance in Living Donor Renal Transplantation," *Transplantation* 73, no. 1 (2002): 248–52; L. K. Kayler, C. S. Rasmussen, D. M. Dykstra, A. O. Ojo, F. K. Port, R. A. Wolfe, and R. M. Merion, "Gender Imbalance and Outcomes in Living Donor Renal Transplantation in the United States," *American Journal of Transplantation* 3, no. 4 (2003): 452–58; S. Inoue, Y. Yamada, K. Kuzuhara, Y. Ubara, S. Hara, and O. Ootubo, "Are Women Privileged Organ Recipients?" *Transplantation Proceedings* 34, no. 7 (2002): 2775–76.

15. W. B. Arnason, "Commentary on 'The Anatomy of a Black Community Based Transplant Education Program: A Model for Community Empowerment,'" in *It Just Ain't Fair* (pp. 241–43), ed. A. Dula and S. Goering (West Port, CT: Praeger, 1994), p. 242. See also C. U. Callender, L. E. Hall, C. L. Yeager, A. W. Washington, and P. G. Smith, "The Anatomy of a Black Community Based Transplant Education Program: A Model for Community Empowerment," in *It Just Ain't Fair* (pp. 234–41), ed. A. Dula and S. Goering (West Port, CT: Praeger, 1994).

16. R. Gaston, I. Ayres, L. Dooley and A. Diethelm, "Racial Equity in Renal Transplantation: The Disparate Impact of HLA-Based Allocation," *Journal of the American Medical Association* 270, no. 11 (1993): 1352–57. See also E. L. Milford, "Organ Transplantation-Barriers, Outcomes, and Evolving Policies," *Journal of the American Medical Association* 280, no. 13 (1998): 1184.

17. L. Cooper-Patrick, J. Gallo, J. Gonzales, H. Thi Vu, C. Nelson, and D. Ford, "Race, Gender, and Partnership in the Patient-Physician Relationship," *Journal of the American Medical Association* 282, no. 6 (1999): 583–89.

18. L. E. Boulware, L. E. Ratner, J. A. Sosa, L. A. Cooper, T. A. LaVeist, and N. R. Powe, "Determinants of Willingness to Donate Living Related and Cadaveric Organs: Identifying Opportunities for Intervention," *Transplantation* 73, no. 10 (2002): 1683–91.

19. "The need for minority donors is critical. For example: African Americans represent 13 percent of the U.S. population, but 32 percent of patients awaiting kidney transplant. Hispanic/Latinos also represent 12 percent of the U.S. population, but 15 percent of patients awaiting kidney transplant. National Minority Awareness Day is observed every August 1 to increase awareness of organ donation among African American, Hispanic/Latino, Asian, Alaskan Native, Pacific Islander and Native American populations. The event also recognizes minority donors and their families." UNOS News Bureau, "National Minority Donor Awareness Day," UNOS, July 31, 2002, http://www.nos.org/news/newsDetail.asp?id=24 (last accessed August 10, 2004); see also "Referrals Less Likely for Blacks," *Transplant Weekly*, December 13, 1999.

20. W. B. Arnason, "Commentary on 'The Anatomy of a Black Community Based Transplant Education Program: A Model for Community Empowerment,'" in *It Just Ain't Fair* (pp. 241–43), ed. A. Dula and S. Goering (West Port, CT: Praeger, 1994), 243. See also W. B. Arnason, "Directed Donation: The Relevance of Race," *The Hastings Center Report* Nov.– Dec. (1991): 13–19.

For further discussion of living kidney donation to strangers, see P. Adams et al., "The Nondirected Live-Kidney Donor: Ethical Considerations and Practice Guidelines: A National Conference Report," *Transplantation* 74, no. 4 (2002): 582–90; A. Spital, "Must Kidney Donation by Living Strangers Be Nondirected?" *Transplantation* 72, no. 5 (2001): 966; W. Cherikh, "Trends in Living Donor Kidney Transplants: Do Minorities Benefit?" *UNOS News Bureau* (2002), September 20.

21. Robert Veatch argues, for example, that a similar case can be made for directed donation on the basis of racial discrimination. All those below the recipient on the waiting list are made better off because of the discrimination. They all move up one on the queue and are thereby more likely to receive an organ, or to receive an organ in a shorter period of time. R. Veatch "Egalitarian and Maximin Theories of Justice: Directed Donation of Organs for Transplant," *Journal of Medicine and Philosophy* 23, no. 5 (1998): 456–76.

On directed donation, see also M. D. Fox, "Directed Organ Donation: Donor Autonomy and Community Values," in *Organ and Tissue Donation: Ethical, Legal, and Pol-*

icy Issues, ed. B. Spielman (Carbondale: Southern Illinois Press, 1996); and W. B. Arnason, "Directed Donation: The Relevance of Race," *The Hastings Center Report*, Nov.–Dec. 1991, 13–19.

22. E. M. Johnson, M. J. Remucal, K. J. Gillingham, R. A. Dahms, J. S. Najarian, and A. J. Matas, "Complications and Risks of Living Donor Nephrectomy," *Transplantation* 64, no. 8 (1997), 1124–28; E. M. Johnson, J. S. Najarian, and A. J. Matas, "Living Kidney Donation: Donors Risks and Quality of Life," *Clinical Transplantation* (1997): 231–40.

23. L. F. Ross, D. T. Rubin, M. Siegler, M. A. Josephson, J. R. Thistlethwaite Jr., and E. S. Woodle, "Ethics of a Paired-Kidney-Exchange Program," *New England Journal of Medicine* 336, no. 24 (1997): 1752–55, p. 1753.

24. See, for example, H. Egawa and K. Tanaka, "Adult Living Donor Liver Transplantation Using Right Lobe," *Transplantation Proceedings* 34, no. 1 (2002): 235–36; J. C. Garcia-Valdecasas, J. Fuster, L. Grande, C. Fondevila, A. Rimola, M. Navasa, E. Bombuy, J. Ferrer, and J. Visa, "Adult Living Donor Liver Transplantation: Initial Results of a Starting Program," *Transplantation Proceedings* 34, no. 1 (2002): 237–38; G. M. Abouna, P. Ganguly, S. Jabur, W. Tweed, H. Hamdy, G. Costa, E. Farid, and A. Sater, "Successful ex vivo Liver Perfusion System for Hepatic Failure Pending Liver Regeneration or Liver Transplantation," *Transplantation Proceedings* 33, no. 12 (2001): 1962–64; G. J. Abouna, "Emergency Adult to Adult Living Donor Liver Transplantation for Fulminant Hepatic Failure—Is It Justifiable?" *Transplantation* 71, no. 10 (2001): 1498–500; J. S. Najarian, B. M. Chavers, L. E. McHugh, and A. J. Matas, "20 Years or More of Follow-up of Living Kidney Donors," *Lancet* 340 (1992): 807–10; M. J. Bia, E. L. Ramos, G. M. Danovitch, R. S. Gaston, W. E. Harmon, A. B. Leichtman, P. A. Lundin, J. Neylan, and B. L. Kasiske, "Evaluation of Living Renal Donors: The Current Practice of US Transplant Centers," *Transplantation* 60 (1995): 322–27; W. H. Bay and L. A. Herbert, "The Living Donor in Kidney Transplantation," *Annals of Internal Medicine* 105 (1987): 719–27.

25. For medical consideration regarding the relative costs and benefits of utilizing living donors, see P. L. Adams, D. J. Cohen, G. M. Danovitch, R. M. Edington, R. S. Gaston, C. L. Jacobs, R. S. Luskin, R. A. Metzger, T. G. Peters, L. A. Siminoff, R. M. Veatch, L. Rothberg-Wegman, S. T. Bartlett, L. Brigham, J. Burdick, S. Gunderson, W. Harmon, A. J. Matas, J. R. Thistlethwaite, and F. L. Delmonico, "The Nondirected Live-Kidney Donor: Ethical Considerations and Practice Guidelines: A National Conference Report," *Transplantation* 74, no. 4 (2002): 582–90; C. O. Callender, M. B. Hall, and P. V. Miles, "Increasing Living Donations: Expanding the National MOTTEP Community Grassroots Model Minority Organ Tissue Transplant Education Program," *Transplantation Proceedings* 34, no. 7 (2002): 2563–64; L. F. Ross, W. Glannon, M. A. Josephson, and J. R. Thistlethwaite Jr., "Should All Living Donors Be Treated Equally?" *Transplantation* 74, no. 3 (2002): 418–21; "Man Donates Portion of Liver to Random Recipient (Curt Bludworth)," *Transplant & Tissue Weekly* (May 28, 2000); "Laparoscopic Kidney Removal Technique Increases Donor Pool," *Transplant & Tissue Weekly* (April 23, 2000).

26. R. A. Epstein, *Mortal Peril: Our Inalienable Right to Health Care?* (Reading, MA: Addison Wesley, 1997), p. 254.

27. R. H. Hauboldt and N. J. Ortner, "2002 Organ and Tissue Transplant Costs and Discussion, A Milliman Research Report," Milliman USA Consultants and Actuaries, 4. http://www.milliman.com/health/publications/research_reports.asp (last accessed August 10, 2004). See also S. J. Mraz, "Why Not Pay Organ Donors?" *Machine Design* 70, no. 22 (1998): 69.

28. L. F. Ross, D. T. Rubin, M. Siegler, M. A. Josephson, J. R. Thistlethwaite Jr., and E. S. Woodle, "Ethics of a Paired-Kidney-Exchange Program," *New England Journal of Medicine* 336, no. 24 (1997): 1752–55.

29. R. A. Epstein, *Mortal Peril: Our Inalienable Right to Health Care?* (Reading, MA: Addison Wesley, 1997), p. 281.

30. M. D. Grossman, P. M. Reilly, D. McMahon, R. V. Hawthorne, D. R. Kauder, and C. W. Schwab, "Who Pays for Failed Organ Procurement and What Is the Cost of Altruism?" *Transplantation* 62, no. 12 (1996): 1828–31.

31. M. A. Schnitzler, C. S. Hollenbeak, D. S. Cohen, R. S. Woodward, J. A. Lowell, G. G. Singer, R. J. Tesii, T. K. Howard, T. Mohanakumar, and D. C. Brennan, "The Economic Implications of HLA Matching in Cadaveric Renal Transplantation," *New England Journal of Medicine* 341, no. 19 (1999): 1440–46. Similarly, kidney transplantation with organs from "expanded criteria" donors, such as organs procured from non-heart-beating donors, is somewhat more expensive than with ordinary donors. In one study, such organs increased expenses from $12,000 to $15,000 per transplant. J. F. Whiting, M. Golconda, R. Smith, S. O'Brien, M. R. First, and J. W. Alexander, "Economic Costs of Expanded Criteria Donors in Renal Transplantation," *Transplantation* 65, no. 2 (1998): 204–7.

32. J. Iglehart, "Canada's Health Care System Faces Its Problems," *New England Journal of Medicine* 322, no. 8 (1990): 562–68, p. 563; R. Wilkins, O. Adams, and A. Brancker, "Changes in Mortality by Income in Urban Canada from 1971 to 1986: Findings of a Joint Study Undertaken by the Policy, Communications, and Information Branch, Health and Welfare Canada, and the Canadian Centre for Health Information," Statistics Canada, *Health Reports* 1, no. 2 (1989): 137–74; R. Wilkins, G. Sherman, and P. A. F. Best, "Birth Outcomes and Infant Mortality by Income in Urban Canada, 1986," Statistics Canada, *Health Reports* 3, no. 1 (1991): 7–31.

33. M. G. Marmot, G. D. Smith, S. Stansfeld, C. Patel, F. North, J. Head, I. White, E. Brunner, and A. Feeney, "Health Inequalities Among British Civil Servants: The Whitehall II Study," *Lancet* 337, no. 8754 (1991): 1387–92; J. E. Ferrie, M. J. Shipley, S. A. Stansfeld, G. D. Smith, and M. Marmot, "Future Uncertainty and Socioeconomic Inequalities in Health: The Whitehall II Study," *Social Science and Medicine* 57, no. 4 (2003): 637–46.

34. M. G. Marmot, G. D. Smith, S. Stansfeld, C. Patel, F. North, J. Head, I. White, E. Brunner, and A. Feeney, "Health Inequalities Among British Civil Servants: The Whitehall II Study," *Lancet* 337, no. 8754 (1991): 1387–92, p. 1392. See also L. Wright, "The Type A Behavior Pattern and Coronary Artery Disease: Quest for the Active Ingredients and the Elusive Mechanism," in *Stress and Coping* (pp. 275–300), ed. A. Monat and R. S. Lazarus (New York: Columbia University Press, 1991), pp. 285–87.

35. M. G. Marmot, H. Bosma, H. Hemingway, E. Brunner, and S. Stansfeld, "Contribution of Job Control and Other Risk Factors to Social Variations in Coronary Heart Disease," *Lancet* 350, no. 9073 (1997): 235–39; S. Taylor, "Health Psychology: The Science and the Field," in *Stress and Coping* (pp. 62–80), ed. A. Monat and R. S. Lazarus (New York: Columbia University Press, 1991), p. 70; D. Goldstein, *Stress, Catecholamines, and Cardiovascular Disease* (New York: Oxford University Press, 1995), p. 397; B. Fletcher, "The Epidemiology of Occupational Stress," in *Causes, Coping and Consequences of Stress at Work* (pp. 3–50), ed. C. L. Cooper and R. Payne (West Sussex: John Wiley & Son Ltd., 1988), p. 27; A. Monat and R. S. Lazarus, "Stress and the Environment," in *Stress and*

Coping (pp. 81–86), ed. A. Monat and R. S. Lazarus (New York: Columbia University Press, 1991), p. 82; A. Monat and R. S. Lazarus, "The Concept of Coping," in *Stress and Coping* (pp. 183–87), ed. A. Monat and R. A. Lazarus (New York: Columbia University Press, 1991), p. 184.

36. M. G. Marmot and M. E. McDowall, "Mortality Decline and Widening Social Inequalities," *Lancet* 2, no. 8501 (1986): 274–76; E. A. Locke and M. S. Taylor, "Stress, Coping and the Meaning of Work," in *Stress and Coping* (pp. 140–58), ed. A. Monat and R. S. Lazarus (New York: Columbia University Press, 1991), pp. 140, 150–55.

37. R. Wilkins, G. Sherman and P. A. F. Best, "Birth Outcomes and Infant Mortality by Income in Urban Canada, 1986," Statistics Canada, *Health Reports* 3, no. 1 (1991): 7–31, p. 8.

38. Office of Technology Assessment, *New Developments in Biotechnology: Ownership of Human Tissues and Cells* (Washington, DC: U.S. Government Printing Office, 1987), p. 12.

39. Ibid., p. 124.

40. Ibid., p. 115.

41. A. tan Alora and J. Lumitao, eds., *Beyond a Western Bioethics* (Washington, DC: Georgetown University Press, 2001).

42. D. Tiong, "Human Organ Transplants," in *Beyond a Western Bioethics* (pp. 89–93), ed. A. tan Alora and J. Lumitao (Washington, DC: Georgetown University Press, 2001), pp. 91–92.

43. N. Daniels, "Equal Liberty and Unequal Worth of Liberty," in *Reading Rawls* (pp. 253–81), ed. N. Daniels (New York: Basic Books, 1975), p. 256; N. Daniels, *Justice and Justification* (Cambridge: Cambridge University Press, 1996).

44. W. Prosser, *Law of Torts* (St. Paul: West, 1971), p. 613.

45. Gillon argues that "respect for autonomy is also of direct relevance in the moral controversy about sale of organs by donors . . . if an autonomous decision to donate a kidney may be respected when a donor is related to the recipient, then I find it hard to understand why the similar decision of an unrelated donor, and/or of one who wishes to sell his kidney for some beneficial purpose, should not similarly be respected as an autonomous decision. The sometimes bruited notion that payment somehow undermines a person's autonomy sufficiently to justify disregard of his or her decision is absurd." R. Gillon, "Transplantation: A Framework for Analysis of the Ethical Issues," *Transplantation Proceedings* 22, no. 3 (1990): 902–3, p. 902.

46. R. Titmuss, *The Gift Relationship* (New York: Vintage Books, 1971), p. 242.

47. J. Feinberg, "Non-Coercive Exploitation," in *Paternalism* (pp. 201–35), ed. R. Sartorious (Minneapolis: University of Minnesota Press, 1983), p. 201; R. Goodin, "Exploiting a Situation and Exploiting a Person," in *Modern Theories of Exploitation* (pp. 166–200), ed. A. Reeve (London: Sage Publishers, 1987), p. 167.

48. A. Wertheimer, "Two Questions about Surrogacy and Exploitation," *Philosophy and Public Affairs* 21 (1992): 211–39, p. 213; A. Wertheimer, *Exploitation* (Princeton: Princeton University Press, 1996), pp. 207–77.

49. Y. M. Ibrahim, "Vote Leaves Iraq as Winner and West at a Loss," *New York Times*, October 18, 1995, p. A1.

50. D. Lamb, *Organ Transplants and Ethics* (New York: Routledge, 1990), p. 137.

51. The categories of "harmful," "mutually advantageous," and "moralistic" exploitation are borrowed from Alan Wertheimer. They have, however, been adopted and altered somewhat for application to the particularities of organ sales. See A. Wertheimer, "Two

Questions about Surrogacy and Exploitation," *Philosophy and Public Affairs* 21 (1992): 211–39; A. Wertheimer, *Exploitation* (Princeton: Princeton University Press, 1996).

52. A. Wertheimer, "Two Questions about Surrogacy and Exploitation," *Philosophy and Public Affairs* 21 (1992): 211–39, p. 215.

53. For further discussion of *ex post* versus *ex ante* assessment of costs and benefits, see Wertheimer, "Two Questions about Surrogacy and Exploitation."

54. Consider, for comparison, commercial surrogacy. Some argue that in addition to the inconvenience and discomfort associated with normal pregnancy, the surrender of the child to the intended parents is psychologically harmful to the surrogate mother. See R. Tong, "The Overdue Death of a Feminist Chameleon: Taking a Stand on Surrogacy Arrangements," *Journal of Social Philosophy* 21 (1990): 40–56.

55. For a similar point regarding commercial surrogacy, see A. Wertheimer, "Two Questions about Surrogacy and Exploitation," *Philosophy and Public Affairs* 21 (1992): 211–39, p. 217.

56. R. Titmuss, *The Gift Relationship* (New York: Vintage Books, 1971).

57. A study conducted in Leeds, for example, found that 67.7 percent of potential blood recipients would be content if the donor had received remuneration, with more than 16 percent more likely to donate if they were to receive payment. R. P. Jones, V. Prasad, J. Kuruvatti, N. Tahir, P. Whitaker, A. S. Dawson, M. A. Harrison, and R. Williams, "Remuneration for Blood Donation and Attitudes Towards Blood Donation and Receipt in Leeds," *Transfusion Medicine* 13, no. 3 (2003): 131–40.

Another study in Germany concluded that of those surveyed, removing all remuneration would result in a 86.1 percent refusal to donate; a full 77 percent would refuse to donate in the future as well. This result appeared to increase with the age of the donor and with the number of donations, but was seen as largely independent of social status. T. Zeiler and V. Kretschmer, "Survey of Blood Donors on the Topic of 'Reimbursement for Blood Donors,'" *Infusionsther Transfusionsmed* 22, no. 1 (1995): 19–24. See also S. Puig, R. Felder, A. Staudenherz, M. Kurz, I. Kolar, and P. Hocker, "Satisfaction of Paid Thrombocyte Donors with Instrumental Thrombocytapheresis," *Infusionsther Transfusionsmed* 22 (1995): 14–18.

58. J. Miskowicz, "Cost Containment through a Hospital-Based Blood Donor Center," *Clinical Lab Management Review* 10, no. 4 (1996): 332–37; C. J. Julius and S. R. Sytsma, "Comparison of Demographics and Motivations of Highly Committed Whole Blood and Platelet Donors," *Journal of Clinical Apheresis* 8 (1993): 82–88; R. G. Strauss, G. A. Ludwig, M. V. Smith, P. J. Villhauer, M. J. Randels, A. Smith-Floss, and T. A. Koerner, "Concurrent Comparison of the Safety of Paid Cytapheresis and Volunteer Whole Blood Donors," *Transfusion* 34, no. 2 (1994): 116–21.

59. Helena Ragoné reports that in the case of commercial surrogacy, many surrogates view their work as a vocation or calling, an important means by which to fulfill themselves. H. Ragoné, *Surrogate Motherhood* (Boulder: Westview Press, 1994), p. 55. See also H. Baber, "For the Legitimacy of Surrogacy Contracts," in *On the Problem of Surrogate Parenthood*, ed. H. Richardson (Lewiston: Edwin Mellen Press, 1987); M. Deegan, "The Gift Mother: A Proposed Ritual for the Integration of Surrogacy into Society," in *On the Problem of Surrogate Parenthood*, ed. H. Richardson (Lewiston: Edwin Mellen Press, 1987); M. Ryan, "Sorting out Motivations: Personal Integrity as the First Criterion of Moral Action," in *On the Problem of Surrogate Parenthood*, ed. H. Richardson (Lewiston: Edwin Mellen Press, 1987).

60. J. E. Roemer, "Should Marxists Be Interested in Exploitation?" *Philosophy and Public Affairs* 14 (1985): 30–65, p. 30. See also J. Reiman, "Exploitation, Force, and the Moral Assessment of Capitalism: Thoughts on Roemer and Cohen," *Philosophy and Public Affairs* 16 (1987): 3–41; D. Miller, "Exploitation in the Market," in *Modern Theories of Exploitation* (pp. 149–65), ed. A. Reeve (London: Sage Publishers, 1987).

61. J. Feinberg, *Harms to Self* (New York: Oxford University Press, 1986), p. 252.

62. D. Josefson, "Selling a Kidney Fails to Rescue Indians from Poverty (News Roundup)," *British Medical Journal* 325 (2002): 795.

63. As Heidi Malm urges regarding commercial surrogacy: "Poor women . . . may feel compelled to enter these arrangements when they would prefer not to do so. Thus we ought to prohibit the arrangements in order to protect poor women from exploitation." H. Malm, "Paid Surrogacy: Arguments and Responses," *Public Affairs Quarterly* 3, no. 2 (1989): 57–66, p. 61. Consider also C. Pateman, *The Sexual Contract* (Stanford: Stanford University Press, 1988); M. J. Radin, "Market-Inalienability," *Harvard Law Review* 100 (1987): 1849–37. As Tavar and Murphy urge: "Compensation can be coercive if it is extravagant relative to the circumstances of the donor's life." R. Tavar and T. F. Murphy, "The Case for Compensation of Tissue Donors," *Archives of Internal Medicine* 161, no. 15 (2001): 1924–25, p. 1924.

64. A. Wertheimer, "Two Questions about Surrogacy and Exploitation," *Philosophy and Public Affairs* 21 (1992): 211–39, p. 223.

65. Marx wrote that capitalism is a system of "forced labor—no matter how much it may seem to result from free contractual agreement." K. Marx, *Capital* (New York: International Publishers, 1967), vol. 3, p. 819. As Cohen encapsulates the point: "Marx defined the proletarian as the producer who has (literally or in effect) nothing to sell but his own labor power (on pain of starvation)." G. A. Cohen, "The Structure of Proletarian Unfreedom," *Philosophy and Public Affairs* 12 (1982): 3–33, p. 3. Where there is no choice, there is coercion.

See also C. B. Macpherson, *Democratic Theory* (Oxford: Oxford University Press, 1973), p. 146; G. A. Cohen, *Karl Marx's Theory of History* (Oxford: Oxford University Press, 1978), pp. 63–77; J. E. Roemer, "Should Marxists Be Interested in Exploitation?" *Philosophy and Public Affairs* 14 (1985): 30–65, p. 30; J. Reiman, "Exploitation, Force, and the Moral Assessment of Capitalism: Thoughts on Roemer and Cohen," *Philosophy and Public Affairs* 16 (1987): 3–41; Onora O'Neill, "Between Consenting Adults," *Philosophy and Public Affairs* 14 (1985): 252–77; T. Carver, "Marx's Political Theory of Exploitation," in *Modern Theories of Exploitation* (pp. 68–79), ed. A. Reeve (London: Sage Publishers, 1987); R. J. Van der Veer, "Can Socialism Be Non-Exploitative," in *Modern Theories of Exploitation* (pp. 80–135), ed. A. Reeve (London: Sage Publishers, 1987).

66. R. Macklin, "Is There Anything Wrong with Surrogate Motherhood?" in *Surrogate Motherhood: Politics and Privacy* (pp. 136–50), ed. L. Gostin (Bloomington: Indiana University Press, 1990), p. 146. See also R. Tong, "The Overdue Death of a Feminist Chameleon: Taking a Stand on Surrogacy Arrangements," *Journal of Social Philosophy* 21 (1990): 40–56.

67. Indeed, given state-legislated donation, it is probably less fair since the donor receives no compensation in return for the value of his organ, in a way analogous to thieves and their victims. See H. Steiner, "A Liberal Theory of Exploitation," *Ethics* 94 (1984): 225–41; H. Steiner, "Exploitation: A Liberal Theory Amended, Defended, and Extended," in *Modern Theories of Exploitation* (pp. 132–48), ed. A. Reeve (London: Sage Publishers, 1987).

68. J. Radcliffe-Richards, "Nephrarious Goings on: Kidney Sales and Moral Arguments," *Journal of Medicine and Philosophy* 21 (1996): 375–416.

69. R. A. Epstein, *Mortal Peril: Our Inalienable Right to Health Care?* (Reading, MA: Addison Wesley, 1997), p. 255. Again, consider the comparison with surrogate motherhood. In 1994 the average family income of married surrogate mothers was $38,700, which was above the national average. The conclusion that surrogates are all poor and desperate is unjustified. H. Ragoné, *Surrogate Motherhood* (Boulder: Westview Press, 1994), p. 54. See also H. Malm, "Paid Surrogacy: Arguments and Responses," *Public Affairs Quarterly* 3, no. 2 (1989): 57–66; H. Malm, "Commodification or Compensation: A Reply to Ketchum," in *Feminist Perspectives in Medical Ethics* (pp. 295–301), ed. H. Holmes and L. Purdy (Bloomington: Indiana University Press, 1992); J. Robertson, "Surrogate Mothers: Not So Novel After All," *Hastings Center Report* 13, no. 5 (1983): 28–34; M. J. Radin, "Market-Inalienability," *Harvard Law Review* 100 (1987): 1849–37.

70. M. Walzer, *Spheres of Exchange* (New York: Basic Books, 1983), p. 120.

71. The claim is that "compensation can be coercive if it is extravagant relative to the circumstances of the donor's life. But, it need not always be. If compensation is scaled correctly, it can appease the donor's sense of entitlement, yet not so much that it induces donors to abandon a rational analysis of the risks and benefits to them of their donation." R. Tavar and T. F. Murphy, "The Case for Compensation of Tissue Donors," *Archives of Internal Medicine* 161, no. 15 (2001): 1924–25, p. 1924. On such grounds, it would be morally appropriate to compensate a rich vendor more significantly than a poor vendor, simply because of their prior state of wealth. Given their relative wealth *ex ante*, the claim is that the monetary increase *ex post* has a less significant impact on the rich vendor than on the poor vendor and thus, it is reasoned, is less likely to overwhelm rational decision making. In short, only those already rich ought to be able to utilize the market for their advantage. Such a result is quite counterintuitive.

72. M. J. Radin, *Contested Commodities* (Cambridge, MA: Harvard University Press, 1996), p. 47.

73. Consider, for example, the ways in which "I was coerced" provides one with an excuse for inappropriate behavior, while "I was manipulated" is generally not enough to excuse. J. Rudinow, "Manipulation," *Ethics* 88 (1978): 338–47, p. 339.

74. H. T. Engelhardt Jr., *The Foundations of Bioethics*, 2nd ed. (New York: Oxford University Press, 1996), p. 309.

75. R. Nozick, "Coercion," in *Philosophy, Science, and Method* (pp. 44–72), ed. S. Morgenbesser, P. Suppes, and M. White (New York: St. Martin's Press, 1969); J. Rudinow, "Manipulation," *Ethics* 88 (1978): 338–47.

76. For an account of negative incentives, see J. Rudinow, "Manipulation," *Ethics* 88 (1978): 338–47; for a discussion of incentives generally, see B. Gert, "Coercion and Freedom," in *Coercion: Nomos XIV* (pp. 30–48), ed. J. R. Pennock and J. W. Chapman (Chicago: Aldine, 1972).

77. D. Zimmerman, "Coercive Wage Offers," *Philosophy and Public Affairs* 10, no. 2 (1981): 121–45, p. 130.

78. J. Rudinow, "Manipulation," *Ethics* 88 (1978): 338–47, p. 347.

79. Similar questions have been discussed in the context of commercial surrogacy. See, for example, K. Oliver, "Marxism and Surrogacy," in *Feminist Perspectives in Medical Ethics* (pp. 266–83), ed. H. Holmes and L. Purdy (Bloomington: Indiana University Press, 1992); G.

Annas, "The Baby Broker Boom," *Hastings Center Report* 16, no. 3 (1986): 30–31; G. Annas, "Baby M: Babies (and Justice) for Sale," *Hastings Center Report* 17, no. 3 (1987): 13–15; G. Annas, "Death without Dignity for Commercial Surrogacy: The Case of Baby M," *Hastings Center Report* 18, no. 2 (1988): 21–24; M. Corea, *The Mother Machine* (New York: Harper & Row, 1985); N. Keane, *The Surrogate Mother* (New York: Everest House, 1981); C. Wilentz, *The Matter of Baby "M,"* New Jersey Supreme Court, N.J., 537, *Atlantic Reporter*, 2nd series (1988): 1234; J. Leibson, *Surrogate Parenting Associates Inc. v. Commonwealth of Kentucky*, Supreme Court of Kentucky, Ky., 704, South West Reporter, 2nd series (1986): 209.

80. H. Frankfurt, "Freedom of the Will and the Concept of a Person," *Journal of Philosophy* 68 (1971): 5–20; H. Frankfurt, "Coercion and Moral Responsibility," in *Essays on Freedom of Action* (pp. 72–85), ed. T. Honderich (London: Routledge and Kegan Paul, 1973); H. Frankfurt and D. Locke, "Three Concepts of Free Action," *Proceedings of the Aristotelean Society, Supplement* 49 (1975): 95–125. See also I. Thalberg, "Motivational Disturbances and Free Will," in *Mental Health: Philosophical Perspectives* (pp. 201–20), ed. H. T. Engelhardt Jr. and S. F. Spicker (Dordrecht: Kluwer Academic Publishers, 1978); C. Whitbeck, "Towards an Understanding of Motivational Disturbances and Freedom of Action," in *Mental Health: Philosophical Perspectives* (pp. 221–31), ed. H. T. Engelhardt Jr. and S. F. Spicker (Dordrecht: Kluwer Academic Publishers, 1978).

81. Second-order desires are desires about the types of desires that one ought to have. Similarly, second-order volitions are volitions about the types of volitions one ought to have.

82. For a detailed discussion of the difference between seductive offers and subtle threats, see V. Held, "Coercion and Coercive Offers," in *Coercion: Nomos XIV* (pp. 49–62), ed. J. R. Pennock and J. Chapman (New York: Aldine-Atherton, 1972).

83. M. J. Radin, *Contested Commodities* (Cambridge, MA: Harvard University Press, 1996), pp. 48–49.

84. G. Dworkin, "Is More Choice Better Than Less?" *Midwest Studies in Philosophy* 7 (1982): 47–61.

85. Office of Technology Assessment, *New Developments in Biotechnology: Ownership of Human Tissues and Cells* (Washington, DC: U.S. Government Printing Office, 1987), p. 96.

86. K. C. Reddy, "Should Paid Organ Donation Be Banned in India? To Buy or Let Die!" *National Medical Journal of India* 6, no. 3 (1993): 137–39.

87. J. Radcliffe-Richards, "Nephrarious Goings On: Kidney Sales and Moral Arguments," *Journal of Medicine and Philosophy* 21 (1996): 375–416, p. 389.

88. R. Nozick, "Coercion," in *Philosophy, Science, and Method* (pp. 44–72), ed. S. Morgenbesser, P. Suppes, and M. White (New York: St. Martin's Press, 1969), pp. 44–50.

89. See also R. Nozick, "Coercion," in *Philosophy, Politics, and Society* (pp. 101–35), ed. P. Laslett, W. G. Runciman, and Q. Skinner (Oxford: Blackwell, 1972), p. 112; R. Goodin, "Exploiting a Situation and Exploiting a Person," in *Modern Theories of Exploitation* (pp. 166–200), ed. A. Reeve (London: Sage Publishers, 1987), p. 171.

90. A. Wertheimer, *Coercion* (Princeton: Princeton University Press, 1987), p. 207; A. Wertheimer, "Two Questions about Surrogacy and Exploitation," *Philosophy and Public Affairs* 21 (1992): 211–39. See also M. Gunderson, "Threats and Coercion," *Canadian Journal of Philosophy* 9 (1979): 247–56.

91. See Hillel Steiner's discussion of a person's monopoly ownership of skilled services versus monopoly ownership of natural resources. H. Steiner, "A Liberal Theory of Exploitation," *Ethics* 94 (1984): 211–41, p. 239.

92. M. Walzer, *Spheres of Exchange* (New York: Basic Books, 1983), p. 120.

93. M. J. Radin, *Contested Commodities* (Cambridge, MA: Harvard University Press, 1996), p. 118.

94. E. R. Gold, *Body Parts: Property Rights and the Ownership of Human Biological Materials* (Washington, DC: Georgetown University Press, 1996), pp. 147–48.

95. M. J. Radin, *Contested Commodities* (Cambridge, MA: Harvard University Press, 1996), p. 10.

96. A. Wertheimer, "Two Questions about Surrogacy and Exploitation," *Philosophy and Public Affairs* 21 (1992): 211–39, p. 218. While market transactions may frequently utilize money as a continuous variable of value, as Locke points out, money is only a placeholder for other goods and values. As Locke claims, "And thus came into the use of money, some lasting thing that men might keep without spoiling, and that by mutual consent men would take in exchange for the truly useful, but perishable supports of life." J. Locke, *Second Treatise of Government*, ed. C. B. Macpherson (Indianapolis: Hackett, 1980 [1690]), p. 28, §47.

97. E. Anderson, "Is Women's Labor a Commodity?" *Philosophy and Public Affairs* 19, no. 1 (1990): 71–92, p. 89.

98. See E. R. Gold, *Body Parts: Property Rights and the Ownership of Human Biological Materials* (Washington, DC: Georgetown University Press, 1996), p. 17.

Richard Posner, for example, is often criticized for applying economic criteria to inappropriate circumstances. See, for example, his discussion of a market in adoption services for young children, in E. Landes and R. Posner, "The Economics of the Baby Shortage," *Journal of Legal Studies* 7 (1978): 323–48; and R. Posner, "The Regulation of the Market in Adoptions," *Boston University Law Review* 59 (1987): 59–72.

99. E. Anderson, "Is Women's Labor a Commodity?" *Philosophy and Public Affairs* 19, no. 1 (1990): 71–92, p. 89.

100. *Moore v. Regents of the University of California et al.*, Supreme Court of California, 51 Cal. 3d 120 (July 9, 1990), at 148. Emphasis in original.

101. E. R. Gold, *Body Parts: Property Rights and the Ownership of Human Biological Materials* (Washington, DC: Georgetown University Press, 1996), p. 36.

102. S. A. Ketchum, "Selling Babies and Selling Bodies," in *Feminist Perspective in Medical Ethics* (pp. 284–93), ed. H. Holmes and L. Purdy (Bloomington: Indiana University Press, 1992), p. 290. For further discussion of surrogate motherhood's supposed commodification of women's bodies, see S. A. Ketchum, "The Moral Status of the Bodies of Persons," *Social Theory and Practice* 10 (1984): 25–38; W. Freedman, *Legal Issues in Biotechnology and Human Reproduction* (New York: Quorum Books, 1991); H. Nelson and J. Nelson, "Cutting Motherhood in Two: Some Suspicions Concerning Surrogacy," in *Feminist Perspectives in Medical Ethics* (pp. 257–65), ed. H. Holmes and L. Purdy (Bloomington: Indiana University Press, 1992); C. T. Sistare, "Reproductive Freedom and Women's Freedom: Surrogacy and Autonomy," *The Philosophical Forum* 19 (1988): 227–40; M. Corea, *The Mother Machine* (New York: Harper & Row, 1985); A. Holder, "Surrogate Motherhood: Babies for Fun and Profit," *Case and Comment* 90 (1985): 3–11; M. J. Radin, "Market-Inalienability," *Harvard Law Review* 100 (1987): 1849–37; P. Werhane, "Against the Legitimacy of Surrogate Contracts," in *On the Problem of Surrogate Parenthood*, ed. H. Richardson (Lewiston: Edwin Mellen Press, 1987); B. Andolsen, "Why a Surrogate Mother Should Have the Right to Change Her Mind: A Feminist Analysis of Changes in

Motherhood Today," in *On the Problem of Surrogate Parenthood*, ed. H. Richardson (Lewiston: Edwin Mellen Press, 1987).

103. R. Fox and J. Swazey, *Spare Parts: Organ Replacement in American Society* (New York: Oxford University Press, 1992), p. 207.

104. Eric Mack notes that the tendency of the market to engage ever wider areas of social life is just that: a tendency. It is not required by the concept or use of the market. E. Mack, "Dominos and the Fear of Commodification," in *Markets and Justice, NOMOS XXXI* (pp. 198–225), ed. J. W. Chapman and J. R. Pennock (New York: New York University Press, 1989).

105. D. Satz, "Markets in Women's Sexual Labor," *Ethics* 106 (1995): 63–85. See also D. Satz, "Markets in Women's Reproductive Labor," *Philosophy and Public Affairs* 21 (1992): 107–31; E. Anderson, *Value in Ethics and Economics* (Cambridge, MA: Harvard University Press, 1993).

106. On objectification, see M. J. Radin, *Contested Commodities* (Cambridge, MA: Harvard University Press, 1996), p. 155.

107. J. Radcliffe-Richards, "Nephrarious Goings On: Kidney Sales and Moral Arguments," *Journal of Medicine and Philosophy* 21 (1996): 375–416, p. 406. Radin echoes these sentiments, arguing that "we are still left with the problem that to the desperate person the desperate exchange must have appeared better than her previous straits, and in banning the exchange we haven't done anything about the straits. It seems to add insult to injury to ban desperate exchanges by deeming them coerced by terrible circumstances, without changing the circumstances." M. J. Radin, *Contested Commodities* (Cambridge, MA: Harvard University Press, 1996), pp. 48–49.

108. R. Titmuss, *The Gift Relationship* (New York: Vintage Books, 1971), p. 198.

109. T. Murray, "Gifts of the Body and the Needs of Strangers," *Hastings Center Report* 17 (1987): 30–35, p. 30.

110. T. Murray, "Organ Vendors, Families, and the Gift of Life," in *Organ Transplantation: Meanings and Realities* (pp. 101–25), ed. S. Youngner, R. C. Fox, and L. O'Connell (Madison: University of Wisconsin Press, 1996), p. 122.

111. Ibid., p. 117.

112. R. Fox and J. Swazey, *Spare Parts: Organ Replacement in American Society* (New York: Oxford University Press, 1992), pp. 8–30.

Advanced immunosuppression has significantly expanded the pool of potentially useful organs as well as of likely recipients. See, for example, S. Tullius, H.-D. Volk, and P. Neuhaus, "Transplantation of Organs from Marginal Donors," *Transplantation* 72, no. 8 (2001): 1341–49; K. Mizutani, Y. Ono, T. Kinukawa, R. Hattori, N. Nishiyama, O. Kamihila, and S. Ohshima, "Use of Marginal Organs from Non-Heart-Beating Cadaveric Kidney Donors," *Transplantation* 72, no. 8 (2001): 1376–80; C. Lama, E. Ramos, J. Figueras, A. Rafecas, J. Fabregat, J. Torras, C. Baliellas, J. Busquets, L. Ibanez, L. Llado, L. Mora, and E. Jaurrieta, "Causes of Mortality after Liver Transplantation: Period of Main Incidence," *Transplantation Proceedings* 34 (2002): 287–89; D. Rodriguez Romano, C. Jimenez Romero, O. Alonso Casado, F. Rodriguez Gonzalez, A. Manrique Municio, E. Marques Medina, I. Garcia Garcia, and E. Moreno Gonzalez, "Liver Transplants in Patients with Alcoholic Cirrhosis-Incidence of Acute Rejection," *Transplantation Proceedings* 34, no. 1 (2002): 243–44; M. D. Navarro, R. Perez, D. Del Castillo, R. Santamaria, and P. Aljama, "Kidney Transplants from Donors Aged Over 65 Years in Comparison with Transplants from Donors Aged Under 65 Years," *Transplantation Proceedings* 34, no. 1 (2002): 241–42;

R. Rull, J. C. Garcia-Valdecasas, D. Momblan, L. Grande, O. Vidal, J. Fuster, F. X. Gonzalez, M. A. Lopez-Boado, K. Cabrer, and J. Visa, "Evaluation of Potential Liver Donors: Expanding Donor Criteria?" *Transplantation Proceedings* 34, no. 1 (2002): 229–30.

113. See A. Spital, "Mandated Choice for Organ Donation: Time to Give It a Try," *Annals of Internal Medicine* 125 (1996): 66–69; A. Klassen and D. Klassen, "Who Are the Donors in Organ Donation? The Family's Perspective in Mandated Choice," *Annals of Internal Medicine* 125 (1996): 70–73.

114. See United Network for Organ Sharing, Presumed Consent Subcommittee of the UNOS Ethics Committee, "An Evaluation of the Ethics of Presumed Consent and a Proposal Based on Required Response" (Rockville, MD, and Richmond, VA: HHS/HRSA/OSP/DOT and UNOS, 1993); United Network for Organ Sharing, Presumed Consent Subcommittee of the UNOS Ethics Committee, "An Evaluation of the Ethics of Presumed Consent and a Proposal Based on Required Response" (Rockville, MD, and Richmond, VA: HHS/HRSA/OSP/DOT and UNOS, 1999).

While such opt-out strategies are gaining in popularity, they may, however counterintuitively, result in fewer organs for transplantation. According to a 1985 Gallup poll conducted for the American Council on Transplantation, approximately three times more individuals would likely consent to the procurement of organs from a deceased relative than would likely donate their own organs. Cited in Task Force on Organ Transplantation, *Organ Transplantation: Issues and Recommendations* (Washington DC: U.S. Government Printing Office, 1986). For additional consideration of such policies, see A. Capron, "Reexamining Organ Transplantation," *Journal of the American Medical Association* 285, no. 3 (2001): 334; D. Wendler and N. Dickert, "The Consent Process for Cadaveric Organ Procurement: How Does It Work? How Can It Be Improved?" *Journal of the American Medical Association* 285, no. 3 (2001): 329; C. H. Fellner and S. H. Schwartz, "Altruism in Disrepute," *New England Journal of Medicine* 284 (1971): 582–85.

115. For example, the UNOS Presumed Consent Subcommittee concluded that "reform of the organ donation process should not be based on the presumed consent model. Ethically, presumed consent offers inadequate safeguards for protecting the individual autonomy of prospective donors. Presumed consent too closely approximates 'routine salvaging' in practice, although in rhetoric it pays homage to the value of individualism inherent in the consent model." United Network for Organ Sharing, Presumed Consent Subcommittee of the UNOS Ethics Committee, "An Evaluation of the Ethics of Presumed Consent and a Proposal Based on Required Response" (Rockville, MD, and Richmond, VA: HHS/HRSA/OSP/DOT and UNOS, 1993).

116. See M. Gumprich, G. Woeste, K. Kohlhaw, J. T. Epplen, and W. O. Bechstein, "Living Related Kidney Transplantation between Identical Twins," *Transplantation Proceedings* 34, no. 6 (2002): 2205–6; R. Emiroglu, M. C. Yagmurdur, H. Karakakayali, G. Moray, and G. Arslan, "Results with Living-Donor Kidney Transplants from Spouses: Fourteen Years of Experience at Our Center," *Transplantation Proceedings* 34, no. 6 (2002): 2060–2061; Office of Technology Assessment, *New Developments in Biotechnology: Ownership of Human Tissues and Cells* (Washington, DC: U.S. Government Printing Office, 1987), p. 117; N. L. Buc and J. Bernstein, "Buying and Selling Human Organs Is Worth a Harder Look," *Health Scan* 1 (1984): 3–5; R. D. Eckert, "Blood, Money, and Monopoly," in *Securing a Safer Blood Supply: Two Views*, R. D. Eckert and E. L.Wallace (Washington, DC: American Enterprise Institute, 1985).

117. "For all its appeal, the gift metaphor has not been especially effective in promoting donation. Despite the degree to which this metaphor pervades transplantation practice,

our studies have demonstrated that 'gift giving' or altruism is not necessarily the primary motivation when families decide to donate. Families often donate for nonaltruistic reasons, for example, a desire to see their loved one live on in the recipient. Moreover, the fundamental incongruity between the surface motivation of altruism in organ donation and the actual situation of donor families at the time of decision can be detrimental to both community and individual. Organ donation does not truly reflect a good freely given, nor a 'Maussean' reciprocal relationship between giver and receiver, in which ongoing ties can be sustained through exchanges of gift and counter gift." L. Siminoff and K. Chillag, "The Fallacy of the 'Gift of Life,'" *Hastings Center Report* 29, no. 6 (1999): 34–41, p. 40.

    For counterarguments, see P. Lauritzen, M. McClure, M. Smith, and A. Trew, "The Gift of Life and the Common Good," *Hastings Center Report* 31, no. 1 (2001): 29–36.

118. Medicare statute 42, U.S.C. 1320a-7b(b). See also Department of Health and Human Services, "OIG Special Fraud Alerts," *Federal Resister*, December 19, 1994.

119. R. A. Epstein, *Mortal Peril: Our Inalienable Right to Health Care?* (Reading, MA: Addison Wesley, 1997), p. 260.

120. M. A. Frutos, P. Ruiz, M. V. Requena, and D. Daga, "Family Refusal in Organ Donation: Analysis of Three Patterns," *Transplantation Proceedings* 34, no. 7 (2002): 2513–14.

121. I. Fukunishi, W. Paris, S. Mitchell, and B. Nour, "Emotional Condition of Donor Families: A Comparison of Japanese and American Outcomes," *Transplantation Proceedings* 34, no. 7 (2002): 2626; I. Fukunishi, W. Paris, S. Mitchell, and B. Nour, "Post-Traumatic Stress Disorder in the Families of Cadaveric and Living Donor Population: A Comparison of Japanese and American Outcomes," *Transplantation Proceedings* 34, no. 7 (2002): 2627.

122. J. Radcliffe-Richards, "Nephrarious Goings on: Kidney Sales and Moral Arguments," *Journal of Medicine and Philosophy* 21 (1996): 375–416, p. 392.

123. R. Titmuss, *The Gift Relationship* (New York: Vintage Books, 1971), p. 240.

124. R. Bell, *Impure Science* (Chichester, NY: John Wiley & Sons, 1992), p. 143; see also M. O'Toole, "Magot O'Toole's Record of Events," *Nature* 351 (1991): 183.

125. R. Bell, *Impure Science* (Chichester, NY: John Wiley & Sons, 1992), pp. 105–6.

126. R. D. Pullan, J. Rhodes, S. Ganesh, V. Mani, J. S. Morris, G. T. Williams, R. G. Newcombe, M. A. Russell, C. Feyerabend, and G. A. Thomas et al., "Transdermal Nicotine for Active Ulcerative Colitis," *New England Journal of Medicine* 330 (1994): 811–15; J. Birtwistle and K. Hall, "Does Nicotine Have Beneficial Effects in the Treatment of Certain Diseases?" *British Journal of Nursing* 5, no. 19 (1996): 1195–202; W. J. Sandborn, W. J. Tremaine, K. P. Offord, G. M. Lawson, B. T. Petersen, K. P. Batts, I. T. Croghan, L. C. Dale, D. R. Schroeder, and R. D. Hurt, "Transdermal Nicotine for Mildly to Moderately Active Ulcerative Colitis; A Randomized, Double Blind, Placebo-Controlled Trial," *Annals of Internal Medicine* 126, no. 5 (1997): 364–71.

127. R. Gray, A. S. Rajan, K. A. Radcliffe, M. Yakehiro, and J. A. Dani, "Hippocampal Synaptic Transmission Enhanced by Low Concentrations of Nicotine," *Nature* 383, no. 6602 (1996): 713–16.

128. Y. Gomita, K. Furuno, N. Matsuka, K. Yao, R. Oishi, M. Nishibori, K. Saeki, H. Nagai, A. Koda, and Y. Shimizu, "Effects of Nicotine and Exposure to Cigarette Smoke on Suppression of Local Graft-Versus-Host Reaction Induced by Immobilization Stress in Mice," *Methods and Findings in Experimental and Clinical Pharmacology* 18, no. 9 (1996): 573–77.

129. B. Fletcher, "The Epidemiology of Occupational Stress," in *Causes, Coping and Consequences of Stress at Work* (pp. 3–50), ed. C. L. Cooper and R. Payne (West Sussex: John Wiley & Son Ltd., 1988); S. Folkman and R. Lazarus, "Coping and Emotion," in *Stress and Coping* (pp. 62–80), ed. A. Monat and R. Lazarus (New York: Columbia University Press, 1991); R. Gray, A. S. Rajan, K. A. Radcliffe, M. Yakehiro, and J. A. Dani, "Hippocampal Synaptic Transmission Enhanced by Low Concentrations of Nicotine," *Nature* 383, no. 6602 (1996): 713–16.

Moreover, in a randomized, double-blinded study of ulcerative colitis, seventeen of the thirty-five patients in the group treated with transdermal nicotine experienced complete remission, as compared to only nine of the placebo group. R. D. Pullan, J. Rhodes, S. Ganesh, V. Mani, J. S. Morris, G. T. Williams, R. G. Newcombe, M. A. Russell, C. Feyerabend, and G. A. Thomas et al., "Transdermal Nicotine for Active Ulcerative Colitis," *New England Journal of Medicine* 330 (1994): 811–15. These results were supported by an independent study conducted by the Mayo Clinic. At four weeks twelve of thirty-one patients, 39 percent, who received nicotine showed clinical improvement compared to only three of thirty-three patients, 9 percent, who received placebo. The study concluded that "transdermal nicotine administered at the highest tolerated dosage (22 mg/d) for 4 weeks is efficacious for controlling clinical manifestations of mildly to moderately active ulcerative colitis." W. J. Sandborn, W. J. Tremaine, K. P. Offord, G. M. Lawson, B. T. Petersen, K. P. Batts, I. T. Croghan, L. C. Dale, D. R. Schroeder, and R. D. Hurt, "Transdermal Nicotine for Mildly to Moderately Active Ulcerative Colitis: A Randomized, Double Blind, Placebo-Controlled Trial," *Annals of Internal Medicine* 126, no. 5 (1997): 364–71, p. 364.

Significant evidence exists that tobacco as a delivery system for a measured dosage of nicotine enhances learning and memory, and has a certain amount of success in treatment to prevent the onset of Alzheimer's disease, as well as Parkinson's disease. As Gray et al. point out, "Nicotine obtained from tobacco can improve learning and memory on various tasks and has been linked to arousal, attention, rapid information processing, working memory and long term memories." R. Gray, A. S. Rajan, K. A. Radcliffe, M. Yakehiro, and J. A. Dani, "Hippocampal Synaptic Transmission Enhanced by Low Concentrations of Nicotine," *Nature* 383, no. 6602 (1996): 713–16, p. 713. The likely mechanism for this effect is that the nicotine enhances or induces neurotransmitter release in the hippocampus. The hippocampus, a center for learning and memory, has rich cholinergic innervation and dense nicotine acetylocholine receptor expression. During Alzheimer's dementia there are fewer of these receptors, and the cholinergic inputs to the hippocampus degenerate. After a cigarette is smoked, nicotine in arterial blood can be delivered to the brain less than ten seconds after absorption in the lungs. Stimulated by nicotine, the hippocampus responds with an increased rate of spontaneous miniature excitatory postsynaptic currents. That is, nicotine stimulates an important part of the brain affected by Alzheimer's disease.

Recent research has also indicated that cigarette smoking is associated with a decreased risk of breast cancer for women who carry the BRAC1 and BRAC2 breast cancer genes. M. Bovsun, "For Women with Breast Cancer Genes, Smoking Lowers Risk," *Biotechnology Newswatch*, June 1, 1998, 14.

130. S. Epstein, *Impure Science: AIDS, Activism, and the Politics of Knowledge* (Berkeley: University of California Press, 1996), p. 11; R. Solvenko, "Homosexuality and the Law: From Condemnation to Celebration," in *Homosexual Behavior: A Modern Reappraisal*, ed. J. Marmor (New York: Basic Books, 1980).

131. S. Epstein, *Impure Science: AIDS, Activism, and the Politics of Knowledge* (Berkeley: University of California Press, 1996), pp. 8–9.

132. D. Rothman and H. Edgar, "Scientific Rigor and Medical Realities: Placebo Trials in Cancer and AIDS Research," in *AIDS: The Making of a Chronic Disease* (pp. 194–206), eds. E. Fee and D. Fox (Berkeley: University of California Press, Berkeley, 1992), p. 204.

133. S. Epstein, *Impure Science: AIDS, Activism, and the Politics of Knowledge* (Berkeley: University of California Press, 1996), pp. 8–9.

134. Consider also the Lysenko controversy in the former Soviet Union. T. D. Lysenko, a soviet agronomist, led an attack in the 1930s through the 1950s against classical genetics, arguing against both the gene concept and the theory of natural selection. He favored a vague Lamarckian notion of the inheritance of acquired characteristics, based in part on the principles of dialectical materialism. Both Stalin and later Khrushchev supported Lysenko. Critics were dismissed from their positions, their laboratories were closed, and at times they were imprisoned. Researchers at times changed their scientific positions based on such nonepistemic political beliefs. Ernan McMullin cites the example of a geneticist Alikhanian who, at a session of the Lenin Academy of Agricultural Science in August of 1948, denounced the genetics he had formally taught, arguing that the support of the Central Committee of the Communist Party for Lysenko must be considered to be valid reason to regard his position as true. E. McMullin, "Scientific Controversy and Its Termination," in *Scientific Controversies* (pp. 49–92), ed. H. T. Engelhardt Jr. and A. Caplan (Cambridge: Cambridge University Press, 1987), p. 81. See also D. Joravsky, *The Lysenko Affair* (Cambridge, MA: Harvard University Press, 1970).

For an additional example, consider the way in which in the eighteenth and nineteenth centuries the moral offense of masturbation was transformed into a disease with somatic rather than just psychological dimensions. Chronic masturbation was considered a serious disorder leading to marked debility and occasionally death. It was held to be the cause of "dyspepsia, constrictions of the urethra, epilepsy, blindness, vertigo, loss of hearing, headache, impotency, loss of memory, 'irregular action of the heart,' general loss of health and strength, rickets, leucorrhea in women, and chronic catarrhal conjunctivitis." H. T. Engelhardt Jr., "The Disease of Masturbation: Values and the Concept of Disease," *Bulletin of the History of Medicine* 48 (Summer 1974): 234–48, p. 236.

The classification of masturbation as a disease incorporated moral assessments concerning deviancy, developed etiological accounts to explain and treat in a coherent fashion a manifold of displeasing signs and symptoms, and provided a direction for diagnosis, prognosis, and therapy. It thereby gave medical and conceptual structure to particular epistemic and nonepistemic values.

135. M. Devita, J. Snyder, and A. Grenvik, "History of Organ Donation by Patients with Cardiac Death," *Kennedy Institute of Ethics Journal* 3 (1993): 113–29, pp. 114–15.

136. A single center study of kidney transplants comparing long-term graft survival of kidneys obtained from non-heart-beating donors versus heart-beating donors observed a significantly higher incidence of delayed graft function among patients who received kidneys from non-heart-beating donors (48.4 percent) versus patients who received kidneys from heart-beating donors (23.8 percent). Yet no significant difference was found in long-term outcomes between the two types of grafts. M. Weber, D. Dindo, N. Demartines, P. M. Ambuhl, and P. A. Clavien, "Kidney Transplantation from Donors Without a Heartbeat," *New England Journal of Medicine* 347, no. 4 (2002): 248–55; see also J. M. Cecka, "Donors Without a Heartbeat," *New England Journal of Medicine* 347, no. 4 (2002):

281–83; Institute of Medicine, *Report on Non-Heart Beating Organ Transplantation*, R. Herdman, Study Director and J. Potts, Principal Investigator (Washington, DC: National Academy Press, 1997); R. Herdman, T. Beauchamp, and J. Potts Jr., "The Institute of Medicine's *Report on Non-Heart Beating Organ Transplantation,*" *Kennedy Institute of Ethics Journal* 8 (1998): 83–90.

137. 42, U.S.C.A. § 274e "Prohibition of Organ Purchases," West Supp. (1985).

138. American Law Institute, *Restatement (Second) of Torts* (St. Paul, Minn.: American Law Institute Publishers, 1965), §282.

139. R. E. Nolan and W. L. Schmidt, "Products Liability and Artificial and Human Organ Transplantation—A Legal Overview," in *Human Organ Transplantation: Societal, Medical-Legal, Regulatory, and Reimbursement Issues* (pp. 137–58), ed. D. H. Cowan, J. A. Kantorowitz, J. Moskowitz, and P. H. Rheinstein (Ann Arbor: Health Administration Press, 1987), p. 138.

140. Ibid., p. 139.

141. W. Prosser, *Law of Torts* (St. Paul: West, 1971), p. 657.

142. R. Wuthnow, *Acts of Compassion: Caring for Others and Helping Ourselves* (Princeton: Princeton University Press, 1991), p. 304.

143. See H. T. Engelhardt Jr. and M. Rie, "Selling Virtue: Ethics as a Profit Maximizing Strategy in Health Care Delivery," *Journal of Health & Social Policy* 4 (1992): 27–35; H. T. Engelhardt Jr., "Virtue for Hire: Some Reflections on Free Choice and the Profit Motive in the Delivery of Health Care," in *Rights to Health Care* (pp. 327–53), ed. T. Bole and W. Bondeson (Dordrecht: Kluwer Academic Publishers, 1991).

144. Elizabeth Anderson notes this circumstance while comparing customer markets with auction markets: auction markets are structured like one-shot prisoners' dilemmas, while customer markets are structured like indefinitely repeated prisoners' dilemmas. "Opportunities for future cooperative interaction provide the parties in customer markets with an extra-legal market-generated incentive to respect each other's interests now. However, the reputational effects of treating others poorly can produce the same incentives in auction markets." E. Anderson, "Comment on Dawson's 'Exit, Voice, and Values in Economic Institutions,'" *Economics and Philosophy* 13 (1997): 101–5, p. 103.

145. For the most recent numbers of member organizations, see www.unos.org.

146. M. Rosenthal, "Swedish Health Policy and the Private Sector," *Milbank Quarterly* 64 (1986): 592–621, p. 595.

CHAPTER 4

1. R. J. Hankinson, "Body and Soul in Greek Philosophy," in *Persons and Their Bodies: Rights, Responsibilities, Relationships* (pp. 35–56), ed. M. J. Cherry (Dordrecht: Kluwer Academic Publishers, 1999).

2. *Phaedo* 64a–67e in Plato, *Five Dialogues: Euthyphro, Apology, Crito, Meno, Phaedo,* trans. G. M. A. Grube (Indianapolis: Hackett, 1981), pp. 100–4.

Similarly, Socrates argues: "such opinion is held by all genuine philosophers, so that they say the following sort of thing to one another: there ought to be some way of escape for us, because while we possess a body and our soul is intertwined with an evil of this sort we shall never sufficiently get hold of what we desire, which we hold to be the truth. For our body distracts us in countless ways because of its need for food. Furthermore, if certain diseases fall upon it, they impede us from the search for reality. It fills us with lusts and desires and fears and every kind of illusion and all sorts of nonsense, so that, as it is said, truly and in reality no thought whatever ever comes to us from it. Rather the body and its desires provide us with nothing other than wars and civil strife and battles; for all wars arise as a result of the acquisition of wealth, and we are compelled to acquire wealth by the body, being held in thrall to its service; and as a result of these distractions we have no time for philosophy. And the absolute limit is that if we ever do find some release from it and turn ourselves towards the investigation of something, it still impinges everywhere upon our investigations, it causes disturbance and confusion and distraction, so that we are unable on its account to see the truth." Ibid., pp. 102–3, *Phaedo* 66b–d.

3. Aristotle, "Nicomachean Ethics," in *The Basic Works of Aristotle*, ed. R. McKeon, trans. W. D. Ross (New York: Random House, 1941), pp. 938–39, book 1, §5.

4. Ibid., pp. 980–83, book 3 §§10–11.

5. Saint Basil, "Ascetical Works: The Long Rules," in *The Fathers of the Church*, ed. R. J. Deferrari et al., trans. Sister M. M. Wagner, C.S.C. (Washington, DC: The Catholic University of America Press, 1962) pp. 330–31.

6. A. L. Smith, "An Orthodox Christian View of Persons and Bodies," in *Persons and Their Bodies: Rights, Responsibilities, Relationships* (pp. 95–110), ed. M. J. Cherry (Dordrecht: Kluwer Academic Publishers, 1999).

7. Saint Cyril of Jerusalem, "Catecheses, Lecture 4," in *The Fathers of the Church*, vol. 61 (pp. 110–11), trans. L. P. McCauley S. J. and A. A. Stephenson (Washington, DC: Catholic University of America Press, 1969), p. 111.

8. As an additional example, suicide was widespread in the ancient world and, particularly among the Romans, was considered acceptable, even laudable and noble. The stoics tended to consider death a matter of indifference; and suicide, at least within appropriate circumstances with an honorable motive, as not merely permissible but praiseworthy. Seneca (4 BC–65 AD), the Roman Stoic who wrote extensively on suicide, eventually aquiesced to the request of his former patron and student, Nero, to put his precepts into practice. According to Tacitus, he died a praiseworthy death of courage and dignity. R. J. Hankinson, "Body and Soul in Greek Philosophy," in *Persons and Their Bodies: Rights, Responsibilities, Relationships* (pp. 35–56), ed. M. J. Cherry (Dordrecht: Kluwer Academic Publishers, 1999), p. 36.

Christians recast these and related concerns, albeit without any acceptance of suicide or any denial of the goodness of the body, as requiring that one turn fully to God. Consider Saint Anthony of the Desert: "Wherefore, children, let us hold fast our discipline, and let us not be careless. For in it the Lord is our fellow-worker, as it is written, 'to all that choose the good, God worketh with them for good.' But to avoid being heedless, it is good to consider the word of the Apostle, 'I die daily.' For if we too live as though dying daily, we shall not sin. And the meaning of that saying is, that as we rise day by day we should think that we shall not abide till evening; and again, when about to lie down to sleep, we should think that we shall not rise up. For our life is naturally uncertain, and Providence allots it to us daily. But thus ordering our daily life, we shall neither fall into sin, nor have a lust for anything, nor cherish wrath against any, nor shall we heap up treasure upon earth. But, as though under the daily expectation of death, we shall be without wealth, and shall forgive all things to all men, nor shall we retain at all the desire of women or of any other foul pleasure. But we shall turn from it as past and gone, ever striving and looking forward to the day of Judgment. For the greater dread and danger of torment ever destroys the ease of pleasure, and sets up the soul if it is like to fall." At. Athanasius [AD 356–362], "Vita S. Anthoni," in *A Select Library of Nicene and Post-Nicene Fathers of the Christian Church*, vol. 4, 2nd ser., ed. P. Schaff and H. Wace (Grand Rapids: Eerdmans, 1978–79 [1890–1900]), p. 201.

9. Council of Nicaea (325), First Council of Constantinople (381), Council of Ephesus (431), Council of Chalcedon (451), Second Council of Constantinople (553), Third Council of Constantinople (680–81), Second Council of Nicaea (787).

10. See, generally, H. T. Engelhardt Jr., *The Foundations of Christian Bioethics* (Lisse: Swets and Zeitlinger Publishers, 2000).

11. Aquinas argues that "consequently the first principle in the practical reason is one founded on the notion of good, viz., that good is that which all things seek after. Hence this is the first precept of law, that good is to be done and pursued, and evil is to be avoided. All other precepts of the natural law are based upon this: so that whatever the practical reason naturally apprehends as man's good (or evil) belongs to the precepts of the natural law as something to be done or avoided. . . . Because in man there is first of all an inclination to good in accordance with the nature which he has in common with all substances: inasmuch as every substance seeks the preservation of its own being, according to its nature: and by reason of this inclination, whatever is a means of preserving human life, and of warding off its obstacles, belongs to the natural law. Secondly, there is in man an inclination to things that pertain to him more specially, according to that nature which he has in common with other animals: and in virtue of this inclination, those things are said to belong to the natural law, which nature has taught to all animals, such as sexual intercourse, education of offspring and so forth. Thirdly, there is in man an inclination to good, according to the nature of his reason, which nature is proper to him: thus man has a natural inclination to know the truth about God, and to live in society: and in this respect, whatever pertains to this inclination belongs to the natural law; for instance, to shun ignorance, to avoid offending those among whom one has to live, and other such things regarding the above inclination." T. Aquinas, *Summa Theologica*, trans. Fathers of the English Dominican Province (Westminster, MD: Christian Classics, 1948), pp. 1009–10, Q I–II, q94, a2.

12. J. Locke, *Second Treatise of Government*, ed. C. B. Macpherson (Indianapolis: Hackett, 1980 [1690]), p. 9, §6.

13. I. Kant, *Critique of Pure Reason*, trans. N. K. Smith (New York: St. Martin's Press, 1965 [1781]), pp. 639–40, A812 = B840.

14. Kant argues that the moral law is a rational imperative; it is a priori and objectively valid for all persons. See, generally, R. C. Walker, "The Rational Imperative: Kant Against Hume," *Proceedings of the British Academy* 74 (1988): 113–33; and J. Hardwig, "Action from Duty but Not in Accord with Duty," *Ethics* 93, no. 2 (1983): 283–90.

As Rawls makes the point, the moral law gives objective, although only practical, reality to the idea of freedom. J. Rawls, "Themes in Kant's Moral Philosophy," in *Kant's Transcendental Deductions: The Three "Critiques" and the "Opus Postumum"* (pp. 81–113), ed. Forster (Stanford: Stanford University Press, 1989).

15. I. Kant, *Critique of Pure Reason*, trans. N. K. Smith (New York: St. Martin's Press, 1965 [1781]), pp. 633–34, A802 = B830. Kant concludes reason commands us to seek to realize the highest good. See L. W. Beck, *A Commentary on Kant's Critique of Practical Reason* (Chicago: University of Chicago Press, 1960), p. 244; J. Silber, "The Copernican Revolution in Ethics: The Good Re-Examined," *Kant-Studien* 51 (1959): 85–101.

16. I. Kant, *The Metaphysics of Morals*, trans. M. Gregor (Cambridge: Cambridge University Press, 1991 [1797]), p. 219, AK 423.

17. Alasdair MacIntyre documents that Thomists in the last hundred years have often ascribed to Aquinas a belief in a set of necessarily true first principles, which any truly rational person is able to evaluate as true. "For this kind of Thomist the rational superiority of Aquinas' overall system of thought does not lie both in its having transcended the limitations of its predecessor traditions, while preserving from them what had withstood dialectical objection, and its since then having not similarly been transcended by any sucessor system of thought, but instead in its argumentative ability to encounter its modern rivals on *their* chosen ground for debate and to exhibit the rational superiority of its claims concerning first principles to theirs." A. MacIntyre, *Whose Justice? Which Rationality?* (Notre Dame: University of Notre Dame Press, 1988), pp. 175–76.

18. T. Aquinas, *Summa Theologica*, trans. Fathers of the English Dominican Province (Westminister, MD: Christian Classics, 1948), Q II–II, q65, a1.

19. For a modern Thomistic defense of this view, see John Finnis, who argues, for example, that biological life is a natural basic good: "A first basic value, corresponding to the drive for self preservation, is the value of life. The term 'life' here signifies every aspect of the vitality (*vita*, life) which puts a human being in good shape for self-determination. Hence, life here includes bodily (including cerebral) health, and freedom from the pain that betokens organic malfunctioning or injury." J. Finnis, *Natural Law and Natural Rights* (Oxford: Oxford Clarendon Press, 1980), p. 86. See also J. Finnis, J. Boyle, and G. Grisez, *Nuclear Deterrence, Morality, and Realism* (New York: Oxford Clarendon Press, 1989).

20. J. Finnis, *Natural Law and Natural Rights* (Oxford: Oxford Clarendon Press, 1980), p. 86.

21. "So the transplantation of a duplicated organ such as the kidney, leaving the whole substantially unimpaired, need not be regarded as doing harm for the sake of good." J. Finnis, *Moral Absolutes: Tradition, Revision, and Truth* (Washington, DC: Catholic University of America Press, 1991), p. 79.

22. Sts. Nicodemus and Agapius, *The Rudder* (Chicago: Orthodox Christian Educational Society, 1957), p. 84.

23. Ibid., p. 163.

24. Ibid., p. 84.

25. Ibid., p. 85.

26. Ibid.

27. Ibid., p. 465.

28. T. Aquinas, *Summa Theologica*, trans. Fathers of the English Dominican Province (Westminster, MD: Christian Classics, 1948), Q II–II, q65, a1.

29. Ibid.

30. Pius XII, "Address to the Delegates at the 26th Congress of Urology, October 8, 1953," in *Papal Teachings: The Human Body* (pp. 277–81), selected and arranged by the Monks of Solesmes (Boston: The Daughters of Saint Paul, 1960), pp. 277–78.

31. P. Finney and P. O'Brien, *Moral Problems in Hospital Practice* (St. Louis: B. Herder, 1956), p. 207.

32. Pius XII, "Address to the First International Congress on the Histopathology of the Nervous System, September 13, 1952" in *Papal Teachings: The Human Body* (pp. 194–208), selected and arranged by the Monks of Solesmes (Boston: The Daughters of Saint Paul, 1960), pp. 198–99.

33. Pius XII, "Address to the Delegates at the 26th Congress of Urology, October 8, 1953," in *Papal Teachings: The Human Body* (pp. 277–81), selected and arranged by the Monks of Solesmes (Boston: The Daughters of Saint Paul, 1960), p. 278.

34. G. Kelly, *Medico-Moral Problems* (Dublin: Clonmore & Reynolds Ltd., 1960), p. 246.

35. B. Ashley and K. O'Rourke, *Ethics of Health Care: An Introductory Textbook*, 2nd ed. (Washington, DC: Georgetown University Press, 1994), p. 75.

36. G. Kelly, *Medico-Moral Problems* (Dublin: Clonmore & Reynolds Ltd., 1960), p. 247.

37. Ibid.

38. Pius XII, "Address to the Italian Association of Blood Donors, October 9, 1948," in *Papal Teachings: The Human Body* (pp. 104–7), selected and arranged by the Monks of Solesmes (Boston: The Daughters of Saint Paul, 1960), p. 105.

39. John XXIII, "Address to the Italian Association of Voluntary Blood Donors," *The Pope Speaks* March 8 (1959): 334.

40. E. F. Healy, *Medical Ethics* (Chicago: Loyola University Press, 1956), p. 125; C. McFadden, *Medical Ethics* (Philadelphia: F. A. Davis, Co., 1961), p. 267; J. Gallagher, "The Principle of Totality: Man's Stewardship of His Body," in *Moral Theology Today* (pp. 217–42), ed. D. G. Macarthy (Braintree, MA: The Pope John Paul Center, 1984). There is additional dispute over whether the surgeon may simply remove the healthy appendix during the course of another abdominal procedure, or whether to justify the incidental appendectomy, he must judge that the appendix's presence after an abdominal operation constitutes a probable danger from adhesions that may render the second operation necessary. See P. Finney and P. O'Brien, *Moral Problems in Hospital Practice* (St. Louis: B. Herder Book Co., 1956), p. 229; J. Shiners, *The Morality of Medical Experimentation on Living Human Subjects in the Light of Recent Papal Pronouncements* (Washington, DC: Catholic University of America Press, 1958), pp. 37–38; M. Nolan, "The Positive Doctrine of Pope Pius XII on the Principle of Totality," *Augustinianum* 3 (1963): 28–44, 290–324; A. Regan, "The Basic Morality of Organic Transplants Between Living Humans," *Studia Moralia* 3 (1965): 320–61; J. Connery, "Notes on Moral Theology," *Theological Studies* 15 (1954): 603; J. Connery, "Notes on Moral Theology," *Theological Studies* 17 (1956): 561; G. Kelly, "Notes on Moral Theology," *Theological Studies* 24 (1963): 628–29.

41. McFadden points out that in unusual cases where it is evident that surgical aid will not be available in the future, it may be permissible, but not obligatory, to undergo elective appendectomy (for example, for missionaries who will be venturing into primitive areas without significant contact with modern medicine). C. McFadden, *Medical Ethics* (Philadelphia: F. A. Davis, Co., 1961), p. 269. See also G. Kelly, *Medico-Moral Problems* (Dublin: Clonmore & Reynolds Ltd., 1960), pp. 253–54; A. C. Varga, *The Main Issues in Bioethics (Revised)* (New York: Paulist Press, 1984), pp. 223–24.

42. As Pope John Paul II stated to a group of blood and organ donors on August 2, 1984: "Above all I appreciate the purpose which has united and mobilized you: namely, to promote and encourage such a noble and meritorious act as donating your own blood or an organ to those of your brothers and sisters who have need of it. Such a gesture is the more laudable in that you are motivated, not by a desire for earthly gain or ends, but by a generous impulse of the heart, by human and Christian solidarity-the love of neighbor, which forms the inspiring motive of the Gospel message, and which has been defined, indeed, as the *new commandment*." John Paul II, "Blood and Organ Donors, Aug. 2, 1984," *The Pope Speaks* 30, no. 1 (1985): 1–2.

In 1991, while acknowledging the benefits of organ transplantation, the pope also encouraged caution: "Among the many remarkable achievements of modern medicine, advances in the fields of immunology and of surgical technology have made possible the therapeutic use of organ and tissue transplants. It is surely a reason for satisfaction that many sick people, who recently could only expect death or at best a painful and restricted existence, can now recover more or less fully through the replacement of a diseased organ with a healthy donated one: We should rejoice that *medicine, in its service to life, has found in organ transplantation a new way of serving the human family,* precisely by safeguarding that fundamental good of the person. . . . Love, communion, solidarity, and absolute respect for the dignity of the human person constitute the only legitimate context of organ transplantation. It is essential not to ignore the moral and spiritual values which come into play when individuals, while observing the ethical norms which guarantee the dignity of the human person and bring it to perfection, freely and consciously decide to give a part of themselves, a part of their own body, in order to save the life of another human being." John Paul II, "Examination of Questions in Greater Depth," *Dolentium Hominum, number 3* (Vatican City: Vatican Press, 1992). See also K. O'Rourke and P. Boyle, *Medical Ethics, Sources of Catholic Teachings* (Washington DC: Georgetown University Press, 1993), pp. 217–22; N. Cummings, "Gene Therapy: Actualities and Possibilities," in *The Twenty-fifth Anniversary of Vatican II: A Look Back and a Look Ahead* (St. Louis: National Catholic Bioethics Center, 1990), pp. 66–67; M. Michejda, "Transplant Issues," in *The Interaction of Catholic Bioethics and Secular Society,* ed. R. Smith (St. Louis: The Pope John Center, 1992).

43. See G. Grisez, *Living a Christian Life,* vol. 2 (Quincy, IL: Franciscan Press, 1993), p. 544.

For discussion of the ways in which contemporary theologians have understood proportionate good to outweigh harmful effects, see B. Hoose, *Proportionalism* (Washington, DC: Georgetown University Press, 1987); R. McCormick and P. Ramsey, *Doing Evil to Achieve Good* (Chicago: Loyola University Press, 1978); L. Cahill, "Contemporary Challenges to Exceptionless Moral Norms," in *Moral Theology Today: Certitudes and Doubts* (pp. 121–35), ed. D. G. Macarthy (St. Louis: The Pope John Center, 1984). For a more traditional account of the doctrine of double effect, see J. Boyle, "The Principle of Double Effect: Good Actions Entangled in Evil," in *Moral Theology Today: Certitudes and Doubts* (pp. 243–60), ed. D. G. Macarthy (St. Louis: The Pope John Center, 1984).

44. C. McFadden, *Medical Ethics* (Philadelphia: F. A. Davis, Co., 1961), p. 268; J. P. Kenny, *Principles of Medical Ethics* (Westminster, MD: The Newman Press, 1962), p. 163; G. Kelly, *Medico-Moral Problems* (Dublin: Clonmore & Reynolds Ltd., 1960), pp. 251–52; P. Finney and P. O'Brien, *Moral Problems in Hospital Practice* (St. Louis: B. Herder Book Co., 1956), p. 233; E. F. Healy, *Medical Ethics* (Chicago: Loyola University Press, 1956), pp. 139–42.

45. J. Boyle, "Personal Responsibility and Freedom in Health Matters: A Contemporary Natural Law Perspective," in *Persons and Their Bodies: Rights, Responsibilities, Relationships* (pp. 111–41), ed. M. J. Cherry (Dordrecht: Kluwer Academic Publishers, 1999), p. 136.

46. Office of Technology Assessment, *New Developments in Biotechnology: Ownership of Human Tissues and Cells* (Washington, DC: U.S. Government Printing Office, 1987), p. 117.

47. J. McHugh and C. Callan, *Moral Theology* (New York: Joseph F. Wagner, Inc., 1960), p. 454.

48. Ibid., p. 495.

49. Pius XII, "Address to a Group of Eye Specialists, May 14, 1956," in *Papal Teachings: The Human Body* (pp. 373–84), selected and arranged by the Monks of Solesmes (Boston: The Daughters of Saint Paul, 1960), pp. 381–82.

50. On the priority one should give the poor see, for example, J. Haas, "Consistent Ethics of Life in Health Care," in *The Twenty-fifth Anniversary of Vatican II: A Look Back and a Look Ahead* (St. Louis: The Pope John Center, 1990); M. Hobgood, "Poor Women, Work, and the U.S. Catholic Bishops: Discerning Myth from Reality in Welfare Reform," *Journal of Religious Ethics* 25, no. 2 (1997): 307–34; D. Finn, "Monologue and Dialogue in Christian Economic Ethics," *Journal of Religious Ethics* 25, no. 2 (1997): 335–42; H. Beckley, "Social Sciences and Theological Ethics," *Journal of Religious Ethics* 25, no. 2 (1997): 343–50; C. Robb, "The Work of Welfare Ethics," *Journal of Religious Ethics* 25, no. 2 (1997): 351–60.

51. Ashley and O'Rourke summarize permissible removal of organs from living persons for transplantation as following five conditions:

1. There is a serious need on the part of the recipient that cannot be fulfilled in any other way.
2. The functional integrity of the donor as a human person will not be impaired, even though anatomical integrity may suffer.
3. The risk taken by the donor as an act of charity is proportionate to the good resulting for the recipient.
4. The donor's consent is free and informed.
5. The recipients for the scarce resources are selected justly.

B. Ashley and K. O'Rourke, *Ethics of Health Care: An Introductory Textbook*, 2nd ed. (Washington, DC: Georgetown University Press, 1996), p. 175.

Only the first four conditions address the removal of healthy organs from living persons. Moreover, each can be plausibly met while compensating donors for the market value of their redundant internal organs. The fifth condition, which derives from neither Aquinas nor the principle of charity, regards justice in allocation of organs as a scarce medical resource. It is a morally distinct concern. One could, for example, utilize a variety of insurance and charitable schemes to ensure that all who need organs would be equally able to purchase necessary organs. See also H. T. Engelhardt, Jr. and M. J. Cherry, eds., *Allocating Scarce Medical Resources: Roman Catholic Perspectives* (Washington, DC: Georgetown University Press, 2002).

52. J. Locke, *Second Treatise of Government*, ed. C. B. Macpherson (Indianapolis: Hackett, 1980 [1690]), p. 19, § 27.

53. Ibid., p. 8, § 4.

54. Ibid., p. 67, §§ 128–29.

55. Ibid., pp. 9–10, § 7.

56. Ibid., p. 98, § 192.

57. Ibid., p. 52, § 95.

58. A. John Simmons identifies two classes of consent: explicit consent, in which persons enter permanently into society, and tacit consent, which grounds more conditional membership. A. J. Simmons, *On the Edge of Anarchy* (Princeton, NJ: Princeton University Press, 1993), p. 81. The varieties of explicit versus tacit consent are detailed in H. Beran, "In Defense of the Consent Theory of Political Obligation and Authority," *Ethics* 87, no. 3 (1977): 260–71; H. Beran, *The Consent Theory of Political Obligation* (London: Croom Helm, 1987); J. Bennet, "A Note on Locke's Theory of Tacit Consent," *Philosophical Review* 88, no. 2 (1979): 224–34; J. Feinberg, *Harms to Self* (New York: Oxford University Press, 1986).

59. J. Locke, *Second Treatise of Government*, ed. C. B. Macpherson (Indianapolis: Hackett, 1980 [1690]), pp. 65–66, § 123.

60. Ibid., p. 67, § 129.

61. See A. J. Simmons, *The Lockean Theory of Rights* (Princeton, NJ: Princeton University Press, 1992), p. 311.
Locke is concerned to protect the natural property that persons bring to society: "to avoid the inconveniences which disorder men's properties in the state of nature, men unite into societies, that they may have the united strength of the whole society to secure and defend these properties." J. Locke, *Second Treatise of Government*, ed. C. B. Macpherson (Indianapolis: Hackett, 1980 [1690]), p. 72, § 136.
As Simmons points out, unless the term "property" changes meaning in this sentence, Locke cannot mean that individuals must surrender their natural property, to receive society's distribution of legal property (however politically determined) on entering society. Simmons, *The Lockean Theory of Rights*, p. 311. See also J. Waldron, "Locke, Tully and the Regulation of Property," *Political Studies* 32 (1984): 98–106; J. W. Gough, *John Locke's Political Philosophy* (Oxford: Oxford University Press, 1950).

62. J. Locke, "A Letter Concerning Toleration" in *The Second Treatise of Civil Government* and *A Letter Concerning Toleration*, ed. J. Gough (Oxford: Basil Blackwell, 1947 [1689]), p. 153.

63. J. Locke, *Second Treatise of Government*, ed. C. B. Macpherson (Indianapolis: Hackett, 1980 [1690]), p. 53, §99.

64. Ibid., pp. 70–71, § 135.

65. Ibid., pp. 72–73, § 137.

66. Ibid., p. 74, § 139.

67. Ibid., p. 74, § 140.

68. Ibid., p. 75, § 142.

69. Ibid., p. 74, § 140.

70. Ibid., p. 67, § 130. See also A. J. Simmons, *On the Edge of Anarchy* (Princeton, NJ: Princeton University Press, 1993), p. 60.

71. J. Locke, *Second Treatise of Government*, ed. C. B. Macpherson (Indianapolis: Hackett, 1980 [1690]), pp. 77–78, §149.

72. Ibid, p. 78.

73. Ibid., p. 91, §176.

74. Ibid., pp. 14–15, §§ 17–18.

75. Ibid., p. 91, §176.

76. J. Locke, *A Letter on Toleration*, in *Great Books of the Western World* (pp. 1–24), ed. C. Sherman (Chicago: Encyclopedia Britannica, 1952 [1689]), p. 8.

77. E. Mack, "Inalienable Rights in the Moral and Political Philosophy of John Locke: A Reappraisal," in *Persons and Their Bodies: Rights, Responsibilities, Relationships* (pp. 143–76), ed. M. J. Cherry (Dordrecht: Kluwer Academic Publishers, 1999), p. 167.

78. J. Locke, *Second Treatise of Government*, ed. C. B. Macpherson (Indianapolis: Hackett, 1980 [1690]), p. 9, §6.

79. Ibid.

80. Ibid., p. 98, §190.

81. A. J. Simmons, *On the Edge of Anarchy* (Princeton, NJ: Princeton University Press, 1993), pp. 115–17; A. J. Simmons, *The Lockean Theory of Rights* (Princeton, NJ: Princeton University Press, 1992), pp. 260–64.

82. J. Locke, *Second Treatise of Government*, ed. C. B. Macpherson (Indianapolis: Hackett, 1980 [1690]), p. 70, §135.

83. Ibid., p. 17, § 23.

84. Locke levies two additional arguments against slavery: First, that licit despotical power cannot be derived from aggression or unlawful conquests. The illegitimate use of force creates a state of war between the aggressor and those he seeks to place under his power. Locke reasons that persons are at liberty to destroy that which threatens them; moreover, "when all cannot be preserved, the safety of the innocent is to be preferred." Ibid., p. 14, § 16.

The natural law permits one to act in defense; this is a right of war, which includes a liberty to kill unjust aggressors. Therefore, rather than yielding new rights of dominion, the aggressor forfeits those rights he has: "because such men are not under the ties of the common law of reason, have no other rule, but that of force and violence, and so may be treated as beasts of prey, those dangerous and noxious creatures." Ibid. These considerations may not forbid taking slaves in a just war.

Second, that licit despotical power cannot be derived from nature: "there being nothing more evident, than that creatures of the same species and rank, promiscuously born to all the same advantages of nature, and the use of the same faculties, should also be equal one amongst another without subordination or subjection." Ibid., p. 8, § 4. Persons are by nature free and equal. Locke's arguments against slavery may only forbid unlimited chattel slavery, which includes the power senselessly to kill one's slaves. After all, in Locke's time there was in England indentured servitude.

85. J. Locke, *A Letter on Toleration*, in *Great Books of the Western World* (pp. 1–24), ed. C. Sherman (Chicago: Encyclopedia Britannica, 1952 [1689]), p. 16.

86. Ibid., p. 14.

87. J. Locke, *Second Treatise of Government*, ed. C. B. Macpherson (Indianapolis: Hackett, 1980 [1690]), p. 13, §14.

88. There is nothing in Locke's argument that would compel any individual, patient, vendor, or physician to participate in such a market. Private providers may legitimately refuse to provide any service are not already contractually obligated to provide. Lockean natural rights define for each person a sphere of moral jurisdiction over himself, his body and property, within which he may do as he sees fit without asking permission of anyone. Such rights define a morally protected domain of choice that holds over against everyone, including the state.

89. I. Kant, *Grounding for Metaphysics of Morals*, trans. J. W. Ellington (Indianapolis: Hackett, 1993 [1785]), p. 30, AK 421.

90. Ibid., p. 36, AK 429.

91. Ibid., p. 38, AK 432. For accounts of the ambiguities among Kant's various formulations of the categorical imperative, see P. Bamford, "The Ambiguity of the Categorical Imperative," *Journal of the History of Philosophy* 17, no. 2 (1979): 135–42; J. B. Schneewind, "Autonomy, Obligation, and Virtue: An Overview of Kant's Moral Philosophy," in *The Cambridge Companion to Kant* (pp. 309–41), ed. P. Guyer (Cambridge: Cambridge University Press, 1993); C. Korsgaard, *Creating the Kingdom of Ends* (Cambridge: Cambridge University Press, 1996), pp. 77–131.

92. I. Kant, *Grounding for Metaphysics of Morals*, trans. J. W. Ellington (Indianapolis: Hackett, 1993 [1785]), p. 36, AK 429.

93. I. Kant, *Lectures on Ethics*, trans. L. Infield (Indianapolis: Hackett, 1963), p. 149.

94. I. Kant, *The Metaphysics of Morals*, trans. M. Gregor (Cambridge: Cambridge University Press, 1991 [1797]), p. 219, AK 423.

95. Kant's indebtedness to the content of Christian mores is striking. He argues with regard to the moral evil of masturbation: "That such an unnatural use (and so misuse) of one's sexual attribute is a violation of duty *to oneself*, and indeed one contrary to morality in its highest degree, occurs to everyone immediately . . . [such] use of one's sexual attribute is inadmissible as being a violation of duty to oneself (and indeed, as far as its unnatural use is concerned, a violation in the highest degree). The ground of proof is, indeed, that by it man surrenders his personality (throwing it away), since he uses himself merely as a means to satisfy an animal impulse. But this does not explain the high degree of violation of the humanity in one's own person by such a vice in its unnaturalness, which seems in terms of its form (the disposition it involves) to exceed even murdering oneself. It consists, then, in this: That a man who defiantly casts off life as a burden is at least not making a feeble surrender to animal impulse in throwing himself away; murdering oneself requires courage, and in this disposition there is still always room for respect for the humanity in one's own person. But unnatural lust, which is complete abandonment of oneself to animal inclination, makes man not only an object of enjoyment but, still further, a thing that is contrary to nature, that is, a loathsome object, and so deprives him of all respect for himself." Ibid., p. 221, AK 425.

Here Kant follows Aquinas, who similarly held that masturbation is an unnatural immoral act. Indeed, Aquinas held that incest, fornication, and rape were lesser sins than masturbation because at least these actions accomplished sexual intercourse in a natural manner. "Therefore, since by the unnatural vices man transgresses that which has been determined by nature with regard to the use of venereal actions, it follows that in this matter this sin is gravest of all. After it comes incest, which, as stated above (A.9), is contrary to the natural respect which we owe persons related to us. With regard to the other species of lust they imply a transgression merely of that which is determined by right reason, on the presupposition, however, of natural principles. Now it is more against reason to make use of the venereal act not only with prejudice to the future offspring, but also so as to injure another person besides. Wherefore simple fornication, which is committed without injustice to another person, is the least grave among the species of lust. Then it is a greater injustice to have intercourse with a woman who is subject to another's authority as regards the act of generation, than as regards merely her guardianship. Wherefore adultery is more grievous than seduction. And both of these are aggravated by the use of violence. Hence rape of a virgin is graver than seduction, and rape of a wife than adultery." T. Aquinas, *Summa Theologica*, trans. Fathers of the English Dominican Province (Westminister, MD: Christian Classics, 1948), Q II-II, q154, a12.

96. I. Kant, *The Metaphysics of Morals*, trans. M. Gregor (Cambridge: Cambridge University Press, 1991 [1797]), p. 219, AK 423.

97. Ibid. The prohibition of suicide asserts an a priori connection between the will of a finite being and actions intended arbitrarily to destroy his life. It is also a claim about the respect owed the subject of morality in one's own person. See M. Gregor, "Kant's Conception of a 'Metaphysic of Morals,'" *Philosophical Quarterly* 10, no. 40 (1960): 238–51.

98. With regard to volunteering to serve in the army and waging war, Kant argued: "For they [the citizens of a state] must always be regarded as colegislating members of a state

(not merely as means, but also as ends in themselves), and must therefore give their free assent, through their representatives, not only to waging war in general but also to each particular declaration of war. Only under this limited condition can a state direct them to serve in a way full of danger to them." I. Kant, *The Metaphysics of Morals*, trans. M. Gregor (Cambridge: Cambridge University Press, 1991 [1797]), p. 152, AK 346. Accordingly, physical life is not as important as "moral life," including courage, devotion, and the other virtues inherent in soldiering. How and why one acts is the focus of morality, rather than the result of one's actions. Soldiers who throw themselves into a hopeless battle die a noble and moral death, whereas those who commit suicide are regarded with disgust as "carrion." As he argues "there is much in the world far more important than life. To observe morality is far more important. It is better to sacrifice one's life than one's morality. To live is not a necessity; but to live honorably while life lasts is a necessity." I. Kant, *Lectures on Ethics*, trans. L. Infield (Indianapolis: Hackett, 1963), pp. 151–52. See also T. Powers, "The Integrity of Body: Kantian Moral Constraints on the Physical Self," in *Persons and Their Bodies: Rights, Responsibilities, Relationships* (pp. 209–32), ed. M. J. Cherry (Dordrecht: Kluwer Academic Publishers).

99. I. Kant, *Grounding for Metaphysics of Morals*, trans. J. W. Ellington (Indianapolis: Hackett, 1993 [1785]), p. 30, AK 428.

100. Ibid.

101. I. Kant, *The Metaphysics of Morals*, trans. M. Gregor (Cambridge: Cambridge University Press, 1991 [1797]), p. 50, AK 223.

102. Kant acknowledges that certain types of distinctions exist among body parts: "to have something cut off that is a part but not an organ of the body, for example, one's hair, cannot be counted as a crime against one's own person." Ibid., p. 219, AK 423.

103. B. Herman, "Mutual Aid and Respect for Persons," *Ethics* 94, no. 4 (1984): 577–602.

104. Thomas Powers argues that "the necessary propaedeutic for a Kantian position on organ transplantation is a clearing away of the prevailing and rather blunt consequentialist sentiments behind the call for increased, compelled, or financially-rewarded organ donation. This is easy enough, since 'pure' consequentialism adopts the unlikely position that consequences are *all* that should matter in moral decisions. So while it is of course true that more people would live if we sacrificed one healthy two-kidney 'donor' for every two patients in need of kidneys, or if we cleared trees from highways so as to reduce traffic fatalities, or even if we *encouraged* motorcyclists to drive without helmets, assuming a greater than 1:1 ratio of organ recipients saved to motorcyclists killed. If the desired consequence is an increase in the number of living human beings, then any of these proposals would be morally required. Clearly they are not. All that a nonconsequentialist position must maintain, Kant's included, is that *something else* matters besides the number of people to be saved by a more vigorous program of organ transplantation. The task for the Kantian is to say what this 'something else' might be." T. Powers, "The Integrity of Body: Kantian Moral Constraints on the Physical Self," in *Persons and Their Bodies: Rights, Responsibilities, Relationships* (pp. 209–32), ed. M. J. Cherry (Dordrecht: Kluwer Academic Publishers, 1999), p. 211. Importantly, such considerations only rule out a market grounded in strictly *consequentialist* reasoning. Yet, as I argue, one can for Kantian nonconsequentialist reasons will the end of a market in organs for transplantation, provided that one wills the health and respect of moral agents as such. It respects agents as persons and promotes the good of the recipients as persons.

105. I. Kant, *Conflict of the Faculties*, trans. M. J. Gregor (New York: Harper & Row, 1957), p. 157.

106. K. Hartmann, "The Profit Motive in Kant and Hegel," in *Rights to Health Care* (pp. 307–25), ed. T. Bole and W. Bondeson (Dordrecht: Kluwer Academic Publishers, 1991), p. 315.

107. I. Kant, *The Metaphysics of Morals*, trans. M. Gregor (Cambridge: Cambridge University Press, 1991 [1797]), p. 136, AK 326. Mary Gregor brings together Kant's account of freedom, duties to others, and private property in "Kant's Theory of Property," *Review of Metaphysics* 41 (1988): 757–87. See also H. Williams, "Kant's Concept of Property," *Philosophical Quarterly* 27, no. 106 (1977): 32–40. For an analysis of Kant's concern for social welfare, see A. Reath, "Two Conceptions of the Highest Good in Kant," *Journal of the History of Philosophy* 26, no. 4 (1988): 593–620.

108. G. W. F. Hegel, *Elements of the Philosophy of Right*, ed. A. Wood, trans. H. B. Nisbet (Cambridge: Cambridge University Press, 1991 [1821]), p. 161, § 134.

109. H. T. Engelhardt Jr., "The Foundations of Bioethics and Secular Humanism: Why Is There No Canonical Moral Content?" in *Reading Engelhardt* (pp. 259–85), ed. B. P. Minogue, G. Palmer-Fernandez, and J. E. Reagan (Dordrecht: Kluwer Academic Publishers, Dordrecht, 1997), p. 260.

110. R. Nozick, *Anarchy, State and Utopia* (New York: Basic Books, 1974), pp. 32–33.

111. Ibid., pp. 57–58. Emphasis is in the original.

112. E. Mack, "How to Derive Libertarian Rights," in *Reading Nozick: Essays on Anarchy, State and Utopia* (pp. 286–302), ed. J. Paul (Totowa, NJ: Rowman & Littlefield, 1981), p. 288.

113. R. Nozick, *Anarchy, State and Utopia* (New York: Basic Books, 1974), p. 118.

114. As Locke notes, governments that use the property of their citizens without permission are not conceptually different than thieves and robbers: "Wherever law ends, tyranny begins, if the law be transgressed to another's harm; and whosoever in authority exceeds the power given him by the law, and makes use of the force he has under his command to compass that upon the subject which the law allows not, ceases in that to be a magistrate, and acting without authority may be opposed, as any other man who by force invades the right of another. This is acknowledged in subordinate magistrates. He that hath authority to seize my person in the street may be opposed as a thief and a robber if he endeavours to break into my house to execute a writ, notwithstanding that I know he has such a warrant and such a legal authority as will empower him to arrest me abroad. And why this should not hold in the highest, as well as in the most inferior magistrate, I would gladly be informed. Is it reasonable that the eldest brother, because he has the greatest part of his father's estate, should thereby have a right to take away any of his younger brothers' portions? Or that a rich man, who possessed a whole country, should from thence have a right to seize, when he pleased, the cottage and garden of his poor neighbour? The being rightfully possessed of great power and riches, exceedingly beyond the greatest part of the sons of Adam, is so far from being an excuse, much less a reason for rapine and oppression, which the endamaging another without authority is, that it is a great aggravation of it. For exceeding the bounds of authority is no more a right in a great than a petty officer, no more justifiable in a king than a constable. But so much the worse in him as that he has more trust put in him, is supposed, from the advantage of education and counsellors, to have better knowledge and less reason to do it, having already a greater share than the rest of his brethren." J. Locke, *Second Treatise of Government*, ed. C. B. Macpherson (Indianapolis: Hackett, 1980 [1690]), p. 103, §202.

115. R. Nozick, *Anarchy, State and Utopia* (New York: Basic Books, 1974), p. 149.

116. Ibid., p. 150.

117. See also J. Paul, introduction to *Reading Nozick: Essays on Anarchy, State and Utopia* (pp. 1–23), ed. J. Paul (Totowa, NJ: Rowman & Littlefield, 1981).

118. R. Nozick, *Anarchy, State and Utopia* (New York: Basic Books, 1974), pp. 265–67.

119. Even if Onora O'Neill is correct in her assessment that Nozick's arguments fail to show how individuals can become entitled to full control over previously unheld resources, such criticism would appear inapplicable to organs. Human organs, unlike other goods, exist initially as part of individual persons. O. O'Neill, "Nozick's Entitlements," in *Reading Nozick: Essays on Anarchy, State and Utopia* (pp. 305–22), ed. J. Paul (Totowa, NJ: Rowman & Littlefield, 1981). See also C. Ryan, "Yours, Mine and Ours: Property Rights and Individual Liberty," in *Reading Nozick: Essays on Anarchy, State and Utopia* (pp. 323–43), ed. J. Paul (Totowa, NJ: Rowman & Littlefield, 1981); L. Davis, "Nozick's Entitlement Theory," in *Reading Nozick: Essays on Anarchy, State and Utopia* (pp. 344–54), ed. J. Paul (Totowa, NJ: Rowman & Littlefield, 1981); I. M. Kirzner, "Entrepreneurship, Entitlement, and Economic Justice," in *Reading Nozick: Essays on Anarchy, State and Utopia* (pp. 383–411), ed. J. Paul (Totowa, NJ: Rowman & Littlefield, 1981).

120. Peter Singer, for example, argues that "utilitarianism has no problem justifying a substantial amount of compulsory redistribution from the rich to the poor. We all recognize that $1,000 means far less to people earning $100,000 than it does to people trying to support a family on $6,000. Therefore in normal circumstances we increase the total happiness when we take from those with a lot and give to those with little. Therefore that is what we ought to do. For the utilitarian it is as simple as that." P. Singer, "The Right to Be Rich or Poor," in *Reading Nozick: Essays on Anarchy, State and Utopia* (pp. 37–53), ed. J. Paul (Totowa, NJ: Rowman & Littlefield, 1981), 50. See also P. Singer, *Practical Ethics* (Cambridge: Cambridge University Press, 1993), pp. 1–54.

121. R. Nozick, *Anarchy, State and Utopia* (New York: Basic Books, 1974), p. 160.

CHAPTER 5

1. Is it appropriate, for example, to spend 1.2 million dollars for six months of ventilator-dependent life for a very ill newborn, who will die regardless of treatment? From a publicity standpoint, care for such children looks like a thick act of compassion. However, there would likely seem to be other appropriate uses for such resources, especially if they come in large measure from tax dollars. See, for example, Fleck's discussion of the Lakeberg twins. L. Fleck, "Just Caring: Health Reform and Health Care Rationing," *Journal of Medicine and Philosophy* 19 (1994): 435–44, pp. 437–39.

2. As Joseph Boyle argues, it seems plausible that patients in PVS can be harmed "by being treated as spectacles or sex objects, by being used improperly for experimental purposes, and so on." Such harms fall into the category of "indignities"—that is, of actions and omissions that do not respect the patient as a person. J. Boyle, "A Case for Sometimes Tube-Feeding Patients in PVS," in *Euthanasia Examined* (pp. 189–99), ed. J. Keown (Cambridge: Cambridge University Press, 1995), p. 193. But do avoiding such harms necessarily require tube-feeding and permanent intubation at significant public expense? How far must clinical treatment extend, at what expense, and for what goals?

3. H. T. Engelhardt Jr., *The Foundations of Bioethics*, 2nd ed. (New York: Oxford University Press, 1996), p. 80.

4. Embryos and fetuses, even late-term fetuses, cannot be experienced as persons from a general secular perspective; thus from a fully secular standpoint their interests are placed within and understood as instrumental to the interests of persons. As a result, abortion, embryo wastage, research, and disposal are generally sanctioned and nearly universally endorsed by the international bioethical community, as well as encouraged by governmental health care policy. Human embryo research has been heralded as very likely leading to significant new treatments for diabetes and Parkinson's disease, immunodeficiencies, cancer, metabolic and genetic disorders, and a wide variety of birth defects, as well as being useful in generating new organs or tissues. The necessary embryos typically either are generated through in vitro fertilization in the laboratory strictly for research purposes or are leftovers from IVF fertility treatments. Since such basic science will likely save lives, reduce suffering, and help to cure disease, from a general secular perspective, it appears decidedly immoral to fail to engage in such research.

In contrast, from a traditional Christian perspective, employing human embryos in research is not resolved through such seemingly straightforward cost/benefit analysis. In vitro fertilization for the purpose of forming embryos, whether for procreation or research, is morally illicit. As Engelhardt argues, "such fertilization removes the procreation of human life from the intimacy of marriage." Moreover, "embryo research involves direct actions against an instance of human life. Although it may not be clear how to regard early embryonic life before it is or could have been in the womb, such life cannot be understood as merely disposable." H. T. Engelhardt Jr., *The Foundations of Christian Bioethics* (Lisse: Swets and Zeitlinger, 2000), p. 261. To treat embryos as merely instrumental and thus disposable is to engage in grave moral evil.

Employing material from already dead embryos raises somewhat different issues. The use of embryonic tissues and cells from dead embryos is governed by similar moral considerations that govern the use of tissue from adult human beings.

"Under circumstances that allow the use of tissues and organs from persons who die accidentally, it is appropriate to use tissues and organs from fetuses who die accidentally. Under circumstances that allow the use of tissues and organs from persons who were murdered, it is similarly allowable to use tissues and organs from fetuses who have been aborted . . . , from 'excess' embryos stored in *in vitro* fertilization clinics, or from embryos that have been formed to produce tissues and organs." Ibid.

Similar concerns are raised regarding use of knowledge derived from such research. One may not employ evil means, encourage their use, or avoid their condemnation; however, insofar as the information exists one may use it to good ends, provided that one is careful neither to endorse nor to encourage such illicit means. Regardless of the hoped for benefits, from a traditional Christian standpoint, one is never permitted to engage or encourage illicit circumstances or means. Here the social, moral, and political clash between the traditional and the post-traditional is stark and forceful.

5. The special accent given to informed consent, for example, is reflective of the manner in which the typical medical encounter is encumbered by moral strangeness. In Western health care, patient and physician typically meet as moral strangers with insufficient common moral grounds for a substantive agreement regarding the other's "best interests" or "good." The formal procedural standards of informed consent help to ensure that patient and physician are only used in ways to which each agrees. These procedures do not, in themselves, convey any particular moral content to the decision reached or to the best interests at stake. The content is that on which agreement is reached.

In other cultures the very process of informed consent may appear unnecessary—or even as in itself harming the patient's best interests. This has been noted among Apache patients within the United States. J. Carrse and L. Rhodes, "Western Bioethics on the Navajo Reservation," *Journal of the American Medical Association* 274 (1996): 826–29. So too, Japanese patients may never raise questions regarding authorizing the physician's acts since the physician is already regarded as established in authority by the underlying moral culture. Similar concerns apply to the Philippines. See A. tan Alora and J. Lumitao, eds., *Beyond a Western Bioethics* (Washington, DC: Georgetown University Press, 2001).

Similarly, within Orthodox Judaism the physician-patient relationship is recast by deep religious understandings. "In the Jewish tradition, informed consent is not always essential. The principle that the physician acts with Divine license to heal may require him, as well as permit him, to do so. Just as it is his duty to heal, so it is the religious obligation of the patient to seek and receive healing. The patient who refuses a reasonable and appropriate medical regimen, whether through willfulness, despondency, invincible ignorance, or irrational fear, is in violation of a Divine trust. The physician . . . would thus not be subject to religious or ethical sanctions for not obtaining consent." Jewish Compendium on Medical Ethics, "The Best Interests of the Patient," in *Bioethics: Readings and Cases* (177–78), ed. B. A. Brody and H. T. Engelhardt Jr. (Englewood Cliffs, NJ: Prentice-Hall, 1987), p. 177.

6. The phrase "culture wars" was made popular by James Hunter. See J. D. Hunter, *Culture Wars: The Struggle to Define America* (New York: Basic Books, 1991).

7. See, generally, H. T. Engelhardt Jr., *The Foundations of Christian Bioethics* (Lisse: Swets and Zeitlinger Publishers, 2000).

8. T. Dagi, "Allocation of Scarce Medical Resources to Critical Care: A Perspective from the Jewish Canonical Tradition," in *Allocating Scarce Medical Resources* (pp. 216–36), ed. H. T. Engelhardt Jr. and M. J. Cherry (Washington, DC: Georgetown University Press, 2002).

9. See J. Peppin and M. J. Cherry, eds., *Regional Perspectives in Bioethics* (Lisse: Swets and Zeitlinger Publishers, 2003); and J. Peppin, M. J. Cherry, and A. Iltis, eds., *Religious Perspectives in Bioethics* (London: Taylor and Francis, 2004).

10. A. tan Alora and J. Lumitao, eds., *Beyond a Western Bioethics* (Washington, DC: Georgetown University Press, 2001).

11. K. Hoshino ed., *Japanese and Western Bioethics: Studies in Moral Diversity* (Dordrecht: Kluwer Academic Publishers, 1997); K. Hoshino, "Bioethics in the Light of Japanese Sentiments," in *Japanese and Western Bioethics: Studies in Moral Diversity* (pp. 13–23), ed. H. Hoshino (Dordrecht: Kluwer Academic Publishers, 1997).

12. K. Hoshino ed., *Japanese and Western Bioethics: Studies in Moral Diversity* (Dordrecht: Kluwer Academic Publishers, 1997), p. xi. See also K. Hoshino, "Gene Therapy in Japan: Current Trends," *Cambridge Quarterly of Healthcare Ethics* 4 (1995): 367–70.

13. The continuing influence of Western bioethics on traditional Japanese bioethics can be seen, for example, in the approach to HIV and AIDS treatment. Consent is becoming much more individual, rather than family, oriented. "HIV+ and AIDS patients seldom disclose the nature of their illness even to their family and intimate friends in Japan. They thus feel very lonely and need a great deal of support medically, physically, mentally, emotionally, socially and economically. Those who do not wish to disclose their illness cannot take advantage of their medical insurance benefit because the type of illness is stated in insurance records. There is no guarantee of confidentiality with the transaction of insurance records." K. Hoshino, "HIV+ /AIDS Related Bioethics Issues in Japan," *Bioethics* 9, no. 3/4 (1995): 303–8, p. 308.

14. As already noted, this position draws on Pope Pius XII's analysis, which recast the principle of totality as allowing that charity might offer sufficient reason to violate the natural good of anatomical wholeness provided that the functional integrity of the body was maintained.

15. R. Tong, "The Ethics of Care: A Feminist Virtue Ethics of Care for Healthcare Practitioners," *Journal of Medicine and Philosophy* 23, no. 2 (1998): 131–52, p. 148.

16. A. L. Carse, "Impartial Principle and Moral Context: Securing a Place for the Particular in Ethical Theory," *Journal of Medicine and Philosophy* 23, no. 2 (1998): 153–69, p. 164.

17. J. H. Penticuff, "Nursing Perspectives in Bioethics," in *Japanese and Western Bioethics: Studies in Moral Diversity* (pp. 49–60), ed. K. Hoshino (Dordrecht: Kluwer Academic Publishers, 1996), p. 55.

18. Part of the difficulty, as Robert Veatch has argued, is that caring is contextual—there is not one theory of care or of what it means to care for someone: "With all of this care-oriented literature, it is increasingly clear that the concept of care is sometimes not sharply defined. Different authors appear to have different notions in mind. It is not clear how care maps onto the more traditional concepts in ethical theory." R. Veatch, "The Place of Care in Ethical Theory," *Journal of Medicine and Philosophy* 23, no. 2 (1998): 210–24, p. 211. Veatch lays out a conceptual geography, comparing care theory with particular cardinal principles of right action, virtues and virtue theory, and various understandings of justice and the role of rules in morality.

19. P. Menzel, "Some Ethical Costs of Rationing," *Law, Medicine & Health Care* 20, no. 1–2 (1992): 57–66, p. 62.

20. A. Gibbard, "When Is the Best Care Too Expensive," in *Bioethics: Readings and Cases* (pp. 192–94), ed. B. A. Brody and H. T. Engelhardt Jr. (Englewood Cliffs, NJ: Prentice-Hall, Inc., 1987), p. 193.

21. I. Kant, *Grounding for Metaphysics of Morals*, trans. J. W. Ellington (Indianapolis: Hackett, 1993 [1785]), pp. 10–13, AK 398–400.

22. M. Midgley, *The Ethical Primate: Humans, Freedom, and Morality* (New York: Routledge, 1994), p. 152.

23. L. Kass, "The Wisdom of Repugnance," *The New Republic*, June 2, 1997, 17–25.

24. E. Keyserlingk, "Quality of Life Decisions and the Hopelessly Ill Patient: The Physician as Moral Agent and Truth Teller," in *Japanese and Western Bioethics: Studies in Moral Diversity* (pp. 103–16), ed. K. Hoshino (Dordrecht: Kluwer Academic Publishers, 1996), p. 113.

25. R. Veatch and F. G. Miller, "The Internal Morality of Medicine: An Introduction," *Journal of Medicine and Philosophy* 26, no. 6 (2001): 555–58, p. 555.

26. Consider Pellegrino, who argues: "Do good and avoid evil is the *primum principium* of all ethics. All ethical systems, medical ethics included, must begin with this dictum, which means that the good must be the focal point and the end of any theory or professional action claiming to be morally justifiable. . . . The good of patients is found to be a quadripartite good, a complex inter-relationship between medical, personal, human, and spiritual good, hierarchically arranged. This concept generates the duties of the clinician. The complexities of its application in medical practice are described. The theory of the good of the patient also has applicability for the ethics of the other healing and helping professions and the virtues and principles pertinent to their practitioners as well." E. D.

Pellegrino, "The Internal Morality of Clinical Medicine: A Paradigm for the Ethics of the Helping and Healing Professions," *Journal of Medicine and Philosophy* 26, no. 6 (2001): 559–80, p. 577.

Miller and Brody present a rather different notion of the internal morality of medicine: "Specification of the goals of medicine is necessary but not sufficient for mapping the normative domain of medicine. In addition to being oriented to a set of proper goals, medicine is guided by a set of internal duties that constrain practices in pursuit of medical goals. We have identified four internal duties incumbent of physicians of integrity: (i) competence in the technical and humanistic skills required to practice medicine; (ii) avoiding disproportionate harms that are not balanced by the prospect of compensating medical benefits; (iii) refraining from the fraudulent misrepresentation of medicine as a scientific practice and clinical art; and (iv) fidelity to the therapeutic relationship with patients in need of care. The IMM (internal morality of medicine) also encompasses a set of clinical virtues—dispositions of character and conduct facilitating excellence in pursuit of the goals of medicine and the performance of professional duties." F. G. Miller and H. Brody, "The Internal Morality of Medicine: An Evolutionary Perspective," *Journal of Medicine and Philosophy* 26, no. 6 (2001): 581–600, p. 583.

27. B. A. Brody, "Medical Futility: Philosophical Reflections on Death," in *Japanese and Western Bioethics: Studies in Moral Diversity* (pp. 135–44), ed. K. Hoshino (Dordrecht: Kluwer Academic Publishers, 1996), pp. 139–40.

28. R. Veatch, "Autonomy and Communitarianism: The Ethics of Terminal Care in Cross-Cultural Perspective," in *Japanese and Western Bioethics: Studies in Moral Diversity* (pp. 119–30), ed. K. Hoshino (Dordrecht: Kluwer Academic Publishers, 1996), p. 120. See also R. Veatch, *Death, Dying, and the Biological Revolution*, rev. ed. (New Haven, CT: Yale University Press, 1989); A. Meisel, "The Legal Consensus About Forgoing Life-Sustaining Treatment: Its Status and Its Prospects," *Kennedy Institute of Ethics Journal* 2 (1992): 309–45.

29. H. T. Engelhardt Jr., *The Foundations of Bioethics*, 2nd ed. (New York: Oxford University Press, 1996), pp. 102 ff.

30. R. Nozick, *Anarchy, State and Utopia* (New York: Basic Books, 1974), pp. 26–35.

31. Witness the recent appointment of bioethicists as special advisors to the U.S. president, the National Bioethics Advisory Committee and former president Clinton's use of bioethicists to sell his health care reformation. Each sought not merely to explain or analyze moral issues but to justify political resolutions. See, for example, G. Khushf, "Ethics, Politics, and Health Care Reform," *Journal of Medicine and Philosophy* 19, no. 5 (1994): 397–406; M. G. Secundy, "Strategic Compromise: Real World Ethics," *Journal of Medicine and Philosophy* 19, no. 5 (1994): 407–18; L. J. O'Connell, "Ethicists and Health Care Reform: An Indecent Proposal?" *Journal of Medicine and Philosophy* 19, no. 5 (1994): 419–24; N. Daniels, "The Articulation of Values and Principles Involved in Health Care Reform," *Journal of Medicine and Philosophy* 19, no. 5 (1994): 425–34.

As Peter Skrabanek documents, the power vested in the medical community is enormous: "they make decisions about employability, fitness to marry and to have children, the right to have an abortion, the time a person is allowed to die, competence to enter into contracts, adopt children or rear one's own children, or about incarceration in mental asylums. Their authoritarian judgment is sought on correct eating, sexual behavior and the use of leisure time." P. Skrabanek, *The Death of Humane Medicine and the Rise of Coercive Healthism* (Suffolk: The Social Affairs Unit, St. Edmundsbury Press Ltd., 1994), p. 146. This is the medicalization of life.

32. See, for example, E. H. Morreim, "Bioethics, Expertise, and the Courts: An Overview and an Argument for Inevitability," *Journal of Medicine and Philosophy* 22, no. 4 (1997): 291–95; K. Wildes, "Healthy Skepticism: The Emperor Has Very Few Clothes," *Journal of Medicine and Philosophy* 22, no. 4 (1997): 365–71.

33. Organisation for Economic Co-operation and Development, *OECD Health Data 2004* (Paris: OECD, 2004), tables 9 and 10.

34. J. Rovner, "U.S. Health Spending Increase Expected to Slow," *Reuters*, Wednesday, February 11, 2004, http://www.reuters.com (last accessed February 11, 2004).

35. Witness the increasingly pervasive use of ideologically directed education of school-children so as to increase organ donation. See, for example, A. Lopez-Navidad, F. Caballero, U. Cortes, J. Martinez, and R. Sola, "Training Course on Donation and Trans-plantation for 16- to 18-Year-Old Schoolchildren in the Hospital de Sant Pau," *Trans-plantation Proceedings* 34, no. 1 (2002): 29–34.

36. K. Bayertz, "The Normative Status of the Human Genome: A European Perspec-tive," in *Japanese and Western Bioethics: Studies in Moral Diversity* (pp. 167–80), ed. K. Hoshino (Dordrecht: Kluwer Academic Publishers, 1996), p. 169.

37. H.-M. Sass, "Introduction: European Bioethics on a Rocky Road," *Journal of Medicine and Philosophy* 26, no. 3 (2001): 215–24, p. 219.

38. Ibid., p. 220.

39. As Catenhusen comments, for example, "in Germany we are particularly sensitive with regard to the application of science and technology to human beings because of our experience with the Third Reich. Human dignity leads to the rejection of positive eugen-ics . . . the attempt to breed the human being." W. M. Catenhusen, "Kodifizierung der Ethik am Beispiel der Gentechnologie," in *Ethik und Gentechnologie* (pp. 37–42), ed. H. Jones (Frankfurt am Main: Gesellschaft Gesundheit und Forschung, 1988), p. 40.

40. H.-M. Sass, "Introduction: European Bioethics on a Rocky Road," *Journal of Medicine and Philosophy* 26, no. 3 (2001): 215–24, p. 220.

41. K. Bayertz, "The Normative Status of the Human Genome: A European Perspec-tive," in *Japanese and Western Bioethics: Studies in Moral Diversity* (pp. 167–80), ed. K. Hoshino (Dordrecht: Kluwer Academic Publishers, 1996), p. 174.

42. I. Kant, *Critique of Pure Reason*, trans. N. K. Smith (New York: St. Martin's Press, 1965 [1781]), pp. 639–40, A812–B840.

43. It is useful to compare this reasoning from sociopragmatic legislation to understand-ings of morality with both natural law and legal positivist accounts of law and morality. Development of legislation in most times and places has been profoundly influenced by the local conventional morality and underlying cultural ideals. For the legal positivist, however, this does not imply any necessary connection between law and morality. See H. L. A. Hart, *The Concept of Law*, 2nd ed. (Oxford: Clarendon Press, 1994), chapter 9. The criterion of the legal validity depends on the legitimate exercise of the legislative process and not upon actual moral norms. The law may at times be influenced by moral-ity, but it does not in itself speak to the licitness of moral norms. According to natural law theory, somewhat crudely speaking, that which is law depends on the correct answer to some moral question. The *locus classicus* for this view is probably Plato's *Laws*, in which he dismisses enactments that are not in the common interest as failing to be true laws. Plato, *Plato in Twelve Volumes*, vols. 10 and 11, trans. R. G. Bury (Cambridge, MA: Harvard University Press; London: William Heinemann Ltd., 1967 and 1968), book 4, 715B. However, the stronger, more typically quoted, versions arose out of Augustine and

Aquinas. Augustine states: "lex mihi esse non videtur, quae iust non fuerit"—"that which is not just does not seem to be a law." J. Finnis, *Natural Law and Natural Rights* (Oxford: Clarendon Press, 1980), p. 363. Modern interpreters shorten Aquinas's stronger version of this to "Lex iniusta non est lex"—"An unjust law is not a law." See N. Kretzmann, "Lex Iniusta Non Est Lex: Interpreting St. Thomas Aquinas," *American Journal of Jurisprudence* 1988: 99–122. An unjust or immoral law is so far removed from the notion of law that it cannot be understood as truly law. One concern worth noting is that given the compromises, special interest groups, and the give and take inherent in any legislative process, it is unlikely that the legislature has enacted the singularly correct moral truth.

44. H. T. Engelhardt Jr., *The Foundations of Bioethics*, 2nd ed. (New York: Oxford University Press, 1996), p. 67.

Index